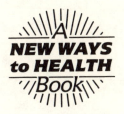

A NEW WAYS to HEALTH Book

Harriet Harvey, Editor

The *New Ways to Health* series

The Magic of Touch
BY SHERRY SUIB COHEN

Your Defense Against Cancer
BY HENRY DREHER

Your Defense Against Cancer

The Complete Guide to Cancer Prevention

Henry Dreher

Created and Edited by
Harriet Harvey

Foreword by Steven Greer, M.D.,
The Royal Marsden Hospital, England

1817

HARPER & ROW, PUBLISHERS, New York
Cambridge, Philadelphia, San Francisco
London, Mexico City, São Paulo, Singapore, Sydney

Grateful acknowledgment is made for permission to reprint:

Chart "How Fats Compare" by Jane E. Brody. Copyright © 1985 by The New York Times Company.

Excerpts from *Healing from Within* by Dennis T. Jaffe. Copyright © 1980 by Dennis T. Jaffe. Reprinted by permission of Alfred A. Knopf, Inc.

Excerpts from *Minding the Body, Mending the Mind* by Joan Borysenko. Copyright © 1987 by Addison-Wesley Publishing Company, Inc., Reading, Massachusetts.

Excerpts from *First Aid for Hypochondriacs* by James M. Gorman. Copyright © 1982 by James M. Gorman. Reprinted by permission of Workman Publishing.

Excerpts from *You Can Fight for Your Life* by Lawrence LeShan. Copyright © 1977 by Lawrence LeShan. Reprinted by permission of the publisher, M. Evans & Co., Inc.

Tables from *Merrill's Atlas of Radiographic Positions and Radiologic Procedures,* sixth edition, by Philip W. Ballinger, St. Louis, 1986. Reproduced by permission from the C.V. Mosby Co.

Excerpts from "Cancer Facts and Figures—1988." Reprinted by permission of the American Cancer Society.

Excerpts from the "University of California, Berkeley, Wellness Letter." Reprinted by permission of Health Letter Associates.

Excerpts from "Ready-to-Eat Cereals." Copyright © 1986 by Consumers Union of United States, Inc., Mount Vernon, NY 10553. Excerpted from *Consumer Reports,* October 1986.

FIRST EDITION

Copyeditor: Margaret Cheney
Designer: C. Linda Dingler
Indexer: Judith Ann Hancock

Library of Congress Cataloging-in-Publication Data

Dreher, Henry.
    Your defense against cancer.

    Includes index.
    1. Cancer—Prevention. 2. Cancer—Nutritional
aspects. 3. Cancer—Environmental aspects. 4. Cancer—
Psychological aspects. I. Title.
RC268.D74 1988   616.99'4052   86-46058
ISBN 0-06-015740-2

89 90 91 92 93 CC/HC 10 9 8 7 6 5 4 3 2 1

To the memory
of my father, Reuben Dreher

Contents

Acknowledgments

The shaping force of the *New Ways to Health* series, and of the concept for *Your Defense Against Cancer,* is Harriet Harvey. Her farsightedness, guidance, and personal support made the writing of this book possible, and I am most grateful. I thank Sallie Coolidge for her important role in getting this project off the ground, and her assistant, Ann Martin-Leff, for all her help. Margaret Wimberger has tended to this book through all its later stages with great care. Harris Dienstfrey also helped make *Your Defense Against Cancer* possible through his early support. I still owe him lunch.

Lawrence LeShan gave me a great deal of his time and the benefit of his experience and profound insight. I greatly appreciate his contribution to this book. Stephanie Simonton-Atchley granted me an interview that was marvelous—both crystal clear and compassionate. I had no initial intention of transcribing it verbatim until I listened to it over again and realized—I can't paraphrase this! Dr. Steven Greer has been most generous. His work is an inspiration, and his encouragement has been extremely gratifying.

Caren Rabbino helped inordinately with her research, and Marion Beckenstein, as always, with her expert typing (not to mention moral support via phone and coffee shop). A great number of individuals—too many to name—helped with bits and pieces of research. One in particular, Amanda Phillips of the Environmental Defense Fund, was of great assistance. Neil Orenstein's technical guidance was invaluable.

Esta Huttner and Richard Huttner planted the seeds for this book by giving me early opportunities as a writer. They also gave me an education in many different arenas which (I hope) they know I value immensely.

Helen Coley Nauts of the Cancer Research Institute has always been available to answer questions and help in numerous personal and professional capacities. But her greatest contribution to this book has simply been her life's work and the inspiration it has provided me. I thank Lloyd J. Old of the Sloan-Kettering Institute and Cancer Research Institute for his support of my work, but also, for his example: his principles, his research, and his remarkable contribution to cancer immunology.

I would like to acknowledge two organizations I have worked for—the Cancer Research Institute and the Institute for the Advancement of Health. Both are dedicated to scientific principles I believe in, and both provided an environment where I could develop my writing and broaden my knowledge.

I wish to thank Deborah Chiel for making the process of writing this book joyful, and for her faith in me. Barbara Miller's affirmations have helped me write and live at the same time, and derive pleasure from both.

Jean Jackson was one of the patients who doctors "give" little or no time—a few months, perhaps. Jean felt she knew what experiences in her life contributed to her cancer, and she worked on them. She also wanted to live and never stopped living. As a result, she survived many years longer than anyone hoped or believed was possible. She helped me personally a great deal during the time of her decline, and also shared with me some of the emotional factors in her own cancer. I am grateful to her for her validation of my developing ideas, and for her openness.

New Ways to Health

When you hear about a new treatment, how can you tell if it will heal you, or harm you, or just plain waste your time and money?

It's not easy. Today's medical and health practices are undergoing major revolutions, and new treatments are being offered to us from all directions. Often, you can receive as many different recommendations as the number of doctors or health practitioners you talk to.

The *New Ways to Health* series brings you new methods *after* they've been well-tested and validated, but *before* they are in general use. These books combine the theories and therapies of Western biomedicine (which is what most of our doctors have been taught) with what has been known until recently as "alternative medicine," but which many modern physicians are now beginning to call "complementary" or "adjunctive" because they think its treatments should be used side by side with our traditional ones. As a result, the *New Ways to Health* series presents what Richard Grossman of Montefiore Hospital likes to call "ecumenical medicine"—unquestionably the medicine of the future.

Many of the new therapies you'll find here—and some of the basic ideas—are coming to us from the ancient and venerable arts of Chinese and Indian medicines. Unlike Western biomedicine, the Eastern systems never separated mind, body, and spirit. Moreover, much of Eastern medicine is directed toward prevention (an area we've badly neglected) and focuses on nutrition, exercises, and meditative practices.

Invaluable age-tested Eastern practices—such as yogic breathing and meditation, exercises from the martial arts, acupuncture, and herbalism—are moving into our modern pharmacopoeia along with some of our own age-old healing arts—such as the power of touch and the laying on of hands—which were swept aside by the scientific revolutions of the past two centuries. But the latest treatments also utilize the quantum leaps forward that "scientific" medicine is making—particularly in genetics and molecular biology.

Interestingly, recent scientific breakthroughs are bringing some of the basic premises of Eastern and Western medicine closer to each other. An entirely new field—with the impossible name of psychoneuroimmunology—is fast proving that the mind/brain and nervous system, the endocrine system, *and*, most important, the immune system are tightly interconnected, thus providing the scientific foundation for the mind/body link that most Eastern medicines have always espoused.

This discovery carries enormous implications—not so much for the infectious diseases, many of which we've tamed with penicillin and other antibiotics—but for our big, unsolved chronic diseases: heart disease, cancer, gastrointestinal diseases, and AIDS. And most especially for those diseases which involve the malfunction of the immune system itself—like cancer, AIDS, and the autoimmune diseases, arthritis and lupus.

What the new breakthroughs reveal is that our emotions and mental states may contribute to—or diminish—our vulnerability to these diseases almost as much as do genes, viral infections, or our exposure to carcinogens. These chronic disorders now appear to be an admixture of many factors, and the psychological factor can no longer be dismissed—in either cause or cure.

The discussion of emotional and mental elements in the cause and treatment of cancer is by far the most controversial section of this *New Ways to Health* book, *Your Defense Against Cancer*. Most physicians—both Old Age and New Age—now accept lifestyle and diet as important factors,* although such was not the case only fifteen years ago. At that time, most doctors completely pooh-poohed any connection between what we eat and the onset of cancer. Now our leading cancer scientists attribute 35 percent of all cancers to nutritional factors.

Just as the nutritional factors were dismissed earlier, the psychological factors are now facing mixed responses, despite research in psychoneuroimmunology and related fields that has scientifically substantiated their role. The idea that the mind actually has considerable control over the body is still a difficult notion for many of us to accept, doctors and laymen alike. However, as veteran science writer Henry Dreher discovered during the two years he studied medical and psychological research coming from Europe, the United Kingdom, and the

*See Part III, "The Diet Factor," about which foods and cooking methods increase our vulnerability to cancer and which foods and vitamins actually decrease it, and Part IV, "The Lifestyle Factor," about which habits—such as suntanning, exercise, or smoking—and which environmental hazards—such as exposure to viruses, air pollution, or household chemicals—increase or decrease our vulnerability.

United States, it's important for all of us to keep an open mind toward the mind-body health field, both because that is where many medical breakthroughs are now occurring and because it gives all of us new ways to take charge of our own health and well-being.

Henry Dreher conducted lengthy interviews with research specialists and medical practitioners in oncology, nutrition, and psychology about such new ways of maximizing well-being, and about other new discoveries that cancer specialists have made. In this book, he brings their impressive research to life so that the latest methods for preventing and fighting cancer will be available to you.

To insure accuracy and to keep in touch with up-to-date scientific research, *New Ways to Health* established a small medical advisory board for its series.

Philip R. Lee, M.D.   University of California, San Francisco, School of Medicine; Health Commission for the City and County of San Francisco

Andrew Weil, M.D.   University of Arizona College of Medicine

Richard Grossman   Albert Einstein College of Medicine, New York

Dolores Krieger, R.N., PhD.   New York University

Lawrence LeShan, PhD.   President of the Association for Humanistic Psychology

Clarence E. Pearson, M.P.H.   Metropolitan Life Insurance Company

Harris Dienstfrey   New York, N.Y.

—Harriet Harvey
Editor, *New Ways to Health*

Foreword

Many people still believe that they can do nothing to avoid cancer. Governmental agencies have done little to correct this misapprehension. Admittedly, there have been occasional antismoking campaigns, but these have been poorly funded and pathetically inadequate compared with the incessant, lavish, and persuasive advertising that extols the pleasures of tobacco. It is not easy to convince people that tobacco kills, when governments continue to allow this drug to be peddled in the marketplace. Since we obviously cannot rely on governments, who is to inform and educate the public? The required information is not easily accessible and is often written in such turgid, jargon-laden prose as to render its meaning impenetrable to all but the learned readers of medical journals and sometimes even to them. Consequently, as Henry Dreher argues, it is up to us to educate ourselves and take our health into our own hands.

That is the central message of *Your Defense Against Cancer* and the reason why the book is so valuable. No other book I know of explains cancer and its risk factors so thoroughly and lucidly, and presents the reader with detailed but easy steps to preventive action.

It is insufficiently appreciated that the majority of cancers are avoidable. Approximately one-third of cancer deaths are due to tobacco. Avoiding (or giving up) smoking is, therefore, the most important preventive action we can take. Other avoidable factors that contribute to cancer include diets that are high in fats or in nitrite-containing foods and low in fiber, heavy alcohol consumption, excessive exposure to sunlight (especially for fair-skinned people) and to x-rays, occupational hazards such as asbestos dust and vinyl chloride, and certain environmental pollutants. Dreher devotes a large part of his book to the effects of nutrition. He provides good evidence linking the diets mentioned above to cancers particularly of the breast, gastrointestinal tract, and prostate. One need not agree with every one of his detailed dietary recommendations to support his main conclusion that—far from being helpless—we can, by altering our eating habits, reduce the risk of developing cancer. This conclusion is of crucial importance, with far-reaching implications for public health.

In the most controversial and stimulating section of the book, Dreher addresses a question that is as old as medicine itself yet that remains unanswered to this day: can psychological attributes contribute to the development of cancer or influence its subsequent course? All too often, this question generates more heat than light. On the one hand are adherents of so-called alternative medicine, whose categorical answer in the affirmative is more an article of faith than a reasoned conclusion. On the other hand are those orthodox scientists and physicians whose scientific objectivity deserts them when this question is raised; they flatly reject any possibility that psychological factors could play a part in the development or progress of cancer. Such knee-jerk reactions, from whatever quarter, are singularly unhelpful. They impede rather than advance knowledge. A more rational, genuinely scientific approach requires a balanced review of such evidence as is available from systematic studies. The author examines that evidence with care.

He describes several studies that have revealed a link between certain personality traits (Type C behavior—suppression of anger, compliance, unassertiveness) and cancer. The reported findings are of considerable interest and suggest the possibility that these psychological attributes may contribute to the development of cancer. But the case should not be overstated. It must be stressed that what has been discovered so far is a *statistical* link. To establish whether there is a *causal* link requires further research. Healthy adult populations have to be assessed psychologically and followed up for a number of years until the relationship between the suspected personality traits and subsequent development of cancer can be determined. The need for such prospective studies, as they are called, is clear. They are not merely of academic interest. If a causal link is found, the next step will be to attempt to reduce the risk of developing cancer by devising methods of altering Type C behavior. Is this a mere flight of fanciful speculation or a realistically attainable goal? Only further research will give the answer.

In the meantime, claims that any kind of psychotherapy—no matter how weird or wonderful—can directly prevent cancer are premature. Dreher suggests that people pursue the goal of psychological well-being primarily because of its intrinsic benefits, and because it promotes physical health as well.

Another intriguing area of research described in the book concerns the possible effect of mental attitudes on the course of cancer. There is evidence from systematic studies that the mental attitudes adopted by patients with early cancer (i.e., where there has been no distant spread of the disease) appear to influence outcome. Patients with an active fighting spirit are more likely to be alive and well up to ten years later than are patients whose attitude is one of helplessness. These results are based on small numbers of patients and should be verified in larger studies. If confirmed, the present results have important practical implications for the treatment of patients with cancer. What is needed now is to devise methods of psychological therapy that will enable patients to adopt a fighting spirit in response to the disease. Research along these lines is currently under way.

It is hardly surprising that the few studies carried out so far have not provided definitive answers to questions about mind states and cancer progression. Nevertheless, these studies have revealed provisional—though by no means conclusive—evidence for a link between psychological factors and the course of cancer. It is not suggested that psychological factors initiate the cancer process but that they may contribute—in certain cases—to the further development of the disease. If psychological factors can influence tumor growth, how is that influence mediated?

The search for biological pathways between the mind and cancer is a new and challenging field of inquiry. Among several possible pathways is the immune system, the complexities of which are described with clarity and simplicity by Dreher. Although still in its infancy and outside the mainstream of cancer research, the field of psychoneuroimmunology, as it is infelicitously called, promises to advance our knowledge about the possible contributory role of psychological factors in tumor growth and restraint. Psychoneuroimmunology has another valuable function. It serves as a salutary reminder that multidisciplinary studies of the whole patient—mind and body—should be an integral part of medical research.

Henry Dreher's *Your Defense Against Cancer* pulls together material from many diverse fields of cancer research and, in doing so, makes a great contribution to the literature of cancer prevention.

STEVEN GREER, M.D.
The Royal Marsden Hospital,
Sutton, Surrey, and London, U.K.

I

CANCER *CAN* BE PREVENTED

1
Cancer *Can* Be Prevented

What is absolutely amazing about the human body is its specialized network of millions of cells that defend us from dangerous outside intruders. Among its ten trillion cells, the body has cells that destroy "aliens" before they can wreak any damage, and cells that marshal other cells and substances to do battle against any invader. Should some clever agents slip by all these defenders and begin to turn our own cells cancerous, we have "soldier" cells that can liquidate the mutant or malignant cells. This remarkable surveillance team—which protects us from invaders like bacteria, viruses, and carcinogens—can also wipe out "subversive" cancer cells arising from within. Our defense system is as ubiquitous and efficient as any defense department could dream of.

I'm not fond of military metaphors but I can think of no other that captures the watchfulness and strength of our remarkable immune system.

But we have to take care of it. We have to keep it in fighting trim. *And* that's what this book is all about:

- Ways not to overwhelm our defense systems with carcinogenic bombardment from the outside.
- Ways to strengthen our defense systems from the inside.

Though the idea is completely contrary to public opinion, each one of us *can* make a tremendous difference in preventing cancer. The prevention potential is so great, in fact, that recent studies suggest that we should shift our national research priorities from treatment to prevention. *At a very conservative estimate, it is now thought that at least 65 percent of all cancers can be prevented.* And Margaret Heckler, former Secretary of Health and Human Services, has gone further: "We now know," she said in 1984, "that fully 80% of cancer cases are linked

3

to lifestyle and environmental factors. And we know that the most important causes of cancer are the ones we can control or influence."

The National Cancer Institute estimates that proper practices would prevent as many as 95,000 cancer deaths a year in the U.S. alone.

Yet very few of us really believe that. And I'm not sure why.

Just last week, when I was catching a quick sandwich between flights at a fast-food restaurant in Chicago's O'Hare Airport, I overheard a conversation between a young couple.

"Don't get a BLT, George," said the woman. "You know bacon is one of the worst things you can eat. Cancer!"

"Aw, honey," replied the man. "If you listen to all that stuff, you couldn't eat a damn thing. You either get cancer or you don't."

This mind set is extraordinarily typical of almost half of U.S. adults. In a 1984 telephone survey made by the National Cancer Institute, 49 percent of the people answered "yes" to this statement: "It seems like everything causes cancer." And 46 percent answered "yes" to this one: "There's not much a person can do to prevent cancer."

Yet nothing could be further from the truth!

Jane Brody, the *New York Times* health columnist, was so impressed by the misunderstanding of the general public that she felt it necessary to state flatly in a recent article: "Contrary to widespread impressions, everything does *not* cause cancer."

All this reminds me of a marvelous list I came across in James Gorman's humorous book *First Aid for Hypochondriacs:*

THE 10,000 CAUSES OF CANCER
(a partial listing)

the sun	saccharin
sadness	hormones
bacon	peanut butter
too much sleep	air pollution
too little sleep	hot foods
the Pill	snuff
cigarettes	color television
water	x-rays
meat	nuclear power
coffee	nuclear war
tea	the nuclear family
too little sex	asbestos
too much sex	pesticides
the wrong kind of sex	crowding

loneliness	Red Dye #2
disco music	glue
PCB's	varnish
PPB's	viruses
DBCP	paint
LSD	science
STP	the Government
STD	doctors
Agent Orange	THEM

Gorman has unquestionably captured the mind set of BLT George—if not that of many others. Fear can cause the line between real and imagined carcinogens to become blurred. Our confusion is partially understandable, because the bio-scientists have changed their minds from time to time about what is carcinogenic and what is not. Nevertheless, every day the nutritionists and bio-scientists learn more and more about what food components (such as fats and nitrates), what substances (such as tobacco, alcohol, and asbestos), what lifestyle factors (such as suntanning and sexually transmitted viruses), put us at greater risk of getting cancer. *And* they learn more about what foods (such as whole grains, broccoli, and carrots) and what emotional states (like joyous involvement in life) actually buttress our cancer defenses.

But even doctors are not paying much attention to these findings. In the same NCI telephone survey mentioned above, 61 percent of the respondents said they would follow prevention advice from their doctors, yet 86 percent said that no doctors had offered them such advice!

It is because of this credibility gap on the part of the layman, and lack of preventive advice on the part of many doctors, that New Ways to Health decided to create this book. I was delighted to be asked to write it, but it was a task that encompassed ever-widening realms of research. I pored over hundreds of studies from many different fields—oncology, molecular biology, immunology, environmental science, toxicology, nutrition, psychology, behavioral medicine, and psychoneuroimmunology. And then I talked with many cancer scientists both in the U.S. and England. As I worked I became more and more convinced that most of us—myself included—don't really appreciate what a profound difference we can make in our own health, what wondrous defense and regenerative abilities are at our command—if we just work to keep them strong and healthy. Our powers are, indeed, formidable.

To use them properly, however, we must look at all aspects of ourselves—body and mind, if not spirit. The new scientific field of psychoneuroimmunology (PNI) is well on its way to showing that mind and body are so intimately connected that many diseases we thought were "purely physical" or "purely mental" are, in fact, an interwoven admixture of the two. We are beginning to see that any program of prevention or therapy must address the needs of both body and mind. This appears to be particularly true of our major unsolved chronic diseases: heart disease, gastrointestinal disorders, and cancer.

Indeed, the mind seems to have powers over the body that few of us (in the scientific-industrial world, at least) ever dreamed possible. It's beginning to look as if all the mind's processes—thinking, feeling, remembering, imagining, experiencing—may profoundly affect all the body's processes—including the immune system itself. The immune system is, of course, the body's major system involved in prevention. And there is more evidence now than ever before that for cancer to occur, there must be a breakdown in the immune system.

Am I talking about psychosomatic and/or holistic medicine? Yes, indeed, I am. But these terms have been so misused in the last fifty years that many people who practice them avoid the terms altogether. It's important to return to their real meanings.

"Psychosomatic" does *not* mean that what goes on in our mind *causes* disease in our bodies. Nor does it mean that such diseases "are *only* in our heads." What it really means, says psychologist Eda LeShan, "is that we are finally coming back to an understanding of human beings that was around through all the ages of history, that there is simply no separation whatever between body and mind—it's only one complete bound package."

With a few additions, the word "holistic"—originally coined in the early part of this century by the biologist-statesman Jan Christian Smuts—means much the same thing: that we are whole human beings and that what happens to one part of us can affect any or all of the other parts. It does *not* mean turning our backs on "traditional" scientific medicine, eating apricot pits, and mumbling weird incantations at the midnight moon. The term has been so misused that Richard Grossman of Montefiore Hospital says, "It won't be long before we have holistic donut shops."

"Holistic" can mean something as simple as that what we eat affects our metabolism *and* our thinking *and* our moods, and that what we think and feel affects what we eat and how it is digested and then utilized by our bodies. The word also suggests that the patient and doctor should work together in addressing the causes of disease and its effects at all levels of experience—mental, physical, and spiritual.

A holistic approach is, of course, just as important in prevention as in treatment—if not more so. If our bodies break down, it means that they have not had the strength or regenerative capacity to protect themselves from outside invaders. Sometimes the invaders are overwhelming. But, more often than not, it means our defenses are weakened; and the strength of those defenses depends as much on our feelings and our attitudes as it does on good nutrition, exercise, and other healthy habits. Almost every disease is multifactoral: part may be caused by outside poisons (like nicotine and tar); part by viruses or germs in the environment; part by poor nutrition; part by the genes we inherit; and part by the emotional stresses in our lives. Studies reveal, for instance, that many people who have suffered a severe loss—such as the death of husband, wife, or child—show a chemical and hormonal imbalance in their bodies for some months afterward, resulting in weakened defenses and a higher vulnerability to disease.

So, just what do we do to keep our defenses strong? And what are the main "outside invaders" that make us susceptible to cancer?

THE CANCER TRIGGERS

The pie chart (see page 8), based on data from the National Cancer Institute, illustrates the approximate percentages of different *risk factors* involved in the incidence of cancer in the U.S.

These are carcinogenic risk factors, *not sole causes*, but some of them are very powerful contributors to cancer. Smoking, in particular, is such an enormous risk that it's not unlike riding a motorcycle at one hundred miles an hour on a narrow, slippery mountain road. Not all smokers get cancer, nor do all speeding mountain motorcyclists fall off cliffs. But the risk is great enough so that we can't allow ourselves to fall back on rationalizations like "Uncle Max smoked like a chimney and was as healthy as a young colt until he died at ninety-seven!"

You will note that 35 percent of all cancer deaths are traced to dietary factors—a tremendous increase from estimates in earlier years. However, there are many different foods involved in diet. Smoking, at 30 percent, therefore, remains the biggest single trigger. Taken together, diet and smoking account for 65 percent of the risk factors.

THE CANCER DEFENSES

Our defense systems are largely kept in order by diminishing the stresses upon them—both physical and emotional. Smoking, as well as being a trigger, weakens many systems—as do overweight, poor diet, and pollution. However, our defenses can be actively buttressed by certain foods and food supplements (described in Chapter 5, "Foods That Are Allies"), by exercise, and by stress-reducing techniques—like meditation and biofeedback which I describe in later chapters.

In addition, our research is beginning to show—and Norman Cous-

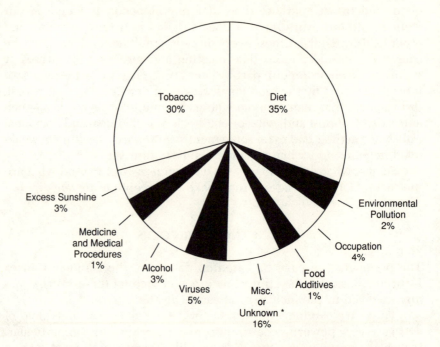

Pie Chart of Cancer Risk Factors. Data derived from National Cancer Institute statistics, cited by former Secretary of Health and Human Services Margaret Heckler, in her March 6, 1984, statement to the press.

*This figure was not directly cited by NCI. A number of cancer scientists and epidemiologists speculate that a variety of factors, including heredity, sources of radioactivity other than medical, and other environmental hazards should be included. Some small percentage of cancers have no known cause.

ins, in his extraordinary books, *Anatomy of an Illness* and *The Healing Heart,* has described it eloquently—that a joyful, active participation in life may be the most powerful support we can give our defenses in prevention as well as in healing. Or, as the cancer psychologist Lawrence LeShan has put it: "How much enjoyment is there in an individual's life? Is there zest, serenity, gusto, and other qualities that will fulfill this (particular) individual's life and make it worthwhile?" As I mentioned before, this is no new idea. It is at least as old as Hippocrates, who believed that a state of harmony between mind and body was essential to health. The great nineteenth-century physician, Sir William Osler, once said he would rather know what sort of person had a disease than what disease the person had.

But how do we start the cancer-prevention process? First, by over-coming fear and resisting apathy.

THE FEAR FACTOR

When something seems dreadful—but is still "out there somewhere" and hasn't directly touched us—we are tempted to deny its existence. This is true of the nuclear bomb threat and it is true of the AIDS crisis. In regard to the latter, it seems absolutely extraordinary that men and women at high risk continue to have unsafe sex, despite the vast media publicity. (This behavior is more prevalent among heterosexuals than homosexuals, who have already been exposed to tremendous firsthand suffering.)

Our view of cancer has also fallen into the trap: "The BIG C is going to get you—or it isn't—and there is nothing you can do about it." But this is a dangerous myth. To those of you who are fearful, I want to say, "Take heart and learn." I repeat: Up to 80 percent of all cancers *are* preventable, no matter what your family history may be—*if* you inte-grate and adopt prevention strategies. Moreover, cancer itself is no longer a death sentence—50 percent of all cancers are now curable. So don't let fear paralyze you. The best thing you can do is to become knowledgeable about carcinogenic triggers, your genetic risks, and the many ways to strengthen your immune defenses. Learn and then go into action and much of your fear will disappear. I want to emphasize: *Cancer is not something we catch from a carcinogen; it only develops when our defenses are incapable of eliminating carcinogens from the body, or cancer cells once they have developed.* Most of us know of people who have had spontaneous regressions of their cancers. It's becoming clearer that these occur not because of some "miracle" but because their immune systems suddenly get back into gear.

To those of you who don't give cancer much thought, and are too happily engaged in other pursuits to be bothered to do so, I recommend you take at least these basic (though sometimes not so simple) steps: (1) Stop smoking by any or all means. (2) Reduce alcohol intake to a maxi-mum of two drinks a day. (3) Remove the cutout section in Appendix 5 of this book, on the "Cancer-Prevention Daily Diet." Post it on your refrigerator and follow its suggestions. WHAT YOU EAT IS VERY IMPOR-TANT. (4) Read the lifestyle chapters that are relevant to you: on recrea-tional or prescription drugs; x-rays or suntanning; viruses or sexually transmitted diseases.

But don't pretend the threat doesn't exist or that cancer will soon be eliminated by some "magic bullet." At the present rate, the American Cancer Society estimates that, in 1988, 985,000 people will have been diagnosed as having cancer and, in the same year, 494,000 will have died of it. All told, about 75 million of the Americans now living will eventually contract cancer—approximately 30 percent of the population. This means that, if this rate continues, cancer will strike about three out of four families over the next few years.

On the other hand, there's good reason *not* to be compulsive about following cancer-prevention recommendations down to the last detail. Trying to do so is self-defeating. Those of us who have tried to diet for years are familiar with the syndrome. One ice-cream cone or plate of pasta can bring on a guilt attack, resulting in self-disgust or, at least, self-disappointment. We feel like failures. The result? Total abandonment of the diet. Cancer-prevention guidelines are not moral laws, and no God-like higher authority will punish us with cancer if we don't follow them. They are—quite simply—based on the best science has to offer as to cancer's causes, and we will feel healthier and safer if we follow them as well as we can.

The risk of cancer is *not* connected to whether we smoke one or two cigarettes a week, or occasionally eat a BLT. Nor is it simply a roll of the dice. The *risk is determined by the balance between exposure to cancer-causing agents on one side and the strength of our defenses on the other.* Both sides of the scale are largely controllable, and both should be weighed carefully so they tip toward prevention.

So set reasonable goals for yourself. If you smoke, work on that first, and don't worry about your diet for the time being. After you've conquered smoking, go on to other lifestyle changes, involving diet, suntanning, etc. Look at your house and your office as possible places for risk factors, and eliminate any suspected carcinogens.

There are, of course, threats from our general environment. The Sierra Club has recently come out with a list of thirty-seven major cities whose air is below the levels of safety set by the U.S. government's Environmental Protection Agency (EPA). All of us should work to help eliminate outside air pollution, nuclear radiation, and other external threats to our life. However, because there are so many knowledgeable, valuable books on these vital public issues, I have limited this book to cancer-prevention techniques that you can undertake for yourself without political action. This in no way means, however, that I do not support attempts to save our planet and ourselves from environmental hazards; it only means that public-action groups cover these issues better than I can. Moreover, in this book, I want to impress upon people the many powerful ways they can make a difference by attending to their own individual lifestyles and habits.

HOW TO USE THIS BOOK

Don't read it all at once. It's too much to absorb. Rather, use it as a reference book to check on your daily routines—in regard to food, stress, smoking, drinking, and other such habits—and find ways to modify them.

The next two chapters, on cancer's origins and our defense systems, aren't easy. They're full of scientific concepts and vocabulary. But try to read them. For, if you begin to have an understanding of just how cancer begins and what amazing capacities our bodies have for defending against it, all the steps you take—from eating broccoli to putting on sunblockers—will take on real meaning, a meaning that you can visualize in terms of your body's interior actions.

Glance through Part III, "The Diet Factor," because no matter how "natural" your diet may be you probably eat some foods that are "enemies" and may yet discover some new nutritional "allies." Above all, make use of Chapter 7, "The Cancer-Prevention Diet Guide." Cut out the duplicate of the Daily Diet provided in Appendix 5 and hang it at some convenient spot where you will see it.

"The Lifestyle Factor"—Part IV—is divided into chapters on specific issues—smoking, x-rays, suntanning, etc. You can skip the chapters that don't apply to you—unless you are trying to help someone else give up a self-destructive behavior. It is my hope that all the advice I give is in no way moralistic but offers compassionate and valid suggestions on how to change habits.

Everyone who spends time in the sun—even a little time—should read the chapter on suntanning. The dermatologists are currently fighting an uphill battle against exposure to ultraviolet rays, which starts in early childhood but doesn't show its effects as cancer until later in life.

Part V, "The Psychological Factor," is for everyone. We are all subject to stress and the wages of loss and disappointment. Our minds and bodies suffer together and the result is a weakened defense system. Moreover, some of us have characteristic ways that make it even harder for our biological systems to bounce back from the inevitable challenges that face them. This part can also be helpful to anyone having difficulty (and which of us doesn't?) with the behavioral changes suggested in earlier chapters. If you encounter problems with diet, smoking, etc., look for clues and possible solutions in Chapters 20 and 21, "Psychological Health and Cancer Prevention" and "New Ways to Mind-Body Health." If you can find new ways to reduce stress and enhance your capacity for pleasure in life, it becomes much easier to stop smoking or change your diet.

I've written this book also as a guide for cancer patients. Although it is primarily focused on prevention, much of the information is valuable for those who are working at overcoming cancer and want to forestall a second or third bout with it.

The early detection of cancer is crucial, because treatment of many cancers is most effective in the early stages. See Appendix 2 for a guide to checkups for early detection.

As the Yale oncological surgeon Bernie Siegel says in his recent book *Love, Medicine and Miracles,*

> We must remove the word "impossible" from our vocabulary . . . when we see how terms like "spontaneous remission" or "miracle" mislead and confuse us, then we will learn. Such terms imply that the patient must be lucky to be cured, but these healings occur through hard work. They are not acts of God. Remember that one generation's miracle may be another's scientific fact. Do not close your eyes to acts or events that are not always measurable. They happen by means of an energy available to all of us. That's why I prefer terms like "creative" or "self-induced" healing, which emphasizes the patients' active role.

There are intangibles in prevention just as there are intangibles in healing. But you can be guided initially by the fact that cancer prevention is not much different from a move toward general health. What prevents cancer promotes well-being in most other areas of life. If significant changes are necessary in our eating habits, lifestyles, and attitudes, these changes will without question benefit our overall vitality. *Your Defense Against Cancer* is no more and no less than a series of clues to help you find your way toward greater health. Once you engage in health awareness, you will be responding to the signals from your own body to guide your preventive actions.

II

UNDERSTANDING CANCER

2

How Cancer Begins

Cancer starts as a form of anarchy.

If you look down at a large city from a low-flying plane, the orderly ebb and flow of human beings and vehicles seems rather remarkable. The easy flow is possible because of the controls that regulate it— streets, signs, lights, policemen, and written and unwritten laws of movement. If one of the controls breaks down, any city dweller knows too well what happens: first congestion in the immediate trouble spot, and then, if the situation isn't remedied, the clog-up spreads to other parts of the city.

With its ten trillion cells, the human body is like a city. Cancer, a disease of the cell, results from a breakdown of the body's regulatory systems. Only one cell needs to change character and go out of control, and if the body's defenses are unable to restore order, that single cell wildly multiplies and eventually becomes a tumor.

Cancer is a multistep process and, fortunately, can be arrested at any number of steps along the way. For prevention, there are two key points: the *trigger* and the *defense.*

For most cancers, scientists believe that something—a chemical agent (carcinogen), a virus, radiation, or unstable molecules within our bodies (free radicals)—triggers one cell or many cells to go awry and become cancerous. Half the story of prevention is about how to eliminate possible triggers from our food, our environment, and our lifestyle.

Whether we like it or not, we are going to be exposed to some carcinogens. Moreover, according to many cancer researchers, all of us harbor some cancer cells at one time or another. Then the crucial question becomes: will our immune system pick up the triggers or the cancer cells and destroy them before a tumor develops? So the second half of the prevention story is about how to keep our defense systems as strong as possible.

15

In this chapter, I will describe how cancer is triggered and how it grows. It's not altogether a simple explanation, but bear with me. I'd like you to be able to visualize cellular process, because it will go a long way toward strengthening your resolve to avoid carcinogens.

In the same way, I hope that the next chapter, "Our Amazing Defense Systems," will help you visualize the array of immune cells and substances that protect us from invading carcinogens and our own cancer cells. Knowing how our great defense systems work will show you how important it is to do everything possible to keep them lively and strong.

WHAT IS CANCER?

Scientists currently believe that the cancer scenario plays like this: every cancer-causing agent—chemical carcinogen, virus, radiation, free radical, etc.—manages, in one way or another, to penetrate the cell and alter a specific gene, called a "cancer gene." The foreign intruder disturbs the DNA that makes up the gene, thus rewriting a portion of the cell's "programming." This is the beginning of the cancerous process within the cell.

Cancer itself starts when that cell or a number of cells radically change character. Normally, cells are uniform and line up in neat rows. When they begin to "transform" into cancer cells, they regress to a more primitive state. Some cells become larger, others smaller. The cell nuclei show obvious irregularities, and the orderly pattern of identically shaped cells is completely disrupted.

Cells turned malignant break most of the rules of cellular organization. For one thing, if not stopped by our immune defenses, they have the audacity to be both prolific and immortal (for as long as the organism survives). As long as nutrients are available, they will multiply endlessly, and they require more than normal shares of food, oxygen, and water from the host. They also attack and invade surrounding normal tissues, and in so doing break the biological law of "contact inhibition," a natural dictate that stipulates that cells stop dividing when they come in close contact with other cells.

Cancer scientists hold many different theories about why and how cancer cells subvert natural regulations. Some theories relate to the processes set in motion when cancer genes are activated (see page 20). Others point to the strategies adopted by cancer cells to avoid controls like contact inhibition.

Normal cells produce specific proteins on their surfaces to stop them from dividing when coming in contact with other cells. It's as if the body had its own means of population control—a mechanism to

prevent overcrowding. One theory holds that cancer cells don't produce these particular proteins, and therefore no longer respond to the
messages from cells around them. Some cancer-cell proteins may actually confound the regulatory signals from other cells.

HOW TUMORS FORM

Tumors form when the multiplying cancer cells clump together into a
small, expanding mass. As cells proliferate rapidly, the mass enlarges,
oblivious of any control signals (cancer cells have a depressing lack of
social awareness). Depending on the character of the cells, the tumor
may be benign, meaning that the mass does not spread to the surrounding tissue. Or, if they are malignant, a "domino" effect will start, as they
invade tissues in the nearby vicinity. In the early stages of growth the
tumor spreads between layers of tissue. During later stages, as they
grow wildly out of control, the malignant cells begin destroying the
tissues.

When doctors speak of a "primary" tumor, they mean the original
tumor mass and refer to it by its locale (lung, bladder, etc.). Secondary
tumors, called *metastases,* result if cancer cells journey from the original tumor to distant sites in the body—other organs, tissues, lymph
nodes. This sojourn begins when a few malignant cells make an exodus
from the primary tumor and manage to find their way into the bloodstream and/or lymphatic system (the network of thin-walled vessels
throughout the body, which carry lymphatic fluid).

On their journey, cancer cells are like the cagiest of enemy agents,
penetrating borders through an array of slips, tricks, and camouflages.
They manufacture enzymes that are their passports into the bloodstream—the enzymes actually dissolve holes through blood-vessel walls.
Traveling through the lymph system, cancer cells usually find their first
shelter at the nearest lymph node. The node might provide a welcome
way station to multiply once again and form another mass. Then they
may continue their journey to even more distant lymph nodes or
glands.

If malignant cells finding their way into the bloodstream *don't meet
resistance from sentries of the immune system,* they will travel through
the larger blood vessels until becoming bottle-necked in a smaller vessel. Under the right circumstances, they break through the vessel and
form a new colony in nearby tissues—the start of a secondary, "metastatic" tumor.

If metastases are widespread and involve distant sites and other
organs, then treatment is usually difficult if not impossible. What begins
as a limited excursion turns into a global war, overcoming all systemic

defense efforts. The "rebellion" has been tragically successful.

Every type of cell—and there are countless types—is susceptible to malignant transformation. Cancers usually take their names from the organs where they arise ("lung," "breast," "colon," etc.) They are also categorized by the types of body tissues in which they originate: sarcomas arise from bone and soft tissues such as blood vessels or muscles; carcinomas arise from the cells that make up the tissues lining the body organs (lung, colon, ovaries, breast, skin etc.); leukemias arise from blood cells; and lymphomas from the blood cells of the bone-marrow or lymph-node cells.

But, because this book focuses on prevention, let's return to the key question of what triggers the *initial changes* within the cell that often lead to cancer.

THE TRIGGERS

We know a lot about triggers and we're learning more every day. They come in the form of (1) chemical agents—carcinogens—that trigger changes in the cell; (2) specific viruses; (3) radiation; (4) hormones—particularly estrogens; and (5) free radicals (more about these later).

There are hundreds of known carcinogens, like nicotine and tar in cigarettes and asbestos fibers. Food is a big source of carcinogens, which is part of the reason one-third of this book is devoted to diet. We all know that carcinogens are also found in air pollution, but the worst of that pollution, surprisingly, is *not outside* but *inside* our homes and workplaces—and we need to pay more attention to that problem. If inhaled, many household and industrial chemicals are carcinogenic.

Some viruses also trigger cancer. At one time some researchers thought that most cancers were caused by viruses. But, as other factors were discovered, that view was largely abandoned. Those viruses that have been proved to initiate cancer—known as oncoviruses—include among others: Epstein-Barr virus, which has been implicated in Burkitt's lymphoma, nasopharyngeal cancer, and possibly Hodgkin's disease; the hepatitis B virus—a certain cause of many (if not most) primary liver cancers; and human papilloma virus—a possible cause of cervical cancer.

If you have been infected with one of these viruses, it does not mean you'll get cancer. It means only that you have a greater risk.

Radiation—including x-rays, gamma rays, and "particulate" radiation (in the form of particles)—can provoke a malignant change in cells. The ultraviolet rays from sunlight, a form of radiation, can cause skin cancers.

Some hormones—particularly the estrogens—can promote cellular changes if there is an imbalance of them, or if excessive drugs containing those hormones are taken.

Some specific carcinogens are known to trigger specific cancers. Smoking is an established cause of lung cancer, for instance, though not all lung cancers are caused by smoking. Such is the case with most cancers: we can identify the triggers of many but not all cancers of a particular type. For many cancers, no cause is known, and speculation about how and why they develop has led to some probing and provocative research.

All the known causes must be considered risk factors, because exposure to any one of them does not mean you will contract cancer. Exposure means that your *risk* of contracting cancer goes up; the greater the exposure, the greater the risk. *But other factors are crucial in determining whether exposure to a cancer-causing agent will lead to disease.*

The most important contributing factors are heredity, diet, and psychological state. Like many other diseases, cancer is multifactoral— with many interacting causes. Some factors have to do with triggers, others have to do with the body's defenses. More than one carcinogen may be necessary for a cell to turn cancerous. In addition, if we contract cancer, our natural defense systems have probably broken down in some way.

Our job is to do all we can to keep those defenses strong.

FREE RADICALS

Another cancer trigger is completely internal, a by-product of normal metabolic responses. *Free radicals* are molecules that contain an extra, unpaired electron. In their attempt to unload the agitated electron, free radicals can damage tissues, which can be a first step to cancer.

Free radicals form in many different ways. One of the most common is for oxygen to react with different chemical substances in the body, including fats. Called "oxidation," this process is what occurs when metals rust or when fats become rancid. Although oxygen is crucial to life, in certain oxidation reactions—such as those involving polyunsaturated fats—oxygen can release the energy of the fats and in doing so create free radicals, known in this case as "oxygen radicals." Oxygen radicals are highly volatile, dangerous molecules, rushing around madly to unload their excess energy, and in the process inflicting damage on proteins, fats, and nucleic acids—including the DNA within cells.

Free radicals can also form when high energy—such as ultraviolet light or ionizing radiation—knocks an electron out of its orbit in an atom. The lost electron is charged with extra energy and quickly seeks a new home in another atom. When it finds one, it latches on quickly, turning its new host into a highly unstable atom with an extra-high-energy electron. Seeking stability once again, these free radicals try to transfer their excess energy wherever they can in the body—which usually means nearby cells, where they can damage the cell membrane and disturb the DNA.

Free radicals are caused by many oxidation reactions: by chemicals, various metals, and high-energy radiation and light. At normal, controlled levels, free radicals don't cause disease; the body's immune and other defenses, including enzymes and the cell membrane itself, can block excess free-radical damage. Uncontrolled free radicals, however, are known to cause brain damage, arthritis, premature aging—as well as cancer. Recent studies have implicated free radicals in more than 60 disorders.

Dietary factors are crucial to the control of free-radical damage, and hence to the prevention of cancer. Particular nutrients—the vitamins and minerals known as antioxidants—block oxidation reactions that produce free radicals. Other nutrients enhance antioxidant enzymes that stop free radicals. Scientists are now testing nutrients and other substances as antiradical therapies for a wide range of physical disorders.*

Antioxidant nutrients—like beta-carotene and vitamins C and E—are great allies in a natural war against enemy molecules formed within, and it is vital that we take advantage of their properties. (For a description of these nutrients, their effects, and recommended intakes, see Chapter 5, "Foods That Are Allies.")

So these are the cancer triggers. But just how do they set off the changes in our normal cells to turn them cancerous?

That's a tale in itself.

THE GENE STORY

Only very recently, molecular biologists made a discovery that has revolutionized cancer research: probably *all cancers begin* within the genetic material of *our own* healthy, normal cells. Because "cancer genes"—known as oncogenes—were first discovered in viruses, many researchers thought that viruses (and only a few viruses at that) triggered cancer. That's why, for a period, much of the scientific cancer community concentrated their study on viruses. Then, a few years ago when biologists discovered oncogenes existed in human and animal cells as well, research turned around. The viruses, it now appears, were only

*The *New York Times* article of April 20, 1988, "Natural Chemicals Now Called Major Cause of Disease," reports on recent breakthroughs in free radical research, including the many diseases involved and the many innovative new forms of antiradical therapy.

"kidnapping" the cancer genes from the animals or humans they infected.

Let's back up a bit.

Within the nucleus of every cell resides the equivalent of a computer chip—strands of DNA (deoxyribonucleic acid), which code for and control all the cell's vital functions. These strands of DNA are organized into paired structures: chromosomes. Human DNA forms twenty-three pairs of chromosomes.

Genes are the tiny molecular units of DNA strung on each chromosome like beads on a string. There are hundreds of genes on a chromosome, and a total of about 50,000 genes in every cell. Each gene—or minuscule bit of DNA—contains a blueprint for the production of one or another protein, each of which performs a different cellular function. As such, genes are the control switches for all of life's functions, and the thousands of genes located on twisting chains of DNA make up the total control panel.

The specific genes that have the ability to turn on the cancer process are called "proto-oncogenes" ("before becoming oncogenes"). In their original form, they probably serve functions vital to the cell's growth, differentiation, and energy metabolism. They also have the ability to switch roles like Jekyll and Hyde. In their Jekyll phase they produce proteins crucial to cell growth, or at least are "asleep" and innocuous. In their Hyde phase something causes their function to become terribly distorted and they begin manufacturing proteins that cause the cell to change character, multiply out of control, and wreak havoc in nearby tissues. In short, the cells become cancerous.

Five years ago, the first human oncogene was isolated from a bladder cancer. Since then, more than twenty oncogenes have been found and implicated in human cancers, including colon, lung, and breast cancers, and certain leukemias and lymphomas (cancers of the lymph system).

Scientists are not completely sure what function the various oncogenes perform in their original, normal (proto-oncogene) identity. There are different theories and perhaps different answers for different oncogenes. One study by Dr. Michael Wigler at the Cold Spring Laboratory in Long Island indicates that one group of oncogenes helps produce a substance vital to cell metabolism, growth, and energy use. Another group may have blueprints for "platelet-derived growth factors"—proteins that help wounds heal.

Some scientists believe that cancer may be a literal form of cell regression. Their theory is that oncogenes "turn on" the rapid growth of cells required earlier by a fetus, after such rapid growth is no longer necessary or desirable. After birth, such genes should become dormant. However, if "switched on" later in life, they might become cancer genes. In fact, cancer diagnosticians use certain "fetal proteins" (shed from cancer cells) as diagnostic "markers" for various cancers (which is an indication that these cells may be controlled by genes responsible for embryonic growth decades earlier). Biochemical blueprints that served their function in infancy but should have long since become dormant are reactivated in adulthood, when their schema is inappropriate and dangerous.

THE GENE AND THE TRIGGER

The basic mechanism of cancer within the cell is the "cancer gene" (oncogene)—but we know that this gene must be "switched on" by an outside entity, the "trigger." Some cancers are probably caused when genes are "switched on" spontaneously, or for unknown reasons. However, this is an exception to the rule; most cancers are caused by known carcinogenic factors.

Oncogenes are triggered in several different ways: Sometimes a cancer-causing substance or virus enters the cell, binds to DNA, and causes a mutation in a susceptible gene. Asbestos is a fitting example: tiny spicules of asbestos penetrate directly into the cell nucleus. Through an electron microscope asbestos fibers have been seen right among the genetic material. In cancer-causing radiation, subatomic particles hit a strand of DNA to cause a defect.

Viruses are believed to bind to the surface of cells, after which they shed their protein "coats." Viruses have their own genes, some of which are dumped right into the cell, combining with DNA and creating or activating cancer genes. Scientists still aren't sure whether viruses have their own oncogenes, or have genes that simply trigger a human cell's oncogenes.

Minor genetic changes and movement can rock the stability of the cell's internal mechanism. In certain cases, a change in only one or two of the thousands of DNA subunits that make up a gene is enough to cause a mutation. The result is an abnormal protein product that initiates malignant changes in the cell.

Another mechanism involves a rearrangement of genes. If a proto-oncogene is thrown into a new position on the chromosome, it may come into contact with another gene that triggers its cancer-causing role. Or it may be removed from the close proximity of a natural "repressor" gene that keeps it in check.

Research at the University of Minnesota Medical School suggests that chromosome breakages activate cancer genes. There appear to be many "fragile sites" on human chromosomes, and if one of them breaks, a rearrangement of genes may occur that switches on cancer genes. The best-documented case of chromosome breakage triggering oncogenes is in the cancer called Burkitt's lymphoma. Scientists have managed to identify the exact breakage point and rearrangement of genes that occur in every case of this disease.

As mentioned, genetic changes or the rearrangement of genes on a chromosome can occur accidentally or for reasons unknown. This fact may account for the small percentage of cancers in which there is no known cause or causes. It may one day be shown that nutritional, environmental, psychological, or other factors alter genetic material in ways that can't now be detected by the modern technology of cancer research.

Recent studies suggest that more than one oncogene must be activated for a normal cell to turn into a cancer cell. Also, more than one carcinogen may be needed to switch on an oncogene and initiate the cancer process.

The first step, *initiation,* occurs when a carcinogen binds to a cell and causes a gene mutation. These cells are now "primed." But nothing crucial may happen unless another agent, a *promoter,* enters the scene. The promoter can prompt initiated cells to proliferate in great numbers: the result is an expanding population of cells that are not yet cancerous, but volatile. Yet another carcinogen, causing an additional mutation, may then be required to launch malignant growth.

The nitrosamines from bacon, and asbestos, are examples of *initiators;* dietary fat is a strong *promoter*—especially in breast and colon tissues. Cigarettes are mini-factories of agents that both initiate *and* promote.

So far, our scenario would seem to be tragically imbalanced on the side of cancer. Oncogenes look like hair triggers that can be set off by any one of hundreds of harmful agents that are all around us. But, as I mentioned earlier, *there are many levels of control and defense that operate to prevent cancer internally. When cancer occurs, it is the result of more than one assault on the cellular level, and more than one breakdown of natural defense mechanisms.*

IS CANCER INHERITED?

The fact that the fundamental mechanism of cancer involves genes *does not mean that cancer is an inherited disease.* It *is* possible to inherit a slightly greater risk of acquiring certain cancers, referred to as a *predisposition.* Such predispositions occur when a person is endowed with a set of genes that, under a host of special circumstances, is more susceptible to the changes that initiate cancer.

Studies show that women with mothers or sisters with breast cancer have a two to three times higher than normal risk of contracting the disease. Other studies show that many more factors come into play to determine whether family history will affect one's risk, including whether or not the family members had breast cancer before or after menopause or in both breasts. Most important, however, is the fact that other variables—including diet and psychological factors—interact with inherited risk to determine the outcome.

Those people with a family background of a type of cancer in which risk can be inherited need only pay more attention to the contributing factors, in order to keep their risks down. Cancer researchers and geneticists are convinced that, in most cases, a few bad genetic cards can be overcome by strong preventive action to eliminate other controllable risk factors.

In very rare instances, family history *is* a strong indicator of increased risk. For example, 50 percent of the offspring of parents with an unusual type of polyp that leads to colon cancer (familial polyposis) will go on to contract the disease. For the most part, however, the increased risk of cancer due to heredity is not nearly as high and preventive action can make an enormous difference.

Lung cancer is the clearest example of genetic and environmental interaction. A recent study indicates that nonsmokers with a history of lung cancer in their family have a four times greater chance of contracting cancer than nonsmokers with no such background. Smokers, of course, have a much higher risk regardless of their inheritance. Those who smoke and have no family history have five times greater risk, but smokers with a family history have *fourteen* times greater risk. By not smoking, those with a family history of lung cancer can keep their risk down from fourteen to four times the risk. Such figures absolutely confirm that our lifestyles make a big difference, even in the face of factors like heredity over which we have no control.

Now let's look at our amazing defense system—that ubiquitous ally in the fight against carcinogens from without and cancer cells from within.

3

Our Amazing Defense Systems

One of the most fascinating figures in modern medicine remains almost unknown. His name is William B. Coley and he was the first to discover what an enormous capacity our immune systems have for combatting cancer.

His was a most important discovery. The front lines of cancer prevention and treatment today are largely engaged in harnessing the power of our immune systems.

A surgeon at Memorial Hospital in New York for forty-six years, Coley began his cancer research in the late 1890s. He discovered in the medical literature cases of spontaneous regression of cancer, in which tumors shrank and disappeared without treatment and for no known reason. He became intrigued by the observation that bacterial infections often coincided with a sudden turnabout of cancer growth. Coley's instincts told him there was a connection. He took a daring step: he purposely infected an inoperable cancer patient with a strain of streptococcal bacteria. Shortly thereafter, the patient came down with a serious infection—replete with chills, sweats, and high fever. Then the tumor shrank and eventually disappeared. The patient, whose large tumor could not be removed, who was deemed beyond hope, had been cured by exposure to another disease!

Coley and many others since have concluded that the bacterial invasion was like a rallying cry. The natural process set in motion to capture and destroy the microbial invaders also jarred the immune system into action against the existing tumor cells. It was the first indication that our own bodies could do the job doctors have been struggling with for centuries. Decades later, in the 1960s, scientists found that bacterial products could be used to prompt regression of animal and human tumors.

During his career, Coley refined his bacterial treatment—using what later became known as "mixed bacterial toxins" or "Coley's toxins." He treated hundreds of patients over several decades, and his rates of cure or amelioration were remarkable for his time. During the 1920s, Coley's toxins moved into disfavor with the powers-that-be at Memorial Hospital, as the seemingly miraculous (at the time) capabilities of radiation and chemotherapy eclipsed them. There may also have been some economic considerations involved, as corporations vied for the production and sale of radium and expensive new drugs. In retrospect, it can be seen that Coley's toxins were successful in treating certain cancers—as effective as radiation or chemotherapy or even more—and should not have been abandoned. Without question, his work should be acknowledged as the forerunner of all current approaches to controlling cancer immunologically.

Since then, research has continued to pile up evidence that cancer can be prevented or controlled internally by our own immune defenses. Rare cases of spontaneous regression of cancer, like those Coley noted in the literature, have been documented for years; people with far-advanced cancers, receiving little or no treatment, suddenly and for no apparent reason become well. Their tumors shrink and disappear, their metastases clear up, their pain subsides. The seeming miracle is confirmed years later when they are found to be in good health, completely free of disease.

Now, in the 1980s, almost all of the new experimental cancer treatments—the ones that are currently making the front pages of newspapers and science magazines—involve stimulating or modifying the immune response against cancer. We have the added advantage today of recombinant DNA technology, which enables researchers to produce immune-cell products outside the body, in a pure form and in very large quantities. Biotechnology is helping us pinpoint cells and substances called "biologicals"—like interferon, interleukin-2, tumor necrosis factor, and specific monoclonal antibodies—that have anticancer properties in the body. They are reproduced through gene splicing and the revolutionary "hybridoma" techniques, and are used to bolster a cancer patient's defense against his own tumor.

Coley began by introducing powerful antigens—his bacterial toxins—into the body, jarring the immune system into action against cancer cells. Probably Coley's method was an amazingly successful way to stimulate natural production of those very "biologicals" that today's immunologists and pharmeceutical companies treasure as the future of cancer therapy. Coley's toxins may have set in motion a network of naturally occurring immune interactions in the body—something that will be hard for immunologists to reproduce in cancer therapy. Someday, it may be found that bacterial products still have great, untapped value in cancer treatment, alongside the biologicals that are in vogue now.

If cancer can be treated by stimulating the immune system to recognize and kill tumor cells, then it follows that cancer can be prevented by keeping our immune systems strong. This is no longer an assumption. Research is bearing out the fact that a healthy immune system is a major cornerstone of cancer prevention. We must try to avoid any and all carcinogens—but there will always be lapses, some of which we cannot help. It is therefore extremely important to take care of that inner network, which so forcefully and brilliantly takes care of us.

REGULATION AND DEFENSE

Regulatory and defense mechanisms exist at almost every stage in the scenario of cancer development. A carcinogen that is breathed in, absorbed through the skin, or ingested, can be picked up in the bloodstream by "scavenger" immune cells—phagocytes. If it's not caught there, the cells themselves have enzymes that detoxify carcinogens. Most of the time, these "detoxification enzymes" break down the molecules of a carcinogen into a form that is excreted in urine.

However, Harry Gelboin of the National Cancer Institute has discovered that individuals may have enzymes that function like double agents. Instead of neutralizing carcinogens, an unfortunate combination of these enzymes works improperly and *activates* carcinogens. The turncoat enzymes give carcinogens access to the cell's inner sanctum—the DNA. Once inside, they have the power to cause a possible mutation. But activated carcinogens still may not bind to DNA; often they bind innocuously to proteins or other parts of the cell.

If an activated carcinogen does bind to DNA, there is still the opportunity for DNA repair before a mutation can take hold. Remarkably, the cell's internal machinery contains a mechanism that is reminiscent of surgery or film editing. Enzymes that perform this repair job cut out the small segment of DNA containing the carcinogen and any resulting defect. Because every unit of DNA exists in a pair (on the "double helix"), the unaffected unit serves as a model for the creation—and insertion—of new, fresh DNA unit(s) to replace those that have been edited out. If the DNA repair mechanism fails, or if the cell divides before repair takes place, the daughter cells will carry the potentially cancer-causing mutation with them.

So carcinogenic initiators can either be vanquished in the bloodstream or rendered harmless by enzymes in the cell. In addition, natu-

ral anticancer substances—some of which come from food sources*
—can counteract the effects of the chemical promoters.

A wound or other injury can also promote cancer-cell development. When an injury occurs within tissues, growth factors are released
locally to aid rapid healing. If initiated cells reside in the area, the
growth factors may also switch on the cancer process in these susceptible cells.

A whole panoply of "ifs" make cancer an improbability: *If* carcinogens get into the body; *if* this agent gets past the immune system; *if*
detoxifying enzymes in the cell act improperly; *if* promoter chemicals
are not neutralized by natural substances; *if* the carcinogen binds directly to DNA; *if* DNA repair either fails or "arrives" too late; and *if*
cancer genes are affected and "switched on." And, *if* normal cells do
transform, the change may only be "benign": a mass of abnormal cells
will develop, but the character of these cells is such that they do not
invade and destroy surrounding tissue.

Finally, if cells do turn fully malignant, there is still one critical line
of defense. The immune system, in all its complexity and power, is able
to detect and destroy cells that have turned cancerous. Sometimes, it
is even able to eliminate a developed tumor.

THE IMMUNE SYSTEM

The body's defense network—the immune system—is about as complicated as the Defense Department. Again, I'm not fond of military metaphors, but they are apropos for the immune system. Its aggressiveness
and ubiquity as an *internal* entity can save us from invasive and destructive external measures, like surgery and radiation.

Except for the nervous system, the immune system is the most
complex biological system we have. It consists of master glands, princi-
pally the thymus; various sites that harbor immune cells; and different
classes of "soldier" cells, which carry out specialized functions—including cells that prompt, cells that alert, cells that facilitate, cells that
activate, cells that surround, cells that kill, even cells that clean up.
Many immune cells also synthesize and secrete special molecules that
act as messengers, regulators, or helpers in the process of defending
against invading elements.

Basically, the immune system functions to keep us healthy. When
it fails, we become susceptible to viruses, bacteria, environmental
agents, and cancer cells. That our immune systems are able to identify
and destroy cancer cells, specifically, is a fairly recent and revolutionary

*Foods rich in anticancer agents are described in Chapter 5, "Foods That Are Allies."

discovery, the result of years of research. Just how does the immune system operate?

ANTIGENS: THE SIGNALERS

Antigens are the fingerprints of immunity. They are identifying molecular markers that reside on the surface of all cells and, like fingerprints, are unique to the cells that bear them. All our body cells have antigens that signal "self-self-self"—a message that they are part of us and therefore are not to be labeled as foreign and are not to be attacked.

Foreign microorganisms, viruses, and just about any outside agent that invades our bodies also have identifying antigens on their cell surfaces, which, when such substances enter our bodies, signal "foreign-foreign-foreign" to the immune system and ready it for immediate attack. That's why organ transplants are difficult; the antigens on the newly-introduced cells sound the "non-self" alarm. To prevent the rejection of transplanted tissues, a patient must be given drugs that suppress the immune system.

If the immune system overreacts to an outside antigen, the result is an allergy. Hayfever, for example, is a hyperresponse to grass or ragweed antigens. When our immune system reacts inappropriately to the antigens on our own cells, the result is called an *autoimmune* disorder. Lupus erythematosus and rheumatoid arthritis are examples of autoimmune diseases, in which, in effect, our own tissues are being attacked from within by the immune system.

If our immune systems *fail* to react to an outside agent—say a virus or bacterium—the result is an infection. Finally, if our immune systems fail to identify and destroy our own cells after they have become malignant, the result is cancer-cell development and, possibly, the growth of tumors. How can the immune system react to our own cancer cells if the antigens on our cells are supposed to signal "self" to ward off any attack? In the answer lies the crux of cancer immunology.

Many cancer immunologists believe that once a cell has transformed, or become cancerous, certain antigens on its surface also change. The altered antigens—known as "cancer-specific" or "cancer-associated" antigens—then signal "non-self" to the immune system. They are the giveaway—the slight change in fingerprints that enables our defenses to pick up on a dangerous inside job. This means that our immune system can be alerted to cancer cells *as if* they were invaders from outside, and respond to them as such—by calling on the troops to move in and wipe out the interlopers.

ANTIBODIES: THE MIRACULOUS FIT

Antibodies are the body's complement to antigens. Think of each antigen as a unique lock, and the protein molecules called antibodies (or immunoglobulins) as custom-made keys for every variation of lock. These molecules are among the minor marvels of the immune system because they can fit, like a complex key, into the specific keyhole of any one of millions of different foreign antigens, including many cancer antigens. Each antigen has a different molecular configuration, and our bodies can produce antibodies that latch into each antigen perfectly.

Antibodies are carried throughout the body by white blood cells called lymphocytes. They are the leading soldiers of the immune system. Lymphocytes come in two main classes—T-lymphocytes and B-lymphocytes (T-cells and B-cells, for short). T-cells are the prime players in the drama of cell-mediated immunity. B-cells are the leaders of humoral immunity, the arm of the immune system involved in antibody production. The latter circulate through the body with antibody molecules on their surfaces. When they pick up the signal of a particular antigen, they multiply and transform into *plasma cells,* which are essentially minifactories with one purpose: to churn out the precise antibodies that will hook onto the antigens of the invader. Antibodies are able not only to neutralize foreign substances or microbes; they also signal other immune sentries into battle. An antigen-antibody bond is a call to arms, and often a "cascade" of immune reactions follow the initial "connection." This cascade—the sum total of activity by the immune system against an invader—is called an *immune response.*

T-CELLS: THE PRIME PLAYERS

T-cells are the prime players in cell-mediated immunity, the arm of the immune system consisting of subgroups of interacting cells. T-cells are so named because they "grow up" in the thymus, a gland the size of a walnut located under the breastbone. Although all immune cells are "born" in the bone marrow, different types follow different developmental pathways. T-cells migrate to the thymus. There, with the aid of various thymic hormones, immature T-cells grow, "learn" to recognize and attack antigens, and develop their "specialties." The thymus is therefore the master gland of cell-mediated immunity, a sort of training school for different classes of T-cells. Mature T-cells are harbored in the spleen and lymph nodes, waiting there for the sound of an alarm signaling an intruder.

The main subcategories of T-cells include:

1. T-helper cells, which alert, stimulate, or enhance the action of other immune cells. They are essential to the performance of their fellow B-cells of the humoral branch; certain antibody reactions depend on help from the helper Ts.
2. Killer T-cells, also known as cytotoxic T-cells, which are able, after being primed by previous exposure, to hook onto the foreign antigen of an invading microbe or cancer cell and instantly destroy it.
3. Suppressor T-cells, which are vital to maintaining a proper balance in immune responses. They are able to suppress or dampen the actions of other immune cells. Without the activity of suppressor Ts, immunity could easily get out of hand, resulting in allergic or auto-immune reactions.

The immune system has a built-in memory. "Memory cells" from the B-cell line remember the first encounter with a specific antigen. As a result, antibodies are produced much more quickly and powerfully the second time an antigen is encountered. The T-cell line also has cells that help strengthen T-cell reactions the second time around. *Immunological memory not only keeps us free of disease agents we've been exposed to, but it is also the mechanism that makes vaccination an effective control of disease.* When we're administered small, harmless amounts of an infectious agent through vaccines, our systems respond and remember. If and when we're exposed again, the immune system is eager for tough and immediate action.

THE BIG EATERS & CO.

The third important class of immune cells are the scavenger cells. Also called phagocytes, they specialize in engulfing microbes or other unwanted products in the bloodstream. Macrophages are a class of phagocytes often referred to as the "big eaters."

For years macrophages were thought to be only the garbagemen of the immune system, checking in after an immune reaction to clean up any remaining wastes. We now know that macrophages play several other key roles in immunity: they often begin the chain reaction of an immune response by processing and presenting any foreign antigens to the lymphocytes. They also release important biological products that help spur on immunity; one of them, called "tumor necrosis factor," has anticancer properties.

There are a host of secondary players in the epic drama of immunity. Among them are a group called "null cells." The most frequently studied and intriguing of the null cells are called "natural killer cells" (NK), which have the uncanny ability to recognize viruses and cancer cells without having ever encountered them before. NK cells are then able to kill their targets without any help from other immune cells.

THE MIRACULOUS "BIOLOGICALS"

Countless protein molecules and enzymes are produced by immune cells, and they provide critical links in the immune response chain. These natural substances perform varied functions; most of them regulate immune-cell interactions. Called "biological response modifiers" ("biologicals," for short), these substances can be either messengers, communicators, helpers, growth inducers or suppressors. And these are the type of substances that Coley probably turned on in the body with his bacterial toxins.

To date, the best-known biologicals are the *interferons,* antiviral proteins that also have anticancer activity. Recently, much publicity has been given to the *interleukins*—especially to interleukin-2 for its ability to aid in cancer-cell destruction. Countless other biologicals are important links in the anticancer defense network, and new ones are now being discovered all the time.

But it is the interferons, interleukin-2, and tumor necrosis factor (TNF) that have shown enough promise in both animal and human studies to warrant synthetic production (through genetic engineering). They are now being tested in full-scale clinical trials on human cancer patients.

Through a remarkable new technology, scientists are also experimenting with manufacturing antibodies themselves, known as "monoclonal antibodies." By fusing a special type of cancer cell with an antibody-producing B-cell, researchers can make mini-factories (called "hybridomas") that relentlessly churn out pure, specific antibodies. Monoclonal antibodies that are specific to certain types of cancer cells are now used to diagnose these cancers. Someday they will be used on a wide scale for cancer therapy.

The hope is that new forms of cancer therapy—utilizing one or more anticancer biologicals—will revolutionize the treatment of cancer. Even further in the future is a time when people will be tested to find out whether or not they lack enough of any of the biologicals. These lacks or imbalances could then be rectified with additional doses of the particular product, thus bolstering immunity and possibly preventing cancer.

HARNESSING OUR IMMUNE POWERS

In the last decade, laboratory research has confirmed that the *immune system can wipe out cancer cells.* Through an electron microscope, scientists have witnessed and photographed the spectacle of T-cells attaching to cancer cells and killing them through a process called "lysis." The cancer cell's membrane is broken open and the cell disintegrates.

Yet questions still exist about why and how the immune system fails when a person contracts cancer. Apparently, cancer cells employ a variety of complex strategies to escape the immune system. They may even shed or mask their cancer antigens so as not to be "recognized." Immunologists have some evidence that cancer cells may even engage the services of suppressor cells to put a damper on an immune attack against them. But, despite cancer cells' clever ploys to fool our defenses, the fact remains that when tumors grow and thrive, the immune system is probably deficient, suppressed, or overwhelmed.

When we embark on an anticancer lifestyle, we are paying attention to the invisible healer inside us, and it requires our cooperation. The cancer-prevention diet can strengthen our immune systems in specific ways that will be described in the chapters on diet. The subtle but powerful ways that psychological well-being may contribute to immunity against cancer and other diseases will be explained in the chapters on psychological factors. Avoiding carcinogens not only reduces the risk of cancer-cell development, but also takes one more load off a system that can become easily overloaded.

Because cancer is a multistep process, we have many opportunities to extinguish cancer cells before they attack us. Some of the guidelines in *Your Defense Against Cancer* are ways to interrupt the various steps of cancer-cell development. Other guidelines involve ways to keep our defense systems healthy and alert—ready for meeting any challenges.

Now let's see what diet can do.

III
THE
DIET FACTOR

4

Diet and Nutrition

It used to be cigarettes. Now it's food. Not that cigarettes have been exonerated—far from it. But as recently as fifteen years ago most cancer specialists thought that anyone who suggested that certain foods could cause or prevent cancer was a faddist or a fanatic. Today, the experts estimate that at least 35 percent of all cancers are either initiated, promoted, or could be prevented by what we eat. Smoking as a cause is estimated at 30 percent. This indicates a monumental change in our awareness of what causes cancer and what we can do about it.

The 35 percent figure for dietary factors may be too conservative. In a 1977 report, researchers Wynder and Gori estimated that more than 40 percent of cancers in men and 60 percent of cancers in women could be attributed to dietary factors. In 1984, the Center for Science in the Public Interest stated that diet plays a key role in approximately 133,000 deaths a year in the U.S.—51,000 from colorectal cancer, 37,000 from breast cancer, 25,000 from prostate cancer, and 20,000 from cancers of the mouth, throat, larynx, and esophagus. Diet is also now thought to be a contributing cause of cancers of the stomach, small intestine, pancreas, liver, ovary, endometrium, thyroid, lung, and bladder. Moreover, many experts today feel it may be indirectly involved in *every* form of cancer.

The big nutrition breakthrough came in 1980, when the National Cancer Institute (NCI), pressed by pioneering biochemists, nutritionists, and cancer specialists on the importance of dietary factors, commissioned the National Research Council to investigate the entire field. A committee of the most distinguished names in nutrition and cancer research was established, drawn from the National Academy of Sciences, and called the Committee on Diet, Nutrition, and Cancer. They published their report in 1982—aptly titled *Diet, Nutrition, and Cancer*—and it is a landmark overview of the field. In retrospect, the claims made in it for dietary cancer prevention seem rather tentative. Nevertheless, it is a striking document—utterly comprehensive and unequivocal in its summary report: "The evidence reviewed by the committee suggests that cancers of most major sites are influenced by dietary patterns." A decade earlier the cancer establishment would have summarily labeled such a claim absurd.

The committee makes another telling point in its summary:

> It has become absolutely clear that cigarettes are the cause of approximately one-quarter of all the fatal cancers in the U.S. If the population had been persuaded to stop smoking when the association with lung cancer was first reported, these cancer deaths would not now be occurring. . . . [W]e are in an interim stage of knowledge similar to that for cigarettes 20 years ago. Therefore, in the judgement of the committee, it is now the time to offer some interim guidelines on diet and cancer.

The cigarette analogy should be our guide. In 1988, the U.S. government issued a landmark report on nutrition and health, wherein the Surgeon General cited dietary fat reduction as a top priority for the prevention of chronic diseases, including cancer. The role of diet in cancer is indisputable, and knowledge of the extent of the connection is being broadened daily.

This means that we must take our diet very seriously—both by eliminating foods that are enemies and by adding foods that are allies. We also must stop smoking. In our diet, however, we don't simply have to give up something; we will be adding foods that will strengthen our bodies and anticancer defenses. There are nutrients in food that can not only nourish us but protect us for a lifetime.

"BUT THEY CHANGE THEIR MINDS EVERY DAY!"

"Ah," you say, like the skeptics in Chapter 1, "but they change their minds every day. If I listened to the experts, I couldn't eat anything."

Yes, the advice does change as scientists learn more about the effects of specific nutrients and their interaction with body chemistry. But their overall thrust is not constantly changing: a low-fat, low-calorie, high-fiber diet, rich in fresh fruits, vegetables, and natural grains, and containing specific vitamins and minerals, is the ticket. This is not being widely questioned. Neither is the existence of established food carcinogens or promoters—especially excess fat—that we should avoid. Such a diet *will* reduce our risk of many cancers. The primary questions left to be answered are:

- How much will these measures reduce our risk?
- What other dietary factors—as yet untested—play a role in cancer development?
- How can we get ourselves to follow these dietary prescriptions?

The last question is the tough one. Just why are we so resistant to new scientific discoveries, and why is it so difficult to make the needed changes? One reason may be the fear factor mentioned earlier: we don't like to worry about the possibility of frightening outcomes—especially long-term ones—that call for immediate changes without immediate tangible benefits. An even bigger factor is that deeply ingrained habits and attitudes are not easily overturned. Our food tastes and habits have been part of our lives since earliest childhood. For many of us, ice cream, candy, and sugary delights were our rewards for eating overcooked vegetables, for being a year older, or for just being "good." Later in life, these same foods are used to make us "feel better" or ease anxiety.

Although our parents may have been aware of the threat of too much sugar, they paid little attention to fat content. The ultimate treat for many children was—and still is—a night out at McDonald's or Burger King, for a feast of charred burgers and greasy french fries. To our parents, these meals seemed nutritious enough: there was protein in the meat, carbohydrates in the potatoes, and a lone slice of tomato or onion for a vegetable. They were unlikely to have been aware of the dangers of fats and cholesterol. Nor was anyone concerned with how the meat was cooked—fried, charbroiled, or grilled—all of which, we now know, are cooking methods that create carcinogens.

The ad men today are cleverly creating images that make us think cancer-promoting foods are actually nutrient-rich and good for us. Fast-food burgers not only look luscious, but shot in closeup to emphasize protruding fresh lettuce and tomatoes, they appear to be complete meals. These ads tap into our childhood food associations while appealing to our adult, health-conscious side. It may be that, within the next decade or so, the government will ban ads that claim (or imply) as "nutritious" those fast and fatty foods, because they are just another form of false advertising. The cigarette T.V. ads of yesteryear had a similar gambit—cigarettes hung from the mouths of hearty, strong cowboys astride their horses.

All this being said, I confess to having had a very hard time resisting the sizzling burgers, fries, pizzas, oily Chinese and Indian dishes, and rich ice creams and whipped-cream delights. Although I learned the facts about the dangers of too much fat in our diet a long time ago—while working for the Cancer Research Institute and having access to wide-ranging research findings—it was hard for me to resist the deep-seated temptations. My early eating patterns, combined with the beckoning appeal of print and TV ads, of restaurants, pizza parlors, and coffee shops, have all conspired to make change a torturous prospect. Nevertheless, when I finally made it, I found the new foods and habits tremendously rewarding. I gained new energy and a feeling that I was at the top of my health. I will present some clues about how to overcome the obstacles and make the necessary changes in Chapter 8, "You Can Change Your Eating Habits."

ADS AND TRENDS

Another word on ads: there is little question that vested interests, such as the beef and pork industries, the dairy and sugar producers, the food-additive manufacturers, will slow down regulatory actions and warnings against the cancer hazards in their products through strong Washington lobbies. Look at the long fight to stop cigarette ads on TV and put warnings on cigarette packs. However, some manufacturers are becoming sensitive to nutritional issues—if not for the public well-being, for their own profit margins. They know that the nation is more health-conscious now than ever. An example is the response of the meat industry to the lowering of meat consumption—they have slowly begun breeding cattle with lower percentages of fat. At the same time, they have stepped up their ad campaigns to recreate images of meat as health-giving sources of all-American protein. In 1988, the National Research Council released a stunning report that argued that not enough is being done by agricultural industries to produce and market lower-fat animal food products. It recommended major changes in the system to discourage high-fat foods and ensure the availability of low-fat products.

Even though some changes are occurring, important regulations have yet to be put into law, and it is up to us to protect our health by resisting the lure of ads and seriously considering the findings of our research scientists. At the same time, we should support the victories of manufacturers like Kellogg, in its fight with the FDA, to advertise their high-fiber cereals as "cancer preventing." High fiber is one valid form of cancer prevention, and the producers of such foods should be encouraged to produce it and advertise it as such. The same could apply to other health-promoting and cancer-preventive foods. We are so glutted with ads inculcating desires for fatty and sugary foods that a bit of subliminal seduction on the side of health is acceptable, as long as the advertising is in good faith. For example, a cereal claiming to be fiber-rich must really be fiber-rich. I will provide guidance on this issue in Chapter 5, "Foods That Are Allies."

At the same time, we should push for bans, or at least warnings, on such foods as nitrite-cured bacon or luncheon meats: i.e., "contains nitrite: may be hazardous to your health." Carcinogenic food additives still on the market should be banned or regulated at safe levels. Health must be directed in the public interest—not in the interest of corporate profit margins.

One final note on current trends of health consciousness: for the most part, they are a positive development. If it takes diet chic to motivate people to change, so be it. Unfortunately though, trends are defined by their inclination to pass. Fad diets eventually give way to those old desires for foods that comfort and appeal to the senses. The clash between health consciousness and old patterns makes us schizoid about diet. How many people do you know (yourself included) who are passionate about healthy eating but still indulge in large quantities of fatty or sugar-saturated or salty foods?

We have to become aware of the sensory and physical satisfactions of healthy eating, and combine this with real knowledge of its health benefits—including cancer prevention—in order to win the war against junk-food influences and childhood patterns of eating. A long-term commitment to changing our eating habits is necessary to cultivate a taste for the natural foods that can protect us.

HOW FOODS PREVENT CANCER

For years, we heard mostly about man-made agents that cause cancer, as in some additives and dyes, and our main concern was "How do we avoid carcinogens in our food?" We knew very little about foods that *prevented* cancer. But more recent nutritional and biochemical research has uncovered just what nutrients—specific vitamins, minerals, and enzymes—can stop cancer's development and how they do it. Now everyone is asking, "What do I eat to prevent cancer?"

In Chapter 5, "Foods That Are Allies," I describe the specific "good" foods, but here I want to impress upon you the many ways nutrients can inhibit cancer growth in our bodies. They may do so by:

- inhibiting the activation of carcinogens
- detoxifying carcinogen molecules
- blocking the action of cancer promoters
- interfering with carcinogens' binding to cells
- helping DNA repair mechanisms after carcinogen damage

- inhibiting tumor growth factors
- scavenging free radicals that cause cancer (antioxidant action)
- bolstering immune-system reactions against carcinogens
- bolstering immune-system reactions against cancer cells
- strengthening the intercellular cement
- inhibiting enzymes produced by cancer cells that make metastases possible
- clearing the system of carcinogens in the lower bowel (fiber).

Obviously, not every anticancer nutrient performs all these functions. Some perform several and some perform only one isolated but vital service. All told, natural foods provide us with an incredible array of protective mechanisms.

THE NUTRITION PIONEERS

From the research on diet and health, entire new fields have begun to spring up, with names like "orthomolecular medicine" (the use of micronutrients for health and healing) and "chemoprevention" (the use of micro- or macronutrients for the prevention of disease), which are beginning to exploit the potential of nutrients for bolstering our body's defenses and maximizing health. How was the diet-cancer connection so suddenly uncovered? What led to this breakthrough, generally unsuspected or unaccepted a mere decade ago?

As is usual with so many medical breakthroughs, the early, and controversial, work of a few pioneering scientists laid the foundation that later led to general medical acceptance and broad-based adoption by the federal government and health organizations.

In the area of diet and cancer, Linus Pauling is one such pioneer. The two-time Nobel Prize-winning biochemist had been ahead of his time before. His discovery of the structure of amino-acid molecules won him his first Nobel Prize, in chemistry, in 1954. His singular contributions during the 1950s to the fight against atomic-bomb testing in the atmosphere set the stage for the test-ban treaty of 1963, and led to his second Nobel Prize, this time for peace.

In the middle 1960s, Pauling became interested in vitamin C, its functions and effects, and its seeming capacity to prevent and ameliorate the common cold and flu. Pauling's wide-ranging studies have helped to confirm the clinical effectiveness of vitamin C in fighting colds, and have explained the myriad ways it works in the body to promote health. To Pauling, vitamin C (ascorbic acid) is a miraculous cog in the biochemical machinery, an "ingredient" essential to our cellular makeup and immune defenses. The vitamin-C-for-colds theory caused endless controversy inside and outside medical circles. Gradually, the value of C in controlling colds and the flu is finally being accepted by a portion of the public and many more doctors.

In the early seventies Pauling extended his work with vitamin C into the realm of cancer. He found that this remarkable micronutrient (the biochemical term generally used for vitamins and minerals) plays a role in warding off cancer's development and could even be used to help slow the growth of tumors and improve the quality of life in cancer patients. The publishing of the book *Cancer and Vitamin C,* which Pauling wrote in collaboration with Dr. Ewan Cameron, brought even more controversy, as Pauling argued that this vitamin has a definite role in the prevention and treatment of cancer.

Pauling and Cameron's studies of the beneficial effects of ascorbic acid on cancer patients have been most hotly debated. Nor were Pauling's less provocative claims for the vitamin's—and nutrition's—role in the prevention of cancer readily accepted at first. In the last few years, a change in attitude has occurred. Since 1982, the NCI has stepped up its support for research on cancer prevention through "chemoprevention" and dietary intervention studies. The recent rapid rise in diet-cancer prevention studies owes a great debt to Pauling's early efforts, though his influence is rarely acknowledged. In Pauling, it is important to be reminded, we have a visionary scientist in our midst, one who has consistently paved the way and charted the course for biomedical breakthroughs. Pauling's overall concept of "orthomolecular medicine" (which began as a new approach to mental-health problems) must be taken seriously as an adjunct or, in special cases, as an alternative to conventional medicine for a spectrum of health problems.

Pauling's work has brought to the fore the question of using supplements—whether we can obtain the vitamins and minerals needed to maintain optimal health from foods alone, or whether we need additional vitamins and minerals. To use Pauling's distinction: the "old" nutrition would have it that balanced meals, including foods from the major food groups, should take care of all our nutritional needs; the "new" nutrition recognizes that we are not likely to fulfill all our vitamin and mineral requirements through foods alone. The "new" nutrition goes even further: judicious use of supplements can help us prevent and cure certain diseases, and in general, help us feel better than we ever thought possible.

Those who oppose the use of supplements invariably invoke the word "nature" to support the view that foods can and should supply us amply with vitamins and minerals. The National Academy of Sciences publishes the Recommended Daily Allowances (RDAs) for levels of vitamins and minerals considered adequate to meet our basic nutritional needs. See pages 44–45 for the U.S. RDAs. Most of us probably

RECOMMENDED DAILY DIETARY ALLOWANCES, REVISED 1980

Food and Nutrition Board, National Academy of Sciences—National Research Council

Designed for the maintenance of good nutrition of practically all healthy people in the U.S.A.

	Age (years)	Weight (kg) (lbs)	Height (cm) (in)	Protein (g)	Vitamin A (IU)*	Vitamin D (μg)	Vitamin E (IU)†	Vitamin C (mg)	Thiamin (mg)	Riboflavin (mg)	Niacin (mg)	Vitamin B₆ (mg N.E.)	Folacin (μg)	Vitamin B₁₂ (μg)	Calcium (mg)	Phosphorus (mg)	Magnesium (mg)	Iron (mg)	Zinc (mg)	Iodine (μg)
								Fat-Soluble Vitamins				Water-Soluble Vitamins						Minerals		
Infants	0.0–0.5	6 / 13	60 / 24	kg × 2.2	2100	10	3	35	0.3	0.4	6	0.3	30	0.5	360	240	50	10	3	40
	0.5–1.0	9 / 20	71 / 28	kg × 2.0	2000	10	4	35	0.5	0.6	8	0.6	45	1.5	540	360	70	15	5	50
Children	1–3	13 / 29	90 / 35	23	2000	10	5	45	0.7	0.8	9	0.9	100	2.0	800	800	150	15	10	70
	4–6	20 / 44	112 / 44	30	2500	10	6	45	0.9	1.0	11	1.3	200	2.5	800	800	200	10	10	90
	7–10	28 / 62	132 / 52	34	3500	10	7	45	1.2	1.4	16	1.6	300	3.0	800	800	250	10	10	120
Males	11–14	45 / 99	157 / 62	45	5000	10	8	50	1.4	1.6	18	1.8	400	3.0	1200	1200	350	18	15	150
	15–18	66 / 145	176 / 69	56	5000	10	10	60	1.4	1.7	18	2.0	400	3.0	1200	1200	400	18	15	150
	19–22	70 / 154	177 / 70	56	5000	7.5	10	60	1.5	1.7	19	2.2	400	3.0	800	800	350	10	15	150
	23–50	70 / 154	178 / 70	56	5000	5	10	60	1.4	1.6	18	2.2	400	3.0	800	800	350	10	15	150
	51+	70 / 154	178 / 70	56	5000	5	10	60	1.2	1.4	16	2.2	400	3.0	800	800	350	10	15	150
Females	11–14	46 / 101	157 / 62	46	4000	10	8	50	1.1	1.3	15	1.8	400	3.0	1200	1200	300	18	15	150
	15–18	55 / 120	163 / 64	46	4000	10	8	60	1.1	1.3	14	2.0	400	3.0	1200	1200	300	18	15	150
	19–22	55 / 120	163 / 64	44	4000	7.5	8	60	1.1	1.3	14	2.0	400	3.0	800	800	300	18	15	150
	23–50	55 / 120	163 / 64	44	4000	5	8	60	1.0	1.2	13	2.0	400	3.0	800	800	300	18	15	150
	51+	55 / 120	163 / 64	44	4000	5	8	60	1.0	1.2	13	2.0	400	3.0	800	800	300	10	15	150
Pregnant				+30	+1000	+5	+2	+20	+0.4	+0.3	+2	+0.6	+400	+1.0	+400	+400	+150	n	+5	+25
Lactating				+20	+2000	+5	+3	+40	+0.5	+0.5	+5	+0.5	+100	+1.0	+400	+400	+150	n	+10	+50

*Calculation from retinol equivalents. †Approximate values due to varying forms of Vitamin E.

RECOMMENDED DIETARY ALLOWANCES, REVISED 1980

Food and Nutrition Board, National Academy of Sciences—National Research Council, Washington, D.C.
Estimated Safe and Adequate Daily Dietary Intakes of Selected Vitamins and Minerals

| | Age (years) | Vitamins | | | | Trace Elements | | | | | | Electrolytes | |
		Vitamin K (µg)	Biotin (µg)	Pantothenic Acid (mg)	Copper (mg)	Manganese (mg)	Fluoride (mg)	Chromium (mg)	Selenium (mg)	Molybdenum (mg)	Sodium (mg)	Potassium (mg)	Chloride (mg)
Infants	0–0.5	12	35	2	0.5–0.7	0.5–0.7	0.1–0.5	0.01–0.04	0.01–0.04	0.03–0.06	115–350	350–925	275–700
	0.5–1	10–20	50	3	0.7–1.0	0.7–1.0	0.2–1.0	0.02–0.06	0.02–0.06	0.04–0.08	250–750	425–1275	400–1200
Children	1–3	15–30	65	3	1.0–1.5	1.0–1.5	0.5–1.5	0.02–0.08	0.02–0.08	0.05–0.1	325–975	550–1650	500–1500
and	4–6	20–40	85	3–4	1.5–2.0	1.5–2.0	1.0–2.5	0.03–0.12	0.03–0.12	0.06–0.15	450–1350	775–2325	700–2100
	7–10	30–60	120	4–5	2.0–2.5	2.0–3.0	1.5–2.5	0.05–0.2	0.05–0.2	0.1–0.3	600–1800	1000–3000	925–2775
Adolescents	11+	50–100	100–200	4–7	2.0–3.0	2.5–5.0	1.5–2.5	0.05–0.2	0.05–0.2	0.15–0.5	900–2700	1525–4575	1400–4200
Adults		70–140	100–200	4–7	2.0–3.0	2.5–5.0	1.5–4.0	0.05–0.2	0.05–0.2	0.15–0.5	1100–3300	1875–5625	1700–5100

can eat enough good food to meet the RDAs, though clearly most of us don't. However, as we shall see in Chapter 5, "Foods That Are Allies," the RDAs represent nutrient levels sufficient only to prevent deficiency diseases—like scurvy, which results from severe vitamin C deficiency—but they are not enough to gain the optimal health benefits possible with supplementation. Without question, one of those additional benefits is the decreased risk of many deadly cancers.

Here I suggest that beneficial, cancer-preventive doses of certain key vitamins and minerals, which though considered large, are not toxic or harmful in any way. A very popular position, taken by some nutritionists and medical experts outside nutrition, is that we should get all our nutrient needs met by adding the proper foods to our diet. Recently, Jane E. Brody, the influential health writer for the *New York Times,* wrote a two-part column coming down on the increasing use of supplements. Like many others, she argued that foods present us with the complete array of interacting nutrient factors we need, and furthermore that taking too many supplements might be dangerous.

The first point is well taken—we should get as much nutrition as we can from food, because various nutrients depend upon each other for proper metabolism and usage by the body. The guidelines I set forth in Chapter 7, "The Cancer-Prevention Diet Guide," emphasize the importance of healthy foods as the first source of nutrients. However, the addition of supplements simply assures us that we get *optimal* amounts of micronutrients that are difficult to obtain from food alone. The point that megadoses of some micronutrients can be toxic is important to consider. Very large doses of certain vitamins and minerals— such as vitamin A and selenium—should *not* be taken. But, as long as clear limits are set, based on scientific research, where there is no risk of side effects, the taking of supplements is not a scary business at all. The supplements I recommend taking in Chapter 7 are well within the bounds of safety, and involve no health risk.

In this culture we are given to popping pills, especially analgesics and antibiotics prescribed by a physician, but we often dismiss as unnecessary, or even harmful, taking nontoxic quantities of nutrients to enhance health. It's true that vitamins are big business, but the cost to the individual of a daily supplement routine pales next to the cost of most prescription drugs needed to combat serious illness.

There are two essential points here: first, the fact is that the modern American diet woefully lacks even minimal amounts of several key nutrients. The overall contribution of fats and refined sugars to our diet has increased 20 percent since the early 1900s. Second, when we take vitamin and/or mineral pills, we are simply ingesting portions of food that are the most biochemically vital to us. Using supplements to prevent and treat disease is a way of amplifying the health-giving properties of the nutrients we ingest in food. The criticism that supplements are somehow unnatural is a contradiction. Is it preferable to rely on over-the-counter and prescription drugs, which are primarily chemicals, to cure our ills when nontoxic doses of nutrients can be used to treat and *prevent* certain diseases without any side effects?

MICRONUTRIENTS ARE LIKE "BIOLOGICALS"

"Biologicals" are natural substances, produced by cells; they have special biochemical and immunological roles in the body. As mentioned in Chapter 3, some biologicals have anticancer activity, and they now comprise the most promising new area in cancer treatment. Thanks to recombinant DNA technology, many of these natural substances can now be produced in the laboratory in large quantities that are both pure and biologically active. This major leap in biotechnology gives scientists hope that cancer therapy with biologicals will soon reduce doctors' reliance on the standard treatments of radiation and chemotherapy. Radiation has severe side effects and most chemotherapy drugs are highly toxic and, tragically, add greatly to the suffering of cancer patients. Biologicals that either enhance the immune response against cancer, or directly kill cancer cells, offer the prospect of far less toxic, painful cancer therapy. Using micronutrients to prevent and treat cancer (and other diseases) is, in some ways, comparable to using biologicals. Biologicals can be extremely potent enhancers of immunity, though not completely free of side effects. In a different way, vitamins, minerals, and proteins are essential to our immune functions and other components of our anticancer defenses. And, in proper amounts they have *no* side effects.

Dr. Robert A. Good, now chairman of the Department of Pediatrics at the University of South Florida, is a pioneer in the field of cancer immunology. He has commented that "we have shown that minerals and vitamins, calorie intake, protein intake, and fat intake can have profound influences on immunity functions." It is now known that the vitamins required for a strong immune system include vitamin A, vitamins B_6 and B_{12}, pantothenic acid, folic acid, vitamin C, and vitamin E. Selenium and zinc are minerals with a definite role in maintaining healthy immunity. Copper has a lesser role, and iron an extremely complex one: too little iron may cause immune deficiency, while too much will almost surely cause immune malfunction. The relationship between vitamins, minerals, fats, carbohydrates, protein, calorie intake, and the ability of the immune system to function will be described fully in Chapter 5, "Foods That Are Allies." Nutrients contribute to other key elements of our anticancer defenses besides the immune system—including the elimination of cancer-causing free radicals. These and other mechanisms by which nutrition bolsters our cancer defenses will be described as well.

DO NATURAL FOODS CONTAIN CARCINOGENS?

There has been a great misunderstanding in both scientific and lay circles about carcinogens in food. In September of 1983, biochemist Bruce Ames, who is chairman of the Department of Biochemistry at the University of California at Berkeley, published an article in *Science* that appeared to upset the applecarts of both environmentalists and the health-conscious public. Ames had, among other accomplishments, developed a simple but widely applicable test—the "Ames test"—that identifies probable carcinogens. His work had formed the basis for regulatory measures to restrict a whole range of environmental and food carcinogens. In his *Science* article, Ames revealed that a large number of highly potent carcinogens may reside in natural food products. He pointed out that, through the course of evolution, plants struggling to survive developed "natural pesticides," which occur in foods as diverse as black pepper, mushrooms, alfalfa sprouts, mustard, figs, parsley, celery, potatoes, lettuce, coffee, black tea, and cottonseed oil. The natural pesticides in these foods are mutagens—molecules capable of damaging the DNA in cells. About 80 percent of all carcinogens are mutagens, and many other mutagens are suspected carcinogens.

Such findings fueled public paranoia about cancer-causing agents being everywhere and in everything we eat. The concept that carcinogens were not strictly horrible man-made aberrations that could therefore be cleaned up or eliminated, but rather could arise from pure Mother Nature, the one seemingly safe realm of reality, was truly terrifying. If natural foods could no longer be a haven from the cancer blight, why not pull out the grill and fry up some bacon?

The answer, fortunately, involves a deeper view of nature and a more thorough understanding of Ames's complex biochemical explorations. The carcinogens found in nature are counterbalanced by the presence of natural anticarcinogens in the same and other plant and animal foods. Dr. Jeffrey Bland, Ph.D., Director of the Nutritional Analysis Laboratory of the Linus Pauling Institute of Science and Medicine, has commented: "I'm not particularly concerned with the carcinogens inherent in fruits and vegetables . . . human beings have lived in balance with plant carcinogens for millennia. The problem is that we're now exposed to so many environmental carcinogens that the ancient balance has been upset. Fortunately, we can strengthen our anticancer defenses with better nutrition."

So there appears to be little rationale for any major restriction on natural foods. It is more crucial to make sure our diets are not weighted in favor of the many fatty or additive-laden foods that we know tip the balance in favor of the cancer process. And a hearty intake of foods that are "allies" should help counterbalance any intake of natural foods that contain some "enemy" molecules. At this time, we have little scientific justification for being overly vigilant about things like alfalfa sprouts and parsley.

DESIGNING YOUR OWN PREVENTION DIET

In Chapter 7, "The Cancer-Prevention Diet Guide," I give simple recommendations, based on the latest knowledge in all areas of research on cancer and nutrition. I have tried to make it as easy as possible for you to come to decisions about diet, based on:

- your personal concerns about cancer;
- risk factors, including family history, psychological factors, and high-risk behaviors (i.e., if you smoke, you may need to take extra vitamin C; if your family has a history of breast cancer, you should cut down more than most on dietary fat);
- what is realistically possible for you to do.

The latter point is especially vital. For example, if you happen to be an ice-cream addict, and realize that the high fat content in your favorite brand is contributing greatly to your fat intake, there's no reason to toss this book out the window and say to hell with it. If your craving has not made you obese and/or miserable, it won't be necessary for you to consign yourself to a lifetime of peering mournfully into supermarket freezers and ice-cream-parlor windows. The percentage of fat in our diets is crucial to cancer risk, but the factors that make up our fat intake are many and varied. It is possible to compensate for such human weaknesses as a passion for ice cream through some creative shuffling and counterbalancing, and keep our overall fat intake low. It may only be necessary to reduce our habits a smidgen, unless they are completely out of control.

Start with Sound Nutrition

Although there are some very specific vitamin and mineral recommendations in the following chapters, it's best to start cancer prevention with a generally sound nutritional diet. A balanced diet with the proper proportion of fats to proteins to carbohydrates, and with the total number of calories involved, is an important part of reducing the risk of cancer. As with a hearty soup, we should start from good stock and then add the other ingredients.

Proteins, fats, and carbohydrates are the backbone of nutrition. Proteins are essential: they build enzymes, build muscle and other tissues, and are a source of energy. Proteins are made up of building blocks called amino acids. Some of the amino acids can be made by the body, and some cannot (histidine, leucine, isoleucine, lysine, methionine, phenylalanine, threonine, tryptophan, and valine). These essential amino acids must be ingested in food, which is broken down by the digestive system and turned back into amino acids for use by the body's cells.

Reduce Protein from Animal Sources

Some studies have suggested an association between high protein intake and an increased risk of breast, colon, pancreatic, kidney, prostate, and endometrial cancers. However, most experts agree that the connection has more to do with fat than protein, since so many of the high-protein-food sources, especially animal proteins and dairy products, are also high in fat content. Still, evidence from laboratory studies indicates that keeping the total percentage of protein in the diet from exceeding 15–20 percent may be cancer preventive. This moderation of protein intake also helps reduce the body's requirement for additional calcium and therefore helps build strong bones. For reasons I will explain more fully in the "fat" section of Chapter 6, "Foods That Are Enemies," it is best to increase the ratio of proteins that come from vegetable sources and reduce those coming from animal sources.

Increase Carbohydrates from Fruits and Vegetables

Carbohydrates, which include the simple kind, sugars (glucose, fructose, and lactose), and the complex kind (starches found in grains or beans), provide most of the energy in our diets. People often mistakenly think of carbohydrates as primarily junk foods. In fact, many nutritionists recommend an increase in overall carbohydrate intake (especially, as opposed to fats). Sugars and starches are more than candy bars, cakes, and bread products. Fruits, vegetables, beans, seeds, and grain provide us with much-needed carbohydrates along with other vital nutrients and fiber.

There is no evidence now to suggest that a diet high in carbohydrates leads to additional cancer risk. There is, however, a body of evidence to suggest that a high-calorie diet increases risk, so we need to watch our carbohydrate intake insofar as it drives up our calories. The most sensible, and healthiest, approach to carbohydrate regulation is this: to lessen the amount of carbohydrates that come from refined or processed sugars (white and brown sugar, honey, candy, and other sweet treats) and increase the amount of complex carbohydrates from fruits, vegetables, beans, nuts, and whole-grain products. The latter foods tend to have less calories, less fat, and more anticancer vitamins and minerals. Both our energy needs and cancer-preventive needs are met more satisfactorily by this kind of carbohydrate regimen.

Fats Are Necessary . . . in Small Amounts

Despite all the negative publicity, fat is part of the triumvirate of essential macronutrients, along with proteins and carbohydrates. Also called "lipids," fats are commonly triglyceride molecules, which are stored in the body and used as needed for fuel. Other categories of fat include cholesterol, the phospholipids and fatty acids. Fats are a key source of metabolic energy; they help the fat-soluble vitamins— A, D, E, and K—enter the bloodstream; they are important components of cell membranes and serve a host of other biological functions. They should certainly not be avoided altogether. But the American diet includes at least 25 percent more fat than is needed for healthy nutrition, and most Americans need to cut back substantially on the number of calories that come from fat. (See Chapter 6, "Foods That Are Enemies.")

There are three different types of fats, which you are probably familiar with but confused by: saturated, monounsaturated, and polyunsaturated. Foods high in saturated fats include animal products such as beef, pork, and lamb; butter and milkfat; coconut and palm oils; and many commercial shortenings found in a range of supermarket food products. Chicken and fish contain saturated fat, but in smaller amounts. Monounsaturated fats include olive oil and peanut oil. Polyunsaturated fats are mainly vegetable oils: corn, safflower, cottonseed, sesame seed, soybean, sunflower oils, and most margarines.

It is certain that saturated fats increase the cholesterol in our bodies, thus increasing our risk of heart disease. Those at risk of heart disease are told to ingest mainly polyunsaturated fats, which not only lack cholesterol but help reduce serum cholesterol. Unfortunately, for different reasons, saturated and polyunsaturated fats both increase our risk of cancers. On the positive side, this makes the task of cancer prevention by lowering fat content less complicated: all kinds of fat need to be restricted in our diet. Also, recent research is providing another solution—monounsaturated fats may be the least dangerous in terms of both heart disease and cancer risk. Olive oil is the purest monounsaturate, and the best choice when we need some oil in our diet. For further details on the whole question of fats and oils, see Chapters 6 and 7.

Calories and Obesity

Fat is also high in calories and therefore a further no-no. Protein and carbohydrate foods have four calories per gram; alcohol has 7; and fat has 9 calories per gram. But what relevance do calories have to cancer prevention? A high-calorie diet, and/or the obesity that can result, may be risk factors for colon and rectal cancers (although the correlation between high fat and these cancers is definitely stronger). Studies with mice show that calorie restriction might inhibit the growth of tumors caused by carcinogens akin to those in cigarettes. Moreover, high-calorie diets lead to obesity, and obesity has been shown to place post-menopausal women at a much higher risk of developing endometrial and breast cancer. Researchers think the reason for this is that obesity tends to enhance the synthesis of estrogens, the female growth hormones that can enhance tumor growth at these sites. In a long-term study of 750,000 men and women by the American Cancer Society, conducted from 1959 to 1972, the rate of death from cancer was significantly higher among those people 40 percent or more overweight. In men, this mainly involved cancer of the colon and rectum; in women, there were higher death rates from breast and endometrial cancers, as well as cancers of the gall bladder and biliary passages and cervix.

Although no definitive statements can yet be made about high-calorie diets and cancer—especially since high fat levels may be involved in these findings—it is still wise to maintain a diet low to moderate in calories. As if we needed another impetus to avoid being overweight!

GENERAL RULES FOR A BALANCED DIET

In 1977, the U.S. Senate Select Committee on Nutrition and Human Needs issued a document on what our nation's dietary goals should be. Although it may be hard to follow percentages, we can take our cues from the committee's recommendations concerning a properly balanced diet:

- To avoid being overweight, consume only as much energy (calories) as is expended; if overweight, decrease energy intake and increase energy expenditure.

- Increase the consumption of complex carbohydrates and "naturally occurring" sugars from about 28 percent to about 48 percent of energy intake.
- Reduce consumption of refined and processed sugars by about 45 percent to account for about 10 percent of total energy intake.
- Reduce overall fat consumption from approximately 40 percent to about 30 percent of energy intake.
- Reduce saturated-fat consumption to account for about 10 percent of total energy intake; balance that with polyunsaturated and monosaturated fats, which should each account for about 10 percent of energy intake.
- Reduce cholesterol consumption to about 30 milligrams a day.
- Limit the intake of sodium by reducing the intake of salt to about 5 grams (2.0 grams of sodium) or less a day.

These dietary prescriptions for balance are well in line with current knowledge about cancer prevention. What isn't there are specifics about what we must add to our diet, such as fresh vegetables, fruits, and whole grains. Let's move on to the food "allies" that can help us further the goal of cancer prevention.

5

Foods That Are Allies

In current nutritional research, the discovery of foods that are allies is fast outpacing the discovery of foods that are enemies. But we mustn't forget that there really are foods that are major enemies. The good news is that, if we eat enough of the food allies, we can indulge occasionally in a few of the delectable enemies without harm—like sirloin steak and french fries. Put simply, the good guys will help fight off the bad guys for us.

In its dry, scientific wording the Committee on Diet, Nutrition, and Cancer stressed "the importance of including fruits, vegetables, and whole grain cereal products in the daily diet." The report continues, "In epidemiological studies, frequent consumption of these foods have been inversely correlated with the incidence of various cancers." On first sight, this doesn't sound like much of a statement. But it's a whopper! Especially for caution-bound scientists who, over ten years ago, saw little connection between food and cancer—either positive or negative.

Some key vitamins—A, C, and E—and minerals—selenium most of all—and the foods they are found in are the major cancer fighters. Vitamins A, C, and E are especially potent. And then there is, of course, fiber for prevention of colon cancer.

The cancer establishment, including the American Cancer Society (ACS) and the government's National Cancer Institute (NCI), has undertaken extensive research, and the early results are demonstrating the power of these vitamins and minerals to prevent cancer. But they still shy away from recommending supplements; the vitamins and minerals should be taken, they say, through foodstuffs, in which the synergistic effect of the other ingredients helps vitamin and mineral absorption.

I am not so conservative about supplements. Nor are many of the important research scientists in nutrition and biology. While I agree that, for the reasons cited above, we should take as many as possible of these vitamins through foodstuffs, I also believe we can't always through food alone obtain levels of certain nutrients high enough for optimal cancer prevention. This is particularly true of vitamin C. The results of some laboratory studies, proving the anticancer benefits of nutrients, suggest the potential value of vitamin consumption at levels that are almost impossible to reach through daily nutrition. And as for the Recommended Daily Allowances (RDAs), they are unquestionably outdated.

Another reason cited by the NCI and ACS for not recommending supplements is that some of the anticancer vitamins and minerals can have toxic effects in megadoses. This is unquestionably true—with several exceptions—but there is tremendous leeway between the amounts I will recommend and the higher levels that may be toxic.

So why not take supplements? *I see no reason not to and every reason to do so.* If taken at safe levels—and I suggest *only very safe levels*—the worst that can happen would be for you to waste a dollar or so by taking a bit more than can be fully used by your body. I think that's better than not taking enough.

The following pages:

- provide a short overview of the research on key vitamins and minerals;
- tell what cancers each nutrient helps prevent;
- list what foods to eat for each vitamin or mineral;
- give recommendations for both foods and supplements.

THE ANTICANCER VITAMINS

Vitamins were first discovered in the early twentieth century and, says Linus Pauling unequivocally, "The recognition that they are essential elements of a healthy diet was one of the most important contributions to health ever made." In his latest book, *How to Live Longer and Feel Better,* he referred to "the recognition, about 20 years ago, that the optimum intakes of several of the vitamins, far larger than the usually recommended intakes, led to further improvement in health, greater protection against many diseases, and enhanced effectiveness in the therapy of diseases."

Although Pauling is perhaps the foremost vitamin enthusiast, there is little question that the full power of vitamins has only begun to be tapped. With regard to cancer prevention, scientists so far may only have scratched the surface. Already, the results of many scientific studies show that the news is very good: there is little question that several vitamins definitely help prevent cancer.

Before proceeding with the vitamins, let me stress that all the recommendations for vitamin and mineral intake in this book are for *adults only.* Vitamin and mineral supplements are suggested for children, but the amounts should be determined by your physician or pediatrician, taking into account the child's age and special requirements. Pregnant women should also consult their physicians about any vitamin-mineral intake, before following these or any other prescriptions for supplements. Now, let's look first at the most potent of these— A, C, and E. This triumvirate is easy to remember: ACE.

VITAMIN A AND BETA-CAROTENE

Recent discoveries about vitamin A and its precursors have caused great optimism in the search for allies in the fight against cancer. No other single nutrient has excited cancer scientists quite as much. It should be noted from the outset that "vitamin A" is a term often used to cover a variety of related substances, some of which are precursors— substances converted into vitamin A in the body. The most important precursor, or "provitamin A," is beta-carotene.

Vitamin A and its precursors offer us some protection against lung cancer, gastrointestinal cancer, and cancer of the esophagus. They may also help ward off colon, rectal, bladder, prostate, breast, cervical, larynx, and skin cancers, among others. The evidence to support these claims comes from worldwide studies of populations with diets full of food rich in vitamin A, as well as from lab studies of the vitamin's ability to prevent cancers in experimental animals.

Vitamin A (and its close cousins) appears to have such powerful anticancer effects that the cancer establishment is starting clinical trials for its use in the *treatment* of cancer as well as for its prevention. This development is particularly surprising since the NCI and the ACS are extremely conservative with regard to new cancer therapies.

But the NCI, ACS, and the Committee on Diet, Nutrition, and Cancer all recommend an increase in our intake of green and yellow fruits and vegetables and other food sources of vitamin A and beta-carotene.

As mentioned, vitamin A is a general term covering several different but related substances. They can be categorized as:

1. Retinol—the form of vitamin A found in animal foods, such as liver and dairy products.

2. Carotenoids—the umbrella term for substances, found in some fruit and vegetable sources, that are converted into vitamin A in the body.
3. Beta-carotene—a particular "precursor" of vitamin A found in dark-green and yellow fruits and vegetables. Beta-carotene is converted into vitamin A as the body requires it. Of all the carotenoids, beta-carotene is the one most efficiently converted to vitamin A.
4. Retinoids—the synthetic chemical versions of vitamin A that are being used in laboratory and clinical studies of vitamin A's capacity to prevent and treat cancer.

If the various terms seem confusing, be comforted by the fact that scientists themselves are confused about some critical differences between types of vitamin A. The main question that has arisen is which form of this vitamin has the anticancer properties. The answer may be that *all forms* of vitamin A help prevent cancer, but thus far the standout for performance appears to be beta-carotene. More on this later.

The Evidence for Vitamin A

A large-scale Japanese study, conducted over twenty years, found that people who ate green and yellow vegetables, rich in beta-carotene, on a daily basis, had a decreased risk of lung, stomach, and other cancers. Smokers who quit smoking and then increased their intake of these vegetables significantly reduced their risk of lung cancer. Apparently, some of the damage from smoking *can be reversed* with the help of provitamin A and its natural food sources.

A study by Richard Shekelle of the University of Chicago followed about two thousand men for nineteen years. Lung cancer was significantly lower in those who ate foods rich in beta-carotene. A Harvard University study of over twelve hundred elderly people found that those with the highest intake of dark-green and yellow vegetables had far less risk of all cancers.

A ground-breaking study by scientists in Norway demonstrated that men who ate vitamin-A-rich foods had one-third as much lung cancer as those who ate far less of these foods. A study of Chinese females in Singapore showed similar results. A group of Italian investigators recently published a report of their study showing that women with diets high in green vegetables and carrots (loaded with beta-carotene) were far less likely to contract cervical cancer.

The lung-cancer studies mentioned above controlled for smoking and other known contributing factors, adding to the weight of their findings. Studies similar to those above have shown that a high intake of foods full of vitamin A or beta-carotene is associated with a lower incidence of all these cancers: larynx, bladder, esophagus, stomach, colorectal, prostate, and others. Furthermore, in three recent reports based on populations in the U.S. and England, investigators noted that the risk of cancer in general was greater in those who measured lower serum levels of vitamin A, and vice versa—cancer risk was down in those with more serum vitamin A.

Finally, a report in the *New England Journal of Medicine,* published in late 1986, told of an unusual study led by researcher Marilyn S. Menkes at Johns Hopkins University. The research team looked at blood samples that had been collected from a group of ninety-nine lung-cancer patients long before they developed the disease. A comparison of these samples with blood taken from a similar group of 196 who did not get cancer, showed a significant difference: the cancer group had generally much lower blood levels of beta-carotene and vitamin E. Specifically, those with low beta-carotene were four times likelier to contract lung cancer than those with normal levels. The researchers refrained from directly linking these low levels to the cause of cancer, but the findings were nonetheless striking.

How Vitamin A Works

Vitamin A and its close relatives are *anticarcinogens.* They also *boost the functioning of the immune system* in many ways. Beta-carotene is a *free-radical scavenger,* putting a stop to the dangerous effects of these highly reactive molecules. These three key properties equal cancer prevention.

Remarkably, vitamin A seems to block the activity of many carcinogenic agents. Numerous studies with rats and mice have thus far produced marked effects. Retinoids (such as the synthetic 13-cis-retinoic acid) inhibit tumor growth after exposure to known chemical carcinogens. Retinoids may be especially adept at blocking the action of chemical promoters of cancer-cell growth.

Beta-carotene is an antioxidant—it can stop or reverse the genetic damage wrought by free radicals that can lead to malignancy. Suntanners take note: the ultraviolet light in sun rays produces the free radicals that probably cause most skin cancers. Beta-carotene is an especially efficient gobbler of these high-energy molecules, and also concentrates highly in the skin. Along with vitamin E, beta-carotene is a critical protector for those who get exposed to too much sun. (See more about this in Chapter 12, "Suntanning.")

The results of vitamin A deficiency also provides additional clues to how and why this nutrient prevents cancer. Vitamin A deficiency can:

- cause a drop in the number of T-cells, which are required to kill any cancer cells that may arise;
- result in lower levels of antibody production (normal antibody responses are necessary for healthy immunity);
- enhance the ability of a carcinogen in tobacco, benzo(a)pyrene, to bind to lung cells, increasing the possibility of cancer;
- cause abnormal changes in epithelial tissues (those that line the inner and outer surfaces of the body and its organs).

The first two points underline vitamin A's importance to anticancer immunity. The third point tells us that vitamin A is needed to block the effects of tobacco smoke in the lungs. Point 4 is especially important to the vitamin-A-cancer connection. Vitamin A is required normally for the proper growth and differentiation of all epithelial tissues. The changes that can occur in these tissues when A is low or absent may presage cancer. Remember that epithelial cancers make up more than half the total cancers in men and women—and occur at a wide variety of sites in the body: skin, larynx, esophagus, cervix, colon, rectum, stomach, bladder, kidney, thyroid, breast, uterus, gall bladder, and prostate. These are many of the same cancers shown, in population studies, to be prevented by a healthy intake of vitamin A. Once again, what has been learned in the lab about a nutrient's effects on cells is confirmed "in the field" by epidemiological research.

How to Get Vitamin A

Vitamin A and its cousins are *all* involved in different aspects of cancer prevention. However, evidence is growing that beta-carotene is the most potent source of anticancer activity, with properties of its own—apart from its conversion to vitamin A—that prevent cancer.

Until this question is fully resolved, it is important that we get a lot of vitamin A from different sources. In this way we cover all our bases. The food sources of both beta-carotene and vitamin A are unequivocally nutritious, and only some of the animal sources should be kept at a low-moderate intake because of their high fat content.

Vitamin A or beta-carotene supplements are a good adjunct to our daily diet. There is one drawback, however: vitamin A is one of the micronutrients for which toxicity is a real issue. It is possible to overdose on vitamin A pills (though it is almost impossible to overdose on vitamin A from food sources. One would probably have to consume several pieces of liver a day—an unlikely prospect). The vitamin, which is fat-soluble, is measured in international units (IU). The RDA of vitamin A for an adult is 5,000 IU—but we need much more. Repeated intakes of well over 50,000 IU could begin to cause nausea, headache, skin conditions, and other symptoms in some individuals. Continued doses of more than 100,000 IU can cause serious toxic symptoms. This problem is one of the main reasons scientists have been using beta-carotene and retinoids, the synthetic derivatives of vitamin A, in their testing with animals and humans. Larger doses of these two forms can be given without significant side effects.

Vitamin A capsules contain a synthetic, "preformed" vitamin A. They are commonly available in 10,000 IU and 25,000 IU dosages. *One 10,000 IU capsule per day is a good dosage for cancer-preventive purposes (and general health), when combined with beta-carotene. This amount is far below toxic levels.* There are two very compelling reasons to consider taking beta-carotene in pill form in addition to supplemental vitamin A. First, as stated, beta-carotene appears to have some special anticancer properties of its own, possibly apart from its conversion into vitamin A, or possibly related to this process of conversion. In either case, any beta-carotene you take *is* converted into usable vitamin A in your body.

Second, beta-carotene can be taken without side effects in much larger doses than Vitamin A pills; it is converted into vitamin A only as the body requires it. All that can happen with very high doses of beta-carotene is that you turn yellow! (Small numbers of people ingesting a lot of beta-carotene have been affected by this naturally occurring pigment; it is responsible for the green and yellow coloration of vegetables it's found in.) Fifteen milligrams of beta-carotene give you 25,000 IU of converted vitamin A. This is a good daily dose for cancer prevention, unlikely to turn your skin yellow. Even higher doses of beta-carotene can be taken if needed—in the form of one or two additional 15-milligram supplements. If the skin does begin to turn yellow, this is not dangerous, just a sign to return to a lower dose. An additional 15 milligrams (total, 30 milligrams) is highly recommended for those who

- smoke,
- suntan at all,
- don't get enough green and yellow fruits and vegetables,
- have been or are exposed, at home or at work, to cancer-causing chemicals.

(For full recommendations for people in these categories, see Chapter 7, "The Cancer-Prevention Diet Guide.")

Food Sources of Vitamin A

I recommend vitamin A and beta-carotene supplementation because it may not always be possible to get a consistent, large intake of these vital anticancer substances from food alone. *Supplemental vitamin A and beta-carotene assure us, on a daily basis, of receiving A's cancer-preventive value, which is enormous. If you smoke, you should be sure to get additional beta-carotene.* Nevertheless, we should get as much vitamin A and beta-carotene as possible from natural food sources. The foods rich in vitamin A provide us with many additional naturally occurring vitamins, minerals, enzymes, fiber, and other nutrients, some of which have a synergistic effect on each other, and make possible greater absorption of individual nutrients. We know how important dietary sources of vitamin A are because most of the population studies cited earlier refer to food intake, not vitamin pills, as the source of cancer protection.

Some animal products are an excellent source of vitamin A. Liver is perhaps the best: a 3½-oz. serving of liver is full of Vitamin A, whether it is lamb (74,500 IU), calf (32,000 IU), beef (53,000 IU), turkey (17,500 IU), or chicken liver (12,000 IU). Butter, margarine, milk products, including cheeses, and egg yolks are relatively high in vitamin A; most meats, fish, and poultry contain some vitamin A. I am not encouraging an increased use of red meat and dairy products (except skim and low-fat variety), because of the very high fat content in most of them. Chicken and fish, which are lower in fat, are also less rich in vitamin A than the other animal foods. Therefore, the general rule is: try to get as much of your vitamin A from fruits and vegetables as possible. As you will see later, many of these same fresh foods also provide other critical cancer-preventive vitamins, minerals, and fiber.

Vitamin A/Carotene in Vegetables

HIGH (MORE THAN 1,000 IU PER SERVING)

Asparagus
Broccoli
Carrots
Dark, leafy greens
   beet
   chard
   collard
   dandelion
   kale
   mustard
   parsley
   romaine lettuce
   spinach
   turnip
   watercress

Endive
Red peppers
Sweet potatoes
Tomatoes
Winter squash

MEDIUM (500–1,000 IU PER SERVING)

Brussels sprouts
Corn
Green beans
Green pepper
Okra
Peas
Summer squash

LOW (LESS THAN 500 IU VITAMIN A PER SERVING)

Cabbage
Cauliflower
Celery
Cucumbers
Lettuce (iceberg)
Kohlrabi
Potatoes

Vitamin A/Carotene in Fruits

HIGH (MORE THAN 1,000 IU PER SERVING)

Apricots
Cantaloupe
Mangoes
Papayas
Peaches
Persimmons
Prunes, dried
Pumpkins

MEDIUM (500–1,000 IU PER SERVING)

Cherries
Watermelon

LOW (LESS THAN 500 IU VITAMIN A PER SERVING)

Apples
Avocados

Grapefruit
Oranges
Pears
Pineapple
Plums
Raspberries
Rhubarb
Strawberries
Tangerines

(List derived from U.S. Dept. of Agriculture publications: *The Nutritive Value of American Foods, Agriculture Handbook No. 456,* and *The Composition of Foods.*)

Recommendations

1. *Choose a vegetable from the high vitamin-A category, preferably twice a day.* Select fruits from the high vitamin-A category often. When in doubt, and this book is not in hand, remember that color is the key: dark green and yellow coloration tell you that beta-carotene is present.
2. Take supplements: 10,000 IU vitamin A *plus* 15 mg. beta-carotene.

See Chapter 7, "The Cancer-Prevention Diet Guide," for more tips on getting vitamin A/beta-carotene in your diet.

VITAMIN C

Vitamin C is a great gift, a miraculous nutrient that performs a dazzling array of functions and protects our bodies in countless ways. Hefty tomes are being written about the powers of vitamin C as more is learned about its benefits and how it works. In the 1970s, the hubbub was all about whether vitamin C prevents or cures the common cold and flu; in the 1980s, the hubbub concerns the vitamin's alleged ability to prevent or cure cancer.

At the center of both controversies is Linus Pauling. Time has borne him out on the question of C and colds; I, for one, have little doubt that it will do so again on the question of C and cancer. In his 1979 book, *Cancer and Vitamin C,* Pauling stressed the vitamin's role as an adjunct in the treatment of cancer. He cited studies—some of them carried out by himself and co-author Ewan Cameron—proving that C alone or in combination with conventional treatment often had a marked effect in improving survival rates, chances of remission, and the quality of life.

Pauling ventured deeply into the realm of vitamin C's modes of action in order to support his case and determine how it halts cancer-cell growth. He discovered many of the key mechanisms, and realized the vitamin's potential for prevention as well. Although there is some connection between the way vitamin C stops cancer after it has developed and the way it prevents cancer from developing, I will concentrate strictly on its preventive role.

The strongest ties between vitamin C and cancer prevention are in cancers of the stomach and esophagus. It is also believed to prevent mouth, larynx, colon, rectal, and possibly lung and bladder cancers. From what has been learned about vitamin C's activities in the body, there is reason to believe that higher quantities of C than is found in the average diet will help prevent cancer.

The NCI, ACS, and NAS's Committee on Diet, Nutrition, and Cancer unequivocally recommend greater consumption of vitamin-C-rich foods and vegetables. Nevertheless, all of these institutions have fallen short of an open-minded assessment of the data, and have refrained from recommending vitamin-C supplements. The RDA for vitamin C is 60 mg., enough to prevent scurvy—the main vitamin-C deficiency disease. It is, however, far from enough to give full cancer-preventive and other health benefits. The argument that we can get enough C from our foods has been convincingly debunked by Linus Pauling. I'll return to this point shortly.

Sixteen years ago, Pauling wrote that he believed the improvements in health from ingesting the optimum amount of ascorbic acid could lead to an increase in life expectancy of two or three years. In 1986, he updated this estimate, "based on an additional 15 years of study in this field," to twenty to twenty-five years of additional health and longevity.

The Evidence for Vitamin C

A handful of major population studies—most of them made in the last decade—have shown that high vitamin-C intake, mainly through eating a lot of fresh citrus fruits, protects against stomach cancer.

Population studies in northern Iran proved that diets very low in fresh fruits and vitamin-C-rich foods were probably responsible for the high incidence of cancer of the esophagus there. A 1981 study showed conclusively that the vitamin C in fruits and vegetables was more strongly linked with protection against cancer of the esophagus than the vitamin A present in those foods.

Vitamin C, together with vitamin A, was found to have a protective effect against cancer of the larynx. The 1981 study that came to this conclusion carefully controlled for the factors of smoking and alcohol, which can lead to laryngeal cancer.

A collaborating group of investigators at St. Mark's Hospital in London and at Memorial Sloan-Kettering Cancer Center in New York reported that high doses of vitamin C can reduce the intestinal polyps characteristic of familial polyposis, an inherited disorder. These polyps can lead to colon cancer, and their reduction with vitamin C may be cancer preventive. The Australian Society of Epidemiology reports that scientists in that country found that high vitamin-C intake significantly lowered the risk of rectal cancer.

How Vitamin C Works

Vitamin C functions to prevent cancer on many different levels at once—its versatility is a biological wonder. Like vitamin A, vitamin C is an antioxidant, blocking free-radical damage. It is an enhancer of the immune system in a variety of ways. In its role as a general detoxifier, vitamin C is a crucial anticarcinogen; it neutralizes carcinogens and even stops their formation. It also strengthens the "intercellular cement," a thick network of collagen and other fibers, that maintains the integrity of the bodily tissues.

Nitrites and nitrates are chemicals found in smoked, pickled, or salt-cured meats, such as bacon, hot dogs, salami, and cured fish. These substances can combine with the amino compounds (amines) in the stomach, to form *nitrosamines.* Nitrosamines are potent carcinogens that can cause stomach and other cancers. When vitamin C is present, it "competes" successfully for the nitrites, preventing formation of the nitrosamine compounds. By blocking nitrosamines, vitamin C puts a stop to one major cause of stomach cancer.

According to Pauling, vitamin C in the body has "rather wide powers to destroy toxic substances." Ascorbic acid collaborates with enzymes in the liver to neutralize these substances, which may include mutagens and carcinogens, and then eliminate them in the urine. Dr. Robert Bruce of the Ludwig Cancer Research Institute in Toronto has reported that vitamin C reduces the amount of mutagens and carcinogens in the intestinal tract, helping to protect against colon cancer.

In laboratory studies with mice, there is always the problem and the question of whether mice and man are really that close. Nevertheless, mouse studies have unlocked biological secrets before, and they will continue to provide invaluable data. One striking study of vitamin C's ability to inhibit cancer formation was conducted in 1980 by W. F. Benedict. A group of mouse embryo cells were exposed in culture to a powerful chemical carcinogen. When vitamin C was added to the culture, the change from normal to cancer was stopped in its tracks. The addition of the C—even *as late as twenty-three days* after treatment with the carcinogen—still resulted in a complete halt to malignant changes. Most remarkable, however, was the fact that in some cases the cells not only stopped changing *but reverted back to their original, normal state.* The mechanism for this effect is still unknown.

Bladder tumors occur with greater frequency among tobacco smokers and chewers. Cigar smokers have the highest rate. A group of investigators found that the ascorbic-acid levels in the urine of those who smoked was abnormally low, and also low in people with bladder tumors. They ran a test using a specific chemical in the bladders of mice, which could produce carcinogenic by-products and cause bladder tumors. The researchers found that bladder tumors did not develop if the mice had extra vitamin C in their drinking water. Apparently, in its antioxidant role, C is able to block the oxidation of the chemical that would have spawned the carcinogenic by-products.

Beyond its capabilities as a detoxifier and anticarcinogen, the properties of vitamin C tell us volumes about why it is a vital ally in the fight against cancer:

1. As an antioxidant: Vitamin C is a powerful antioxidant, blocking "lipid peroxidation," or the rancid breakdown of fatty foods that leads to free-radical formation (and cancer).
2. As an immune enhancer: Vitamin C stimulates the action of phagocytes, and especially of macrophages, which are key soldiers in the anticancer chain reaction. It may also stimulate the transformation of T- and B-cells, and it appears to induce the body to manufacture more interferon.
3. As an antiviral: Vitamin C protects the body against viruses. Because there are a number of known cancer-causing viruses, C may be an indirect preventer of cancers from such viruses.
4. As a collagen strengthener: Collagen is the fibrous substance that constitutes most of the "intercellular cement," or glue that maintains the integrity of our tissues. Vitamin C is essential to the synthesis of collagen, which undoubtedly helps us to resist invasion by cancer cells.

The interferon connection is especially telling. The federal government and many research institutes throughout the country are spending enormous sums on interferon production and research, in order to test its promise as an anticancer agent. In all probability, large intakes of vitamin C help us produce higher quantities of our own interferon— perhaps saving us the terrible misfortune of ever having to seek out cancer treatment with synthetic interferon.

How Much Vitamin C Do We Need?

Perhaps of all the vitamins, very large supplements of vitamin C—in addition to the vitamin from food sources—are most justified. The reason is twofold: Unlike vitamin A, we can't overdose on C (although there can be some "bowel toxicity"; I'll return to this later). If we take too much, it is simply excreted in the urine. Second, unlike the other vitamins, human beings no longer know how to make their own C.

Through the course of evolution, claims Pauling, the human species lost the ability to synthesize its own vitamin C. We are in interesting company. Of all the mammals in the animal kingdom, only humans, guinea pigs, and fruit-eating bats depend on extra vitamin C because they can no longer make their own. Why and how could we lose this ability? Pauling thinks that, in an earlier epoch, there was an abundance of vitamin-C-rich foods in the natural environment, and we were able to "shuffle off" the genetic/molecular machinery needed to synthesize our own. However, the same availability of large quantities of vitamin C in our natural diets no longer exists. For this reason and because we are unable to make our own, we need to ingest a lot of vitamin C.

Other researchers, as well as Pauling, tried to calculate how much extra vitamin C we really need. They've done this by discovering how much C is manufactured by an animal that can make its own, and then extrapolating a figure for humans based on body weight. For example, cats, dogs, cows, sheep, and rabbits all make about the same amount of vitamin C per pound of their own body weight. If you translated their C production into the equivalent for a 150-pound person, it would average 10,000 mg. per day (10 grams).

Many people ask whether taking large doses of C is fruitless because so much of it is eliminated in urine. It is true that a higher percentage of the vitamin is lost with higher dosages, but it is still relative: the more we take, the more is available for use by the body. It is advisable, however, to break down a large dose into several smaller doses so that larger percentages of ascorbate are retained with each. I suggest three equal doses spread throughout the day.

We are each a unique individual, and our nutrient needs vary from person to person. This phenomenon is often referred to as "biochemical individuality." Depending on the amount of vitamin C we are getting in our diet, on what kinds of toxins, infectious agents, or chemicals we are commonly exposed to, and other unique features of our biochemical systems, we may need more or less extra vitamin C. Pauling has stated that, at present, "it is very difficult to determine the nutritional needs of an individual person except by trial of various intakes, but we hope that reliable clinical tests that show the individual needs will be developed before long."

I strongly suggest a range of supplemental vitamin C be given, from low to high, and that you place yourself within that range based on your own perception of your health needs. Based on Pauling's conclusions and my readings of the literature on vitamin C and cancer, *I recommend between 2,000 and 5,000 milligrams (2–5 grams) per day for cancer prevention.* For your information, Pauling recommends between 6,000 and 18,000 milligrams per day. My more modest recommendation is based not on disagreement with the Nobel laureate, but rather on my personal experience with people's great hesitancy to consider such supposedly mammoth doses. (Five grams is a good dose on the high end, and, if you have reason to believe you would benefit from more, up to 18 grams will bring no risk of toxic side effects, except in very rare cases—see below.) You may consider starting at the low end (2 grams) if you are in good health. You may consider working toward the high end (5 grams), if you have specific health or cancer-related concerns, or if you:

- smoke,
- drink alcohol regularly,
- eat foods containing nitrates.

Smokers have between 30 and 50 percent less vitamin C in their blood than nonsmokers. It isn't certain why this is the case—whether the C is somehow destroyed by tobacco-smoke constituents, or whether the C is used up in the processes of detoxification. In any case, it is imperative that smokers get extra vitamin C to fortify their defenses against the toxic and carcinogenic agents in smoke, and to keep their ascorbic-acid level from dropping down to a point where all aspects of health based on vitamin C are threatened.

People who both smoke and drink alcohol have an increased risk of cancers of the mouth and esophagus. These individuals must take additional vitamin C, which will directly help prevent these dreadful cancers.

Clearly, if you are eating a lot of foods filled with nitrites and nitrates—such as bacon, ham, sausages, other luncheon meats, or smoked fish (really, *anything* that is smoked or cured)—you should take more vitamin C to block formation of nitrosamines in your stomach. Both C and E are powerful in blocking nitrosamine formation. (See Chapter 6, "Foods That Are Enemies," for a further discussion of foods that contain nitrates and nitrites.)

Are there side effects to high dosages of vitamin C? Hardly— most people can tolerate even 20 or more grams of vitamin C without any side effects, and cancer patients have been known to take over 100 grams without toxicity. This vitamin is considered one of the *least* toxic nutrients, and is certainly safer than almost any over- or below-the-counter drug available. One of the few—and basically harmless—symptoms from very large doses of vitamin C is some looseness of the bowel, or diarrhea. For this reason, it is a good idea to work your way up to larger doses gradually (i.e., move from 2 to 5 grams by starting at 2 and adding 1 gram a day). If and when any laxative action occurs, you have probably reached your "bowel tolerance" and should come down a gram or so and stay there as your daily dose. Also, don't suddenly stop taking a large dose of C. If you need to lower your dose, *do so gradually*—a gram a day or so. Otherwise, you may experience a "rebound" effect, where your body reacts as if there's a vitamin C deficiency.

The only other significant problem cited in the literature is vitamin C's alleged capacity to cause kidney-stone formation. This appears as a highly unlikely possibility, except in people who are prone to a particular class of stones (primarily, those composed of calcium oxalate) that form in urine that is acidic. These people may still be able to take moderate amounts of C in the form of sodium ascorbate or calcium ascorbate, which does not acidify the urine. Also, people prone to such stones should take adequate doses of magnesium and vitamin B_6 (see supplement recommendations), which prevent their formation. In any event, you should consult your doctor about taking large doses of vitamin C if you have a tendency to develop stones that form in acidic urine.*

People with ulcers or stomachs that are inclined to be acidic should take vitamin C in the form of calcium ascorbate, which is less acidic and will not irritate the lining of tender stomachs. The same doses apply, and can be taken in powdered or crystalline form as well. Powder or crystals can be mixed with tea or fruit juice, allowing you to take large doses without having to pop a lot of pills.

Food Sources of Vitamin C

It is important to get as much vitamin C as possible from fresh foods, because the full complement of other vitamins, minerals, enzymes, bioflavonoids (nutrient substances found in vitamin-C-rich foods), and fiber create a perfect biochemical context for proper absorption and utilization of ascorbic acid. However, I've stressed supplements in this section because, without doubt, *we need a lot more vitamin C than we can get from food alone.*

The optimal cancer-preventive intake of vitamin C involves both food sources and supplements.

---

*One other circumstance requires caution and consultation with your physician. A very few individuals suffer from a deficiency of the enzyme G-6-PD. There is a slim possibility that people with a G-6-PD deficiency (who may suffer hemolytic anemia as a result) could be susceptible to complications from a very high C regimen.

Vitamin C in Vegetables

HIGH (MORE THAN 20 MG. PER AVERAGE SERVING)

Asparagus
Broccoli
Brussels sprouts
Cabbage
Cauliflower
Dark, leafy greens
   beet
   collard
   kale
   kohlrabi
   mustard
   turnip
   watercress
Green pepper
Peas
Red pepper
Spinach
Sweet potatoes
Tomatoes

MEDIUM (5 TO 20 MG. PER AVERAGE SERVING)

Bean sprouts
Beets
Carrots
Corn
Dark, leafy greens
   chard
   dandelion
Green beans
Lima beans
Lettuce (iceberg)
Okra
Onions
Parsnips
Potatoes
Summer squash
Winter squash

LOW (LESS THAN 5 MG. PER AVERAGE SERVING)
Celery
Cucumber
Parsley

Vitamin C in Fruits

HIGH (MORE THAN 20 MG. PER AVERAGE SERVING)
Avocado
Cantaloupe
Grapefruit
Lemons
Limes
Oranges
Papayas
Pineapple
Raspberries
Strawberries
Tangerines

MEDIUM (5 TO 20 MG. PER AVERAGE SERVING)
Apricots
Bananas
Blackberries
Cherries
Mangoes
Peaches
Persimmons
Rhubarb
Watermelon

LOW (LESS THAN 5 MG. PER AVERAGE SERVING)
Apples
Grapes
Pears
Plums
Pumpkins

(List derived from U.S. Department of Agriculture publications: *The Nutritive Value of American Foods, Agriculture Handbook No. 456* and *The Composition of Foods.*)

Recommendations

1. Two or three servings of fruits or vegetables from the high category each day. An easy way to accomplish this is to think in terms of one fruit and two vegetable servings, or two fruits and one vegetable per day.
2. Vitamin-C supplements: 2,000 to 5,000 milligrams (2–5 grams) per day, taken in at least three doses: morning, noon, and night. Smokers, drinkers, and those who eat foods containing nitrites should take amounts closer to the 5,000 mark. See Chapter 7, "The Cancer-Prevention Diet Guide," for more tips.

VITAMIN E

Although not yet proved to be as powerful as A and C, vitamin E's anticancer potential seems to be increasing steadily. Currently, there is little epidemiological data to support vitamin E's capacity to prevent cancer. The vitamin is found in such a wide variety of food groups that it is hard to identify populations with different intakes. Therefore, scientists can't clearly determine associations between E and cancer incidence.

Nevertheless, vitamin E (the chemical term is "tocopherol") continues to reveal unexpected potential, now in the realm of cancer prevention. Like vitamins A and C, it is a potent antioxidant. Vitamin E is especially proficient at blocking the free-radical formation that comes from the oxidation of fats—the process by which fatty foods and oils turn rancid. This particular form of oxidation ("lipid peroxidation") and the free radicals that result are especially dangerous. This process is thought to be a leading contributing cause of colon and breast cancer, and *vitamin E is a major ally* against lipid peroxidation.

Vitamin E also blocks the formation of nitrosamines, which are potent carcinogens. Like vitamin C, vitamin E competes for nitrites or nitrates with the amines in the stomach, and can stop them from coupling to form dangerous nitrosamines.

One recent, exciting study underlined the potential of vitamin E. As mentioned in the section on beta-carotene, researchers at Johns Hopkins University, under the direction of Marilyn Menkes, analyzed blood samples of patients who had gone on to develop lung cancer. They found that, among the 99 cancer patients, there were very low blood levels of both vitamin E and beta-carotene, as compared to the 196 who did not have cancer. The low level of vitamin E appeared to increase the risk of lung cancer by two and a half times.

In laboratory studies, vitamin E has been shown to stop or slow the growth of some cancer cells. It may be able to prevent a number of chemical carcinogens from damaging the genetic material in cells, though this research is still preliminary. Researchers at the University of Colorado have conducted laboratory tests showing that vitamin E can halt the growth of prostate cancer cells. It's too early to tell because more studies need to be done, but there may be a role for vitamin E in the prevention and treatment of prostate cancer.

"Fibrocystic disease" is a very common condition among women. It is a benign disease, in which cysts develop in the breasts that are often accompanied by some tenderness and pain. Some experts believe that women with fibrocystic disease may be at increased risk of breast cancer. Vitamin E can be used very effectively to ameliorate this disease. In recent studies, between 75 and 85 percent of women with cysts who were given 600 IU of vitamin E showed improvement. The effects ranged from some relief of pain to reduced size of cysts to the actual disappearance of cysts.

Since vitamin E can ameliorate fibrocystic disease, there may be an indirect role for this vitamin in the prevention of breast cancer. Maurice Black, M.D., of New York Medical College, has used vitamin A and vitamin E in follow-up clinical tests of women who have had one bout with breast cancer. Before the tests, these women had shown no immune response against their cancer cells. Black demonstrated that both A and E alone stimulated the immune system into action against breast-cancer cells in 50 to 60 percent of these women. Both vitamins together resulted in an 80 percent response. This still isn't proof of vitamin E's capacity to prevent breast cancer, but it is intriguing evidence.

Vitamin E, again like A and C, is crucial to proper immune-system functioning. When we don't get enough vitamin E, our ability to produce antibodies, proliferate T- and B-cells, and to resist infection is compromised.

E also seems to work in concert with the other anticancer vitamins and minerals—especially A, C, and the antioxidant selenium. *Vitamin E in combination with selenium increases the power of both to boost immunity and fight free radicals.* It must be included in any anticancer diet, and I recommend supplements—between 200 and 600 IU—to make sure we have a consistent, daily intake.

Dark-green, leafy vegetables, whole-grain cereals, and wheat germ are the best sources of vitamin E. These foods are also rich in fiber, vitamins A, C, and the B vitamins, and anticancer minerals. The nut and oil sources of E are high-fat foods and therefore should not be the source for most of our vitamin E.

Food Sources of Vitamin E

Dark-green, leafy vegetables
Whole-grain cereals
Wheat germ
Liver and some other organ meats
Walnuts, almonds, and peanuts
Vegetable oils

Recommendations

1. Include one of the nonfatty vitamin E food sources in your daily diet. Dark-green, leafy vegetables and whole-grain cereals are especially recommended.
2. Supplements: take 200–600 IU per day

THE B VITAMINS

The entire complement of B vitamins—B_1 (thiamin), B_2 (riboflavin), B_3 (niacin), B_6 (pyridoxine), B_{12} (cyanocobalamin), folic acid, and pantothenic acid—are essential to health. Although there is not yet a great deal of data on the relationship of B vitamins to cancer, there is limited interest in some of the Bs for their value in cancer prevention.

Vitamins B_6 and folic acid are currently grabbing most of the attention. Folic acid, which plays a key role in the normal maturation of cells, has been of particular interest. One recent study involved 47 women with abnormal Pap smears (indicating precancerous changes in the cervix), who were taking oral contraceptives. Some were given oral folic acid, while the rest received a placebo. The placebo group showed no change, while those taking folic acid showed marked improvements of the tissue slides—precancerous cells beginning to return to normalcy. A 1988 study at the University of Alabama demonstrated similar effects with folic acid and vitamin B_{12} in a group of male smokers with precancerous lung cells.

Vitamin B_6, of all the B vitamins, plays the most crucial role in maintaining healthy immunity. Both arms of the immune system—humoral (involving B-cells and antibody production) and cell-mediated (led by T-cells and involving a network of immune cell interaction)—suffer greatly if there is a deficiency of B_6. Part of the cancer-preventive potential of B_6 is due to its immune-enhancing properties.

Investigators at the University of Freiburg have demonstrated the potential of vitamin B_6. A group of women with cancer of the cervix, breast, and uterus were being treated by radiation. Some of them also received a large dose of B_6. Forty-one percent of the women who only had radiation survived after five years, whereas 56 percent of those who also received vitamin B_6 reached the five-year mark. The primary investigator in the study believed that B_6 helped to restore some of the crucial enzymes destroyed by radiation and helped strengthen weakened immune functions, thus improving survival rates.

Vitamins B_6, B_{12}, folic acid, pantothenic acid, and to a lesser exent B_1 and B_2, are part of the legion of micronutrients that keep our immune system alert and strong. All the water-soluble B vitamins, which are interdependent in their actions, are needed for healthy energy metabolism, red-blood-cell formation, nervous-system and immune-system functioning.

Because it is difficult to keep track of our food intake of the specific members of the B family, it is hard to count milligrams in our daily diet. Some foods contain much more of one B vitamin than another. For that reason alone, it's a very good idea to take a super B-complex vitamin pill. These supplements usually contain the full range and proper distribution of B vitamins.

Food Sources of Vitamin B Include

(containing a range of the B vitamins in varying amounts)

Whole-grain cereals
Liver
Meats, fish, and poultry
Eggs
Beans and peas
Milk products
Brewer's yeast

Recommendations

1. Eat food sources of vitamin B, especially whole-grain cereals; meats, fish, and poultry; beans and peas; and brewer's yeast.
2. Take one super B-complex pill daily, preferably one that has 50 or 100 mg. values of most of the B vitamins (often marketed as "B-50" or "B-100").

THE ANTICANCER MINERALS

Minerals represent a whole new territory of discovery in the search for cancer-preventive nutrients. As nutritional research becomes more sophisticated, the vital biochemical role of minerals is being laid bare.

At present, three key minerals are known allies in cancer prevention: calcium, and the trace elements selenium and zinc. "Trace minerals" are those found in minute quantities within our bodies, which, nevertheless, play a critical role in our physiological processes.

For general health, we require major minerals, such as phosphorus, magnesium, potassium, and sodium. In addition to selenium, other trace minerals are needed in smaller amounts: copper, chromium, iodine, iron, manganese. Some trace minerals, like cadmium and lead, can be cancer-*causing*, if ingested in high concentrations.

Although we require all the minerals listed above for good health, I will discuss here only the three minerals that to date have been proven to have definite value in cancer prevention.

Selenium

The trace metal selenium is the mineral with the clearest and most compelling cancer-preventive capabilities. Like vitamin C, it has been the source of some controversy. Also like vitamin C, its protective powers are only beginning to be understood, and the early results are extremely promising.

The Evidence for Selenium

G. N. Schrauzer of the University of California, San Diego, collected data for more than twenty-seven countries and nineteen states in the U.S. He and his colleagues found that the higher the selenium intake from food sources, and the higher the blood levels of selenium, the lower the incidence of breast, colon, rectal, prostate, and several other cancers, including leukemias.

In a 1965 study of U.S. and Canadian populations, R. J. Shamberger and his group showed that the higher the crop level of selenium the lower the death rate for cancer—especially for cancers of the gastrointestinal and genitourinary tracts. Selenium deficiency is also more common among cancer patients than healthy people. This finding is intriguing although it may be a result of having cancer rather than a causal factor.

How Selenium Works

Selenium is a component of a major antioxidant, one of the most potent free-radical scavengers in our diet. It protects cell membranes from free-radical attack, maintaining the integrity of the cell nucleus and its genetic contents. Selenium is especially good at protecting the body against cancer-cell growth caused by by-products of the breakdown of polyunsaturated fats. In recent studies with mice, selenium was added to their drinking water, resulting in lower incidence of breast and colon tumors. Selenium has also been found, in numerous studies, to reduce the incidence and progression of cancer in animals that have been given a wide range of chemical carcinogens. Selenium may interfere with the metabolism of these agents.

Selenium can protect us from some of the toxic effects of heavy metals such as mercury, cadmium, and arsenic, which we may be exposed to through food or the environment. It is possible that selenium shields us from the cancer-causing effects of these and other heavy metals by turning them into inert compounds that can be excreted.

Selenium is a biological switch that helps turn on a powerful antioxidant factor—the enzyme *glutathione peroxidase.* This enzyme is a very effective free-radical scavenger and may work together with selenium for optimal anticancer effects. Selenium and vitamin E also work in concert and increase each other's effectiveness as antioxidants.

The immune system benefits from dietary selenium as well. This mineral promotes humoral immunity (B-cells and antibodies) and helps white cells (lymphocytes) and macrophages (the scavenger cells) in their antibacterial and tumor-cell-killing functions.

How Do We Get Selenium?

Selenium is found in fish (especially sardines), meats, whole wheat, wheat germ, grain (barley, oats, and rye), asparagus, mushrooms, and garlic. These are all wholesome, robust sources of selenium—they can safely be included in our diet.

Because of selenium's defined anticancer properties, and because counting micrograms of this mineral in food sources is a difficult and highly unlikely task, we should take a daily supplement of selenium. The National Research Council recommends between 50 and 200 micrograms per day. *For cancer-preventive purposes, I think 100–200 micrograms per day is best.* Selenium can be toxic in high doses: prolonged amounts of more than 2,400 micrograms per day can cause serious side effects. *More than 500 micrograms per day should not be taken.* The 100–200-micrograms dose per day is perfectly safe.

Food Sources of Selenium

Fish (especially sardines)
Whole wheat
Wheat germ
Grains (barley, oats, and rye)

Asparagus
Mushrooms
Garlic

Recommendations

1. Eat foods rich in selenium every day, especially fish, wheat products, and other grains (that are rich in fiber, too).
2. Supplements—take 100–200 micrograms daily.

Calcium

Calcium has been a media star of late, for its alleged ability to prevent osteoporosis, the degenerative bone disease common among post-menopausal women. The publicity about calcium now includes claims for its capacity to prevent high blood pressure and colon cancer.

The evidence that calcium helps prevent colon cancer is starting to pile up. The *New England Journal of Medicine* published a 1985 study in which calcium supplements were given to ten people at high risk for familial colon cancer, all of whom had some abnormal colon cells. A few months after taking daily doses of calcium, the colon cells of all ten actually began to revert to normal.

Another provocative study was also reported in 1985, in the British medical journal *Lancet.* Beginning in 1957, dietary histories and physical exams were taken for 1,957 men. Nineteen years later, follow-ups determined that 29 of these men had developed colon cancer, while 20 had contracted rectal cancer. The men who developed colorectal cancer did not differ appreciably from those who did not, as far as calories, animal protein, or fat and carbohydrate intake was concerned. They did, however, differ in one respect. Those with colorectal cancer had less calcium and vitamin D in their diets.

Death rates from colon cancer in the U.S. are highest in populations exposed to the least amount of sunlight (those who live in urban areas or northern rural areas). These people, who get less sun, produce less vitamin D internally, and therefore absorb less calcium (vitamin D is necessary for calcium absorption in the intestine).

How does calcium halt the growth of colon cancer? At this stage of research, scientists are not sure. There is speculation that calcium binds up fatty acids and bile acids that can irritate the colon and initiate abnormal cell growth.

Based on this compelling preliminary evidence, and because calcium is very important for healthy bone development and the prevention of osteoporosis, adequate amounts of this mineral should be present in our diets and through supplements.

The food sources of calcium are simple and inexpensive: milk products, preferably of the skim and low-fat variety; dark-green vegetables; shellfish; sardines; and salmon (fresh or canned) eaten with the bones.

There are several reasons to take calcium supplements, foremost of which is that we don't get enough calcium in our diets. Milk products, among the richest sources of calcium, include whole milk, which is also high in fat content. Skim-milk products, though encouraged, are not to everyone's taste. Shellfish are far from a dietary staple, and although dark-green vegetables are often a good source of calcium, one or two servings a day are unlikely to reach even the RDA.

Postmenopausal women and people at risk for colon cancer should take calcium supplements. I suggest 800 mg. (the RDA) for adults and 1,200 milligrams for older women (to prevent osteoporosis); 1,200 milligrams is also suggested for those at special risk of colon cancer—either because (1) it runs in the family, or (2) they have had colonic polyps, or (3) because they have had high-fat, low-fiber dietary tendencies. These dosages have no side effects.

Food Sources of Calcium

Whole- and skim-milk products
Shellfish
Dark-green, leafy vegetables

Magnesium is another crucial nutrient, required for a range of metabolic functions. It helps regulate the metabolism of calcium, and should be taken with calcium at a 2:1 ratio—for example, if you take 800 milligrams of calcium, take 400 milligrams of magnesium.

Recommendations

1. Eat calcium-rich foods daily, particularly dark-green, leafy vegetables or shellfish. High-fat whole-milk products are not recommended; select skim-milk or low-fat products.
2. Supplements:
   For adults: 800 milligrams calcium and 400 milligrams magnesium. For postmenopausal women and those who have a family history of colon cancer, those who have colonic polyps, those who have a tendency to high-fat, low-fiber diets: 1,200 milligrams and 600 milligrams magnesium.

Zinc

Zinc is a metal needed for growth, protein synthesis, the production of essential enzymes, and a healthy immune system. We still don't know whether zinc plays a direct role in preventing cancer, but, without question, it helps indirectly by keeping our immune defenses strong.

Some studies have reported low levels of serum zinc in patients with esophagus, lung, and other cancers. These low levels may have existed before the development of cancer, or may be a result of the cancer itself. Population studies have also correlated low dietary zinc with an increase in the rate of esophageal cancer.

There have been contradictory reports about the effects of zinc in animals exposed to chemical carcinogens. Nevertheless, in several experiments with hamsters and rats, zinc has suppressed the growth of chemically caused tumors.

Robert A. Good, the cancer immunologist, points out that zinc is absolutely essential to T-cell immunity, the most active arm of the immune system in the fight against cancer cells. Zinc is needed for a healthy thymus gland (which harbors and matures T-cells) and for adequate numbers of active, fully developed T-cells. A healthy ratio of T-helpers to T-suppressors—a crucial index of a properly balanced immune system—may depend on zinc levels. However, too much zinc may *suppress* the function of phagocytes, including macrophages, white cells that are also important subsidiary soldiers in fighting bacteria and cancer. For this and other reasons, moderation is required in taking zinc supplements. (When you have a bacterial infection, you should refrain temporarily from taking extra zinc because of its suspected role in inhibiting the phagocytes that neutralize bacteria.)

Zinc-rich foods include seafood, organ meats, brewer's yeast, soybeans, peas, spinach, wheat bran and wheat flour, and mushrooms.

Such foods are often lacking in our diets. While we should try to eat more seafood and whole-wheat products and beans, many of us still won't get enough zinc. Moreover, other dietary factors deplete zinc levels in our body, notably alcohol (whose intake we should diminish) and high-fiber foods (whose intake we should increase).

To offset these factors—especially an increased intake of fiber—and to keep our T-cell immune system healthy, *I recommend a 25-milligram supplement of zinc every day.*

Copper is a mineral worth mentioning here for two reasons: (1) there is evidence that copper plays a role in maintaining healthy immunity and is involved in various healing processes; and (2) recent literature points to the fact that zinc supplements can deplete the level of copper in our bodies. Although copper is not itself a known cancer preventor, it is still important in small amounts (too much copper can also be harmful). *Therefore, 3 milligrams of copper—no more—is recommended when 25 milligrams of zinc is taken.*

Foods Rich in Zinc

Seafood
Organ meats
Brewer's yeast
Soybeans
Peas
Spinach
Wheat bran and wheat flour
Mushrooms

Recommendations

1. Eat zinc-rich foods daily, especially seafood, foods containing wheat bran or wheat flour, soybeans, peas, spinach, or mushrooms.
2. Supplements: Take one 25-milligram tablet of zinc daily. Take 3 milligrams of copper with zinc.

FIBER

The discovery that fiber in our diets decreases our risk of colon cancer is a great example of modern medical science's pointing us increasingly in the direction of natural living. With all of the sophisticated medical technology involved in research and development of new drugs, nothing quite like fiber could ever be concocted to prevent colon cancer and treat a number of other conditions, like diverticular disease, irritable bowel syndrome, and diabetes.

Fiber is a term covering a group of different substances, all components of the cell walls of plants. Most forms of fiber are complex carbohydrates that can't be digested by enzymes in the intestine. There are two types of fiber: soluble and insoluble. Both types have healthful properties. Some scientists believe that the insoluble fibers (those that don't dissolve in water), are the most effective against colon cancer. They create bulk in the digestive tract, bind up carcinogenic agents, and move fecal material through the colon faster (quicker "transit time"), preventing the inner lining of the colon from prolonged exposure to carcinogens.

Insoluble fibers include:

- Cellulose: found in bran
- Hemicellulose: found in whole-grain foods
- Lignin: found in fruits, vegetables, and grains

The soluble fibers include mucilages and gums, found in certain legumes, fruit, and vegetables; and pectins, which are also derived from fruits and vegetables. *Bran is, without question, the best bulk-producing fiber and the most highly recommended dietary source of fiber for cancer prevention.* There is also a spectrum of whole grains, fruits, and vegetables that are good sources of fiber (see page 87).

There is little controversy about fiber. The NCI, ACS, and NAS's Committee on Diet, Nutrition, and Cancer all recommend a high-fiber diet for prevention of colon cancer. Yet they are still cautious in their statements about the "direct role" of fiber, because of some contradictory findings in population studies. Despite these contradictions, an overview of the data leaves me convinced that some component of fiber is nature's way of protecting us from abnormalities in the colon, including colon cancer, which is the second leading cause of death from cancer in the U.S.

The Evidence for Fiber

Denis Burkitt, a British physician who worked in Africa from 1946 to 1966, was one of the first to popularize the notion that fiber halts the growth of colon cancer. He noted that many rural Africans excreted stool that was bulkier and weighed more than twice that of the average British subject. This was clearly based on their much higher intake of unrefined fiber foods. Burkitt saw a relationship between the African diet, bulk in the stool, and their remarkably low incidence of colon cancer—especially as compared to British and other Western populations. The diet of these rural Africans provided over 50 grams of crude fiber a day, while most Western diets contain approximately half that or less.

Worldwide studies have been conducted since the late 1970s, correlating high-fiber intake with low colorectal cancer rates and low-fiber intake with high rates of this cancer. In 1977, an Indian investigator, S. L. Malhotra, noted differences among northern and southern populations in India. People in the North had diets high in roughage and vegetable fiber (these fibers were abundant in their stool) and virtually no incidence of colon cancer. There was no vegetable fiber in the stools of subjects from the South, where the colon-cancer rate was much higher.

The Harvard Medical School *Health Letter* recently pointed out, by way of example, a study in which "New Yorkers, who eat little fiber, have been compared with people from Finland, who eat twice as much fiber. The Finns develop about one-quarter as many bowel cancers as the New Yorkers."

The Committee on Diet, Nutrition, and Cancer rightly points out that population studies and "case-control" studies (where the dietary patterns of colon-cancer patients and normals are compared) have not been completely unanimous in relating total fiber intake to lowered risk of colon cancer. Research is needed to determine whether a low dietary fat content is a superseding factor, more important than fiber. There is also strong evidence that, because certain food sources of fiber (like bran) are better protectors than other sources, some *component* of fiber may be the real anticancer ally.

How Fiber Works

Animal studies have provided data and insight on the mode of action of fiber. Burkitt's belief that fiber in the diet moves fecal matter through the lower bowel more quickly, minimizing contact between the colon wall and cancer-causing agents, is still widely held today. The additional bulk may simply dilute carcinogens, and some types of fiber can bind directly to potent carcinogens, such as steroid hormones, making possible their removal from the intestine.

Fiber also absorbs and binds bile acids in the colon. Free-floating bile acids can aid in the formation of carcinogens when interacting with intestinal bacteria, and may irritate the intestinal lining, making tissues more susceptible to cancerous changes. By moving bile acids out of the colon, fiber prevents these dangers. Fiber also binds to cholesterol and lipids and eliminates them in the stool. We know about the contribution of fat to colon cancer (see Chapter 6, "Foods That Are Enemies"); fiber could be the strongest antidote available to the effects of fat in the intestinal tract.

Another theory about the protective action of fiber has been advanced, one involving a controversial component—phytic acid. Some nutritionists have stated the concern that the phytic acid in fiber robs the body of its ability to use iron and zinc. Dr. Ernst Graf of Pillsbury and Dr. John Eaton of the University of Minnesota have analyzed the problem, by comparing the cancer rates and eating habits of people of Finland and Denmark. The Finns have less colon cancer. The key difference the researchers uncovered is in the sources of fiber: the Finns got their fiber from bran foods, seeds, nuts, and beans, all high in phytic acid; while the Danes got theirs mainly from fruits, vegetables, and starches, which have little phytic acid. Graf and Eaton believe that phytic acid can bind excess iron in the colon. If there's too much iron in the colon, it can oxidize and lead to the release of cancer-causing free radicals. This iron-binding effect could be another mechanism of fiber's protection and another reason to prevent intake of too much iron (see page 116 in "Foods That Are Enemies" on the problems with iron). These researchers argue further that it's unlikely we could ingest enough phytic acid to keep us from getting sufficient zinc and iron.

How to Get Fiber

The simplest, most efficient way to put fiber in your diet is to eat whole-grain foods, especially bran. Bran cereals are an excellent way to start the day. Half a cup of *100 percent whole-bran cereal* provides more than 6 grams of fiber—a healthy portion of our daily requirement, *which should range between 30 and 40 grams per day.* Today's average American diet is about 15–20 grams or less.

Because fiber is currently such a hot anticancer subject, the cereal companies in particular have begun fiber advertising campaigns and many cereal boxes brandish big labels "high in fiber" or name their products "Bran ——."

What you're looking for is a cereal truly high in fiber. The words "bran," "wheat," and certainly "natural" do not necessarily mean the cereal is full of fiber. Check the box labels to be sure of the actual fiber content—your cereal should contain at least 4 and preferably over 5 grams per one-ounce serving. Unfortunately, however, some cereal box labels don't tell you how much fiber they contain. To make life easier for you, the following list, derived from a 1986 *Consumer Reports* investigation of the nutrient value of ready-to-eat cereals, gives the fiber content of the major cereals in order of most fiber to least fiber. (Within each category of number of grams of fiber, the cereals are listed in the order they were rated by *Consumer Reports* in terms of overall nutrient value—high in fiber and protein; low in sugar, sodium, and fat. For instance, if you choose a cereal in the 4-grams column and also want the most nutritious, you would pick Nabisco Shredded Wheat 'N Bran over Kellogg's Cracklin' Oat Bran.)

*Grams of Fiber per 1-oz. Serving of Cereal**

12 GRAMS

Fiber One (General Mills)

*Two recent cereal products, not rated in 1986 *Consumer Reports,* are very high in fiber and worth trying: Nabisco's 100% Bran (10 grams) and Kellogg's Bran Buds (8 grams).

9 GRAMS

All-Bran (Kellogg)

5 GRAMS

Post Natural Bran Flakes
Quaker Corn Bran
Bran Chex (Ralston Purina)

4 GRAMS

Nabisco Shredded Wheat 'N Bran
Familia Swiss Birchermuesli (Biofamilia)
Kellogg's Bran Flakes
Fruit & Fibre Harvest Medley (Post)
Fruit & Fibre Mountain Trail (Post)
Fruit & Fibre Tropical Fruit (Post)
Fruitful Bran (Kellogg)
Post Natural Raisin Bran
Kellogg's Raisin Bran
Cracklin' Oat Bran (Kellogg)

3 GRAMS

Nabisco Shredded Wheat Spoon Size
Nabisco Shredded Wheat
Frosted Mini-Wheats (Kellogg)
Familia Genuine Swiss Muesli (Biofamilia)

2 GRAMS

Nutri-Grain Wheat (Kellogg)
Grape-Nuts (Post)
Wheat Chex (Ralston Purina)
Nutri-Grain Corn (Kellogg)
Cheerios (General Mills)
Grape-Nuts Flakes (Post)
Total (General Mills)
Wheaties (General Mills)

1 GRAM

Nutri-Grain Wheat & Raisins (Kellogg)
Sun Country Granola with Raisins (International Multi-Foods)
Life (Quaker Oats)
Raisin Life (Quaker Oats)
Almond Delight (Ralston Purina)

TRACE

Special K (Kellogg)
Sun Flakes Crispy Wheat & Rice Flakes (Ralston Purina)
100% Natural Cereal Raisin & Date (Quaker Oats)
Crispix (Kellogg)
Kellogg's Corn Flakes
100% Natural Cereal (Quaker Oats)
Product 19 (Kellogg)
Rice Chex (Ralston Purina)
Rice Krispies (Kellogg)
Super Golden Crisp (Post)
Corn Chex (Ralston Purina)
Honey Smacks (Kellogg)

Corn Pops (Kellogg)
Apple Jacks (Kellogg)
Froot Loops (Kellogg)
Cocoa Krispies (Kellogg)
Crispy Wheats 'N Raisins (General Mills)
Frosted Flakes (Kellogg)
Honey Comb (Post)
Lucky Charms (General Mills)
Cocoa Pebbles (Post)
Fruity Pebbles (Post)
Golden Grahams (General Mills)
Honey Nut Cheerios (General Mills)
Trix (General Mills)
Cocoa Puffs (General Mills)
Cap'n Crunch (Quaker Oats)

(List derived from *Consumer Reports,* October 1986, pages 628–37.)

You'll note how few cereals actually have more than 5 grams of fiber per serving; how most using the term "bran" have an average fiber content of 4 grams; and how so many cereals using the words "natural" and "wheat" have very little or no fiber. Who'd have ever thought that Quaker Oats's 100 percent Natural Cereal would have no fiber to speak of—on a par with other crunchy delights like Cap'n Crunch, Cocoa Krispies, and Froot Loops!

There are a number of cereals marketed to appear highly nutritious and full of fiber, with package designs highlighting natural grains and fresh fruit. In fact, many of these are only modestly nutritious and fiber-containing. Kellogg's Nutri-Grain line (Almond and Raisin, Brown Rice, and Corn Whole Grain Cereal) is an example, with only 1–2 grams of fiber per ounce. However, the Nutri-Grain line has little sugar and no preservatives and does contain an array of necessary vitamins and minerals. If you like the taste of such a cereal and prefer it to the truly high-fiber products, you can make your breakfast delight high in fiber by adding at least 2 tablespoons (2.7 grams) of pure unprocessed bran.

I have a friend who, to make sure he meets his daily fiber requirements, every morning eats 2 tablespoons of unprocessed bran straight from the spoon, washing it down with a tart glass of grapefruit juice. This is a bit like eating sawdust. However, Quaker's Unprocessed Bran has some good suggestions on its box for including bran in baking and cooking and offers a free bran recipe booklet. If one acquires the habit of adding bran to things like meatloaf, pancakes, and rolls, it's not a bad way to go.

There are many other creative ways to include fiber in our diets. Whole grains, fruits, and vegetables high in fiber are also rich in anticancer vitamins and minerals. They counteract some of the effects of fats and carcinogenic agents via their fiber and micronutrient contents.

The following table provides a list of high fiber foods other than the breakfast cereals already listed. Use this chart to help yourself get more fiber into your diet.

FIBER CONTENT OF FOODS*

The dietary fiber content of many foods is still unknown, so this is not a comprehensive list of the fiber content of foods. (Fiber content for vegetables and fruits that can be eaten with their skins includes fiber content for the skins.)

Rich Sources of Food Fiber
4 grams or more per serving

	Serving	Calories (Rounded to the nearest 5)
Legumes (cooked portions)		
Kidney beans	½ cup	110
Lima beans	½ cup	130
Navy beans	½ cup	110
Pinto beans	½ cup	110
White beans	½ cup	110
Fruits		
Blackberries	½ cup	35
Dried prunes	3	60

*For cereals, see the chart on page 84.

Moderately Rich Sources of Food Fiber
1 to 3 grams of fiber per serving

	Serving	Calories (Rounded to the nearest 5)
Breads and cooked cereals		
Bran muffins	1 medium	105
Popcorn (air-popped)	1 cup	25
Whole-wheat bread	1 slice	60
Whole-wheat spaghetti	1 cup	120
Oatmeal, cooked	¾ cup	110
Legumes (cooked) and Nuts		
Chick peas (garbanzo beans)	½ cup	135
Lentils	½ cup	105
Almonds	10 nuts	80
Peanuts	10 nuts	105
Vegetables		
Artichoke	1 small	45
Asparagus	½ cup	30
Beans, green	½ cup	15
Broccoli†	½ cup	20
Brussels sprouts	½ cup	30
Cabbage, red and white	½ cup	15
Carrots	½ cup	25
Cauliflower	½ cup	15
Corn	½ cup	70
Green peas	½ cup	55
Kale	½ cup	20
Parsnip	½ cup	50
Potato	1 medium	95
Spinach, cooked	½ cup	20
Spinach, raw	½ cup	5
Summer squash	½ cup	15
Sweet potato	½ medium	80
Turnip	½ cup	15
Bean sprouts (soy)	½ cup	15
Celery	½ cup	10
Tomato	1 medium	20
Winter squash†	½ cup	65
Fruits		
Apple	1 medium	80
Apricot, fresh	3 medium	50
Apricot, dried	5 halves	40

	Serving	Calories *(Rounded to the nearest 5)*
Banana	1 medium	105
Blueberries	½ cup	40
Cantaloupe	¼ melon	50
Cherries	10	50
Cranberries†	½ cup	20
Dates, dried	3	70
Figs, dried	1 medium	50
Grapefruit	½	40
Orange	1 medium	60
Peach	1 medium	35
Pear	1 medium	100
Pineapple	½ cup	40
Raisins	¼ cup	110
Raspberries†	½ cup	35
Strawberries	1 cup	45

Low Sources of Food Fiber
Less than 1 gram of fiber per serving

	Serving	Calories *(Rounded to the nearest 5)*
Breads and Cereals		
White bread	1 slice	70
Spaghetti, cooked	1 cup	155
Brown rice, cooked	½ cup	90
White rice, cooked	½ cup	80
Vegetables		
Lettuce, shredded	1 cup	10
Mushrooms, sliced	½ cup	10
Onions, sliced	½ cup	20
Pepper, green, sliced	½ cup	10
Fruits		
Grapes	20	30
Watermelon	1 cup	50

	Serving	Calories (Rounded to the nearest 5)
Fruit Juices		
Apple	½ cup-4 oz	60
Grapefruit	½ cup-4 oz	50
Grape	½ cup-4 oz	80
Orange	½ cup-4 oz	55
Papaya	½ cup-4 oz	70

†Author's additional entries.
Table adapted from U.S. Dept. of Health and Human Services, NIH Publication No. 85-2711, *Diet, Nutrition, and Cancer Prevention: A Guide to Food Choices.*

(For more tips on increasing fiber in your diet, see Chapter 7, "The Cancer-Prevention Diet Guide.")

THE CABBAGE FAMILY AND SOYBEANS: THE MIRACULOUS VEGETABLES

Quite apart from a high content of vitamins, minerals, and fiber, all the cabbage family contains additional cancer-blocking powers. Known as "the cruciferous vegetables" because their flowers form a cross, the most common among them are cabbage, broccoli, Brussels sprouts and cauliflower. For cancer prevention, they are the vegetables of prime choice.

The cruciferous vegetables are abundant in substances called "indoles." In experiments with mice, indoles were added to their diets before and during the administration of carcinogens (like those in cigarettes); they stopped the growth of tumors developing in the stomach and lung. In some way not yet clear, indoles deactivate carcinogens or block them from damaging cells, acting at several different stages of carcinogenesis to stop both "promoters" and "initiators." It may be that indoles buttress the enzyme system responsible for metabolizing carcinogens, and, in all probability, they increase the antioxidant action of glutathione compounds. However this works, the cruciferous vegetables have proved to be terrific anticancer nutrients.

So are soybeans, chick peas, and lima beans, for a different reason. They—and a few other plants and seeds—contain powerful tumor-blocking substances called "protease inhibitors" (soybeans and chick peas have by far the highest content of these). Rats exposed to radiation, then fed a diet rich in protease inhibitors, had far less incidence of breast cancer. Protease inhibitors are highly skillful at stopping chemical promoters, possibly by preventing free radicals from being formed by these carcinogen-activating agents. Soybean products, including tofu and miso, also have this ability. Soybean oil is not especially recommended because it is high in polyunsaturates.

Cruciferous	*Protease Inhibitors*
Broccoli	Soybeans and their related products,
Brussels sprouts	including tofu, miso
Cabbage	Lima beans
Cauliflower	Chick peas
Chinese cabbage	
Collards	
Horseradish	
Kale	
Kohlrabi	
Mustard	
Radish	
Rutabaga	
Turnip	
Watercress	

Recommendations

Eat as many cruciferous vegetables as you can—every day, if possible. *In addition to having their special properties, many of them are high in vitamins A, C, and E; some contain anticancer minerals; and most are high in fiber.*

Eat soybean products frequently. Their cancer-prevention properties are different from those of the cabbage family, so they are not a cabbage substitute. As you know, soybeans are also an excellent source of protein.

OTHER ANTIOXIDANT FACTORS

Glutathione (a peptide), cysteine (an amino acid), and superoxide dismutase (SOD, an enzyme) all have antioxidant properties and may contribute to cancer prevention. Although these are available in supplement form, there is at this time not enough evidence to warrant taking additional glutathione, cysteine, and SOD as separate dosages.

However, several nutrient companies market antioxidant combination supplements, which contain some or all of these substances in addition to vitamins A, C, and E, beta-carotene, selenium, and zinc. These combination products are often excellent for simplifying the whole supplement routine. They are a way to get reasonable dosages of the complete range of antioxidant nutrients. I stress the use of this type of product because it contains more of the essential anticancer nutrients than most multivitamin, multimineral supplements, and thus enables you to take fewer pills each day. *I must also emphasize that, if you take an antioxidant combination pill, you should not take a multivitamin in addition. You may be adding too much to your intake of Vitamin A, selenium, and zinc. If you do start taking combination pills—antioxidants or multivitamins—always make sure you're not doubling up and getting more than is recommended here.*

In Chapter 7, "The Cancer-Prevention Diet Guide," I present a simple daily plan for eating protein, fruits, vegetables, dairy and grains, and lists of foods to choose from that are rich in anticancer nutrients. I will also repeat the supplement list below. So if you want to use this book in a hurry, refer to Chapter 7.

Nature offers us a breathtaking array of allies for maintaining healthy immune systems and vital cells and tissues. In the case of vitamins, minerals, and fiber, the evidence is striking and the conclusions are firm, although we are still not certain about the optimal amounts; they may be higher than we think. Nor are we sure what the full benefits really are. The recommendations I have made reflect our knowledge to this point and provide guidance on how to receive *some* anticancer benefits without danger of overdosing.

I also want to emphasize that the laboratory approach to nutritional research—exemplified by the reports of the Committee on Diet, Nutrition, and Cancer Prevention—has its advantages and its limitations. Laboratory studies have opened a world of discovery about cancer-preventive nutrients. However, when each individual substance is isolated, purified, and used for testing, remember that it is being taken out of its rich natural context. Macronutrients and micronutrients work together and, through their synergism, complement and augment each other's biological activities. We may not be learning all there is to know about potential anticancer vitamins and minerals by removing them from their natural context and giving them to mice that have been exposed to carcinogens.

Nutritional biochemists may have to heed some of the lessons taught to us by the holistic health movement. The ultimate key to cancer prevention through nutrition must come through a diet rich in the major cancer-preventive substances, yet replete with a wide variety of nutrients acting together as an allied force.

DAILY SUPPLEMENT LIST

The way to achieve the best balance of vitamins and minerals is to take (in addition to the food sources, of course) the supplements individually at the recommended levels. However, it is a lot of trouble to ingest that many different pills. Some people don't like taking pills and others can't remember to. I can't. So I offer three options, but I recommend the first system for anyone at risk.

System 1: Ideal

Take in the A.M.:

Vitamin A—10,000 IU and 15 mg. beta-carotene
Vitamin B—B-complex pill (high B-50 or B-100)
Vitamin C—2–5 grams (2,000–5,000 mg.)*
Vitamin E—200–600 IU
Selenium—100–200 mcg.
Calcium—800–1,200 mg.
Magnesium—400–600 mg.
Zinc—25 mg.
Copper—3 mg.

Use a multivitamin, multimineral pill if you prefer to take fewer pills. Try to avoid those that contain iron. (See section on iron in Chapter 6, "Foods That Are Enemies.")

System 2: Good

In the A.M.: Take an antioxidant combination that includes beta-carotene, C, E, selenium and zinc. Back this up with a Super B-complex, one or more grams of C, and additional E. (That brings you down to 4+ pills in the morning, depending on how much extra C you take.)

In the P.M.: Take the additional C you need to meet your daily requirement. Divided doses can be taken at noon and after dinner.

System 3: Okay

In the A.M.: Take an antioxidant combination with a B-complex pill and a gram of C. This keeps you down to 3 pills in the morning.

In the P.M.: Take the additional C you need to meet your daily requirement in one or more additional doses when most convenient.

*Divide doses of C as needed and take additional quantities in the P.M.

Let the contents of your antioxidant pill be your guide. Check the values of A, C, E, selenium, and zinc it contains against my ideal recommendations and see how well it fares. Shore up this pill with B, C, or E according to Systems 2 or 3. Try to include calcium-magnesium, and zinc-copper. *Watch that your total values don't exceed the recommendations in System 1.* Of course, if you can hack it, System 1 is ideal; come as close to it as you can within your pill-taking capabilities.

6

Foods That Are Enemies

Yes, there really are foods that contain cancer-causing substances. But there are not *that* many of them and avoiding them is not *that* difficult.

One of our biggest enemies is fat—fats of all kinds, including polyunsaturated oils. In 1988, the U.S. Government issued its most comprehensive report ever on nutrition and health. In it the Surgeon General cited fat as a leading cause of chronic diseases such as heart disease, some cancers, diabetes, hypertension, and strokes. According to the *New York Times,* "it was the first time the government has identified reduction of fat intake as the No. 1 dietary priority of the nation."

For many of us, reducing our fat intake may be the hardest switch we have to make—especially if we're used to the "normal" American diet, which contains at least 25 percent too much fat, and usually more. Some fat is necessary; but diets high in fat promote the growth of certain tumor types. If you are eating high off the hog, you need to make a basic change in your habits. I will give you guidelines to make it as easy for you as possible.

However, there is absolutely no reason to be paranoid about every morsel you ingest. We will never eliminate all carcinogenic traces from our diets, and scientists don't believe that minor traces are likely to lead to cancer anyway. But we do need to eliminate known carcinogens and pay careful attention to the balance—or imbalance—between foods that are allies and those that are enemies, and tip the scales heavily toward the allies. With the support of a good diet, our defense systems can nullify carcinogens and even halt cancer-cell growth.

Food additives and contaminants that may cause cancer have had a lot of publicity and some of them have been banned by the FDA (see below). Overall, it is hard to estimate the role of food additives, contaminants, molds, and minerals, because population studies showing the effects of prolonged intake may be impossible to conduct or extrapolate from. Scientists have to rely on laboratory tests and animals, which can only provide rough estimates of cancer risks to humans. I am not contending that, because the data are imprecise, we should ignore the problem. On the contrary—because the data are imprecise, many food constituents that should be banned by the FDA have not been. We need to be aware of what chemicals in our food might be carcinogenic.

The FDA's Food, Drug, and Cosmetic Act includes the Delaney clause, for regulation of carcinogens in food and drugs. Several substances have been banned under this clause, and others have been restricted to "safe" levels. However, we can't leave it up to the FDA or any agency to fully take care of regulation. They should, of course, but we know enough about federal red tape not to completely rely on them.

All this being said, the chemical food additives now on the market do not seem to be responsible for much of the incidence of cancer in the U.S. By one estimate, they are thought to comprise only about 1 percent of all cancer-risk factors. This could be an underestimation, and additives may combine with other carcinogenic factors to increase risk. Based on what we know about additives (and what we don't know), I suggest that, on the continuum from complacent to concerned to compulsive, you find your way toward "concerned." In this chapter, I will help you evaluate substances still on the market that are suspect, and it is up to you to consider the evidence and avoid them when possible.

Below, I will describe the enemies: those foods that contain naturally occurring or man-made constituents that can cause cancer. Some are *real enemies*—powerful, proven carcinogens that should be avoided at all costs. Others have a lesser effect or are just suspect; they should be eaten sparingly if at all. For the less we are exposed to dietary carcinogens, the more likely our natural defenses—supported by the anticancer nutrients—will be able to eliminate other carcinogens and developing cancer cells.

Do your best to avoid the enemies. In instances where intake is unavoidable, I will suggest some specific "allied" antidotes.

DIETARY FAT

As I mentioned above, you should be *most* concerned about fat in your diet. The Committee on Diet, Nutrition, and Cancer, usually so circumspect in its conclusions, went out on a limb with regard to fat: "Of all the dietary components [the committee] studied, the combined epidemiological and experimental evidence is most suggestive for a causal relationship between fat intake and the occurrence of cancer." Translation: Of all the things in our diet that could promote cancer, fat is the most worrisome.

In 1977, the U.S. Senate Select Committee on Nutrition and Human Needs recommended a decrease in the average American intake of fat from 40 percent of energy intake to 30 percent. At that time, not a great deal was known about the extent of fat's contribution to certain cancers; and their recommendation was based on general health considerations and, in particular, on prevention of heart disease. In 1982, a mere five years later, the Committee on Diet, Nutrition, and Cancer made the same recommendation: cut your fat intake from 40 percent of overall calories to 30 percent or less—this time based on cancer prevention alone. The goal is reasonable, in that it is attainable without undue restriction; and consequential: it should make a great difference in lowering our risk of cancer.

Fats in food include the saturated animal fats in meats, fish, and poultry, the solid fats in butter and margarine, the fats in milk and dairy products, the polyunsaturates in most vegetable oils, and the fats in processed snack foods and rich sauces. We must reduce our consumption of these fatty foods.

The Evidence Against Fats

High-fat diets increase the risk of colon, breast, and prostate cancer. Take note of how unequivocal this statement is, because it reflects the results of global studies and the opinions of investigators all over the world—not just the Committee on Diet, Nutrition, and Cancer. Furthermore, there is also some evidence—albeit less compelling—that high-fat diets add to the risk of ovarian, endometrial, and pancreatic cancers.

The three cancers linked most strongly to a high-fat diet—colorectal, breast, and prostate cancers—accounted for an estimated 381,900, or *39 percent* of all new cancer cases in 1988. *When the statistics are in, some 131,800 people will have died of these types of cancers in 1988, which represents 27 percent of all cancer deaths.* Colon, breast, and prostate cancers follow lung cancer as numbers 2, 3, and 4 respectively on the list of cancers resulting in the most deaths.

These tragically prevalent cancers may be prevented by a simple task: lowering the percentages of fat in our diets. Not all colon, breast, and prostate cancers will be prevented this way, nor is lowering fat the only approach to preventing them. However, there is no doubt that tens of thousands of lives would be saved if we all took this one recommendation to heart.

Here are a few representative examples of population studies showing the relationship between high fat and cancer:

The connection between dietary fat intake and breast cancer is very strong. On a broad scale, many international correlation studies have shown that countries where the per capita fat intake (measuring total fat consumption) was high had higher rates of breast cancer. The United States is decidedly a high-risk country, because our diets are characterized by a lot of cholesterol and saturated and unsaturated fats. Our breast-cancer rate is tragically high.

The Japanese diet is relatively low-risk, with 20 percent of calories derived from fat (half of the U.S. average). Correspondingly, the incidence of breast and colon cancer in Japan is much lower. Further proof that the fat factor is the crucial difference came with studies showing that Japanese who have come to this country and adopted our eating habits eventually developed breast and colon cancer at the same high rate as Americans, after living here for only twenty years.

Researcher R. L. Phillips followed Seventh-Day Adventists, whose primarily vegetarian diets make them a bona-fide low-fat group. He found that their breast-cancer mortality rate was between one-half and two-thirds of the overall rate in the U.S. Both Seventh-Day Adventists and Mormons, another low-fat group, have far less colorectal cancer.

Although all types of fat are associated with a higher risk of cancer, the saturated fats in meat may have an even greater effect on colon cancer. In the study comparing Finnish and New York City populations, it was found that the total fat intake was similar, though the Finns got most of their fat from dairy foods and the New Yorkers from meat products. The New Yorkers had a considerably higher rate of colon cancer, though their lesser intake of fiber was also a factor. Reviews of colon-cancer rates and meat intake per capita from many countries throughout the world show consistent correlations.

The international data on prostate cancer shows a connection between fat intake and death from prostate cancer, though not for incidence. However, studies of individual countries do show that high fat is often associated with more prostate cancer. Since 1950, the fat intake in Japan has gone up, and so has the rate of prostate cancer—dramatically. In the U.S., one group of investigators looked at the relationship between fat and prostate cancer on a country-by-country basis. They found that countries with a high risk for prostate cancer among whites had relatively high-fat diets.

Although far less population research has been conducted on ovarian and endometrial cancers, a handful of studies tell us these cancers, and pancreatic cancer (which, although not common, is usually fatal), may be related to fats in our diet.

One final note about fats and colon cancer: a few studies have shown that people with colon cancer have lower blood serum levels of cholesterol. When these findings were publicized, it was another seeming cause for throwing in the cancer-prevention towel: "You mean I'm supposed to lower my fat to prevent colon cancer, and lower my cholesterol to prevent heart disease, but by lowering my cholesterol I'm increasing my risk of colon cancer?!"

If you heard this report and were similarly confused, don't be. Although the reasons for the findings have not been fully clarified, several other studies contradicted the idea that low cholesterol is related to colon cancer.* Furthermore, a recent article in the *Journal of the American Medical Association* reviewed cases of cancer seemingly associated with low cholesterol in a group of participants in the famous Multiple Risk Factor Intervention Trial. The researchers concluded that the drop in serum cholesterol was a result, not a cause, of the cancers. They went further by suggesting that the low cholesterol found in patients before they developed symptoms of cancer was probably caused by cancer that was not yet detectable. Many nutritionists do believe that too little cholesterol can have a negative effect on health, but there is still no strong evidence to associate low cholesterol with cancer.

How Fat Promotes Cancer

Diets high in fat—*all fats,* whether of the meat or dairy variety, saturated or polyunsaturated—increase your risks of cancer in a myriad of insidious ways.

With regard to breast cancer, laboratory studies with mice are extremely consistent: fatty diets enhance cancerous growth, whether the tumors are chemically caused, occur spontaneously, or are transplanted from other mice. These experiments have also helped reveal the specific role of fat in cancer causation. Breast-cancer growth is enhanced in these mice when high-fat diets are fed to them after—*not before*—chemical carcinogens are given. This confirms the widely held idea that fat is a cancer *promoter,* not an initiator. Fat itself is not a carcinogen; rather, excess fat can act to promote cancerous growth in cells that are, for whatever reason, so predisposed.

Fat can also facilitate the growth of breast cancers in another way— via its effect on female hormones. It is known that high estrogen and prolactin levels can overstimulate breast tissue and trigger cancer. Apparently, a high-fat diet causes women to produce more estrogen. Women who are overweight and ingest a lot of fat have reduced levels of a protein substance that is responsible for binding estrogen. Without enough of this protein, greater amounts of "unbound" estrogen can circulate and do their damage to breast tissue. A similar mechanism may also be responsible for the connection between fat and ovarian and endometrial cancers. Another telling factor is that obesity is clearly

*In fact, two recent reports in the *New England Journal of Medicine* showed a direct association between high cholesterol and *increased* risk of colon cancer.

associated with high risk of breast, ovarian, and endometrial cancers. Prostate cancer may be influenced by fat intake in a similar manner. Male hormone levels are probably affected by high fat in a way that can promote changes in prostate cells.

Our risk of colon cancer can be elevated by a variety of mechanisms. Fats—especially saturated fats—increase the production of bile acids and bile salts in the large bowel. Bacteria are plentiful in the intestine, as they should be; we need bacteria there for proper digestion. Yet anaerobic bacteria, the type that doesn't need O_2 to survive, can combine with bile acids in the bowel, which together produce colon-cancer-causing chemicals. The bile acids alone may initiate or promote tumor-cell growth by injuring the lining of the large intestine.

Remember that *a high-fat diet together with a low-fiber intake is a potentially lethal one-two punch.* * The carcinogenic potential of bile acids, bacteria, and various by-products of fat metabolism in the large bowel can be nullified by fiber. Fiber may bind bile acids and carcinogens and move them quickly out of the intestine before the damage can be inflicted that leads to cancer.

Most dietary fat is stored in the body in the form of triglycerides. These are made up of fatty acids of three different types: saturated, monounsaturated, and polyunsaturated. Fatty acids are composed of chains of molecules, on which there is room for hydrogen atoms to be attached. Saturated fats have no room for any more hydrogen atoms; monounsaturated fats have room for two; and polyunsaturated fats have room for four or more hydrogen atoms. A fat is categorized based on whether *most* of its constituent fatty acids are saturated, monounsaturated, or polyunsaturated. You've seen the term "hydrogenated" on a wide variety of food labels—the more "hydrogenated" a fat, the more saturated it is. There is quite a lot of confusion about whether to choose foods or oils containing mostly saturated, polyunsaturated, or monounsaturated fats. First, here's a short list of fats indicating which type of fat they are predominantly composed of:

MOSTLY SATURATED:

milkfat	coconut and palm oils
butter	most shortenings (hydrogenated
animal fats (beef, lamb, pork)	oils)

MOSTLY POLYUNSATURATED:

corn oil	sunflower oil
sesame oil	soybean oil

---

*A recent study in the *British Medical Journal* compared 50 colon cancer patients to 50 matched controls without cancer. The cancer patients differed only in their consumption of more high-fat, low-fiber, sugary foods.

safflower oil
most margarines (though partially converted into saturated fats via
  hydrogenation)

MOSTLY MONOUNSATURATED:

olive oil	avocado oil
peanut oil	some margarines

Fats may increase the risk of cancer through another mechanism—
"lipid peroxidation" (the breakdown of fats through oxidation; it's the
process by which fats turn rancid). When oxygen reacts with fats, free
radicals are formed as by-products and these radicals go on to produce
hydroperoxides, which produce more free radicals. Polyunsaturated
fats have been recommended for years as the best fats to prevent heart
disease, because they lower blood cholesterol. *Unfortunately, polyunsaturates are the most likely to produce free radicals that can damage
cell structures and cause malignant transformation.* In other words,
the fat that has been considered all right for the heart may be the worst
for cancer prevention.

Indeed, when overall fat intake is low, *polyunsaturated fats are an
even stronger risk factor for cancer than are saturated fats!* When the
fat intake is high, the effects of saturated and polyunsaturated fats
appear to be about the same. With regard to breast cancer, some studies
tell us that polyunsaturated fats are riskier than saturated fats (though,
the opposite is true of colon cancer—saturated fats are considered the
more likely culprit).

At this stage of research, enough is known about polyunsaturated
fats and oils, and the dangerous, extremely reactive free radicals they
spawn, to recommend cutting down on them. For years TV commer-
cials and news reports have told us to use polyunsaturated vegetable oils
and margarines as a way of cutting down on cholesterol and lowering
our risk of heart disease. Now it is up to us to lower our intake of *both*
saturated (animal) and polyunsaturated fats and oils in order to reduce
our risk of both heart disease and cancer.

Before you throw up your hands (thinking, how can I cook?) there
is one very good alternative to saturated and polyunsaturated fats—a
way out of the trap. *The answer is monounsaturated fats.*

By "answer" I mean that it is a safer fat to ingest than saturated or
polyunsaturated, not that you should go ahead and overindulge. All
types of fat contain some saturated, monounsaturated, and polyunsaturated fats (a fat is designated in one category or other because it
contains much more of one that the other). *Olive oil is the best monounsaturated fat because it has the highest percentage of monounsaturates.*
Here's a quick look at six types of fat and how they compare, in terms
of percentages.

Type	Saturated	Monounsaturated	Polyunsaturated
Butter	66.0%	30.0%	4.0%
Corn oil	14.5%	27.6%	57.9%
Olive oil	17.1%	72.3%	10.6%
Peanut oil	20.4%	48.1%	31.5%
Safflower oil	9.2%	13.1%	77.7%
Soybean oil	15.6%	23.4%	61.0%

From "Personal Health," Jane E. Brody, *New York Times,* April 24, 1985.

As you can see, *olive oil is the monounsaturate of choice,* peanut oil a distant second (peanut oil is also less preferable because it has been found to promote artery damage in some animal studies). What makes monounsaturates better? First, recent research has uncovered the fact that monounsaturated fats can be even more effective than polyunsaturated fats in reducing cholesterol, and therefore, the risk of heart disease. A collaboration between researchers at the University of Texas and the University of California at San Diego found that, in a group of people fed special liquid diets, both polyunsaturated and monounsaturated fats reduced blood cholesterol equally. However, the monounsaturates lowered the portion of cholesterol (the low-density lipoproteins, or LDLs) that damages arteries—the so-called "bad cholesterol." But, unlike polyunsaturates, they leave alone the "good cholesterol" (high-density lipoproteins, or HDLs), which actually protects arteries from damage. This may be why Greeks and Italians, who use mostly olive oil, have low rates of heart disease. The researchers concluded that olive oil offers the best protection against heart disease.

Second, because of their chemical structure, monounsaturates are less prone to turn rancid and produce cell-damaging free radicals than the polyunsaturated fats. They are therefore less likely to increase cancer risk than the polyunsaturates. This finding has yet to be proven definitively, but research is leading toward this conclusion. Additional evidence comes from population surveys of Greeks and Spaniards, who both use a lot of olive oil: they have unusually low rates of breast and colon cancer.

Therefore, as part of your fat-cutting regime, I strongly recommend that you select olive oil. It's crucial to keep your overall fat intake below 30 percent, so don't overdo it; it's still fat and carries with it some deleterious effects. The trick is to substitute olive oil where once you used butter or vegetable oils. It tastes great, and should do the trick for most users. Researchers are now trying to develop corn, sunflower, and safflower oils that are mainly monounsaturated, but until they're available, stick with olive oil. Extra-virgin and virgin are the highest quality, made from the first pressing of olives without added chemicals. If extra-virgin is too expensive, the less costly olive oils are okay and better than other oils. Olive oil may not be practical for deep frying (if you must deep fry, use peanut oil), but it will take higher heat than butter, so it is fine for sautéing.

It would be difficult to completely eliminate polyunsaturated vegetable oils from the diet. Although it is important to keep intake of polyunsaturates low, and best to use olive oil instead whenever possible, there is no reason to be paranoid about a low intake of polyunsatures. Remember, polyunsatures themselves do not directly cause cancer: it is only when they are oxidized in the body that they can cause dangerous free radicals. *The antioxidant nutrients—beta-carotene, vitamins C and E, and selenium—help block the oxidation of polyunsaturates. Adequate intake of these nutrients can protect us from the damage that might be caused by any polyunsaturated fats in our diet. So keep intake of them low, use olive oil where possible, and get your antioxidants for the best protection.*

The benefits of margarine, once thought to be *the* alternative to butter for lowering cholesterol, have been questioned in recent years. First, most margarine is made of polyunsaturated vegetable oils, which we now realize are problematic in terms of cancer risk. Some of these polyunsaturates are converted into saturated fat during the manufacture of margarine, thus negating some of margarine's supposed ability to reduce the risk of heart disease. This process of converting liquid oils to solid fat, called hydrogenation (the spaces for hydrogen atoms on the fat chain are being filled), also carries with it additional risks. Chemical changes are wrought, producing what are known as *trans* fatty acids. In some animal studies, trans fatty acids have caused increased incidence of cancer. Margarine may reduce blood cholesterol, but not as effectively or as safely as scientists once believed. Given what we know about polyunsaturates and trans fatty acids, I recommend you use little or no margarine. Don't consider margarine a safe and surefire alternative to butter, to be used liberally on breads, in sauces, and for cooking. If you must, use a little butter here, a little margarine there. Best of all, substitute olive oil when and where you can.

Heating oil—especially polyunsaturated oil—is ill-advised. Heat increases oxidation processes that produce free-radical by-products. The higher the heat, the greater the danger, and reheating oil steps up this process even further. Although some oil is needed for sautéing or quick frying, *don't overheat oil and never reuse it,* once it has been heated and let cool. Avoid fast-food joints, which not only cook foods in tremendous quantities of saturated or polyunsaturated fat but also heat and reheat oil in huge vats. Stay away from these places; they produce foods cooked in ways that maximize the potential harm of the fats they contain.

Remember, it is not O.K. to eat a lot of fat if we take antioxidant supplements. It simply means that we have an additional shield against the cancer-promoting effects of fat. The best approach is to replace some of the fatty foods in our diet with fresh foods rich in antioxidant nutrients, in order to restore a healthy balance and substantially reduce the risk of colon, breast, and prostate cancer.

How to Lower Fat Intake

The task at hand, then, is to lower our fat intake from 40 percent of our total calories to 30 percent or, preferably, even less. In the first week or two, it is best to aim for a goal of 20 percent.

Fat is measured in grams, and each gram of fat has 9 calories (protein and carbohydrates have 4 calories per gram). One way to determine if a food is high-fat is to find out what percentage of calories in that food are derived from fat. This can be determined by the following formula:

Grams of fat per serving × *9* ÷ by the total calories per serving

By referring to Appendix 1 in this book or by carefully reading the labels on food, you can determine the grams of fat and total calories per serving, and then, by using this formula, the percentage of calories from fat. In oils, fats, butter, and margarine, 100 percent of the calories come from fat. Well over one-half the calories in foods like eggs, cheeses, pork, hot dogs, and peanut butter come from fat. Almost zero percent of the calories from fruit and vegetable juices come from fat.

There is one way to determine carefully the number of grams of fat that should be your daily maximum if you are to keep at the 30 percent mark. First, find out approximately what your daily intake of calories is. If you're not a dieter or not nutrition-conscious and don't know, spend three days with a calorie counter and find out. Once you've done so, determine the number of calories from fat you should not exceed, by answering the mathematical question: what is 30 percent of X (total number of calories you take in each day)? Take this number of calories, divide by 9, and you have the number of grams of fat per day that you should not exceed. Here are examples of different-calorie diets, and the number of calories and grams of fat to stay under to remain under the 30 percent mark:

Daily Calories	No. of Calories from Fat to Stay Under	No. of Grams of Fat to Stay Under
1,000	300	33
1,250	375	42
1,500	450	50
1,750	525	58
2,000	600	67
2,250	675	75
2,500	750	83

Locate yourself on the above chart, or if you need to be more precise, make your own calculation. Once you figure out how many grams of fat you should take in each day to stay at 30 percent, you'll have your guidepost. Then use Appendix 1 of this book (which gives the number of grams of fat and calories for some foods) to determine your intake, and stay at or below your proper threshold. For those foods not included in the Appendix, *read labels.*

I'm not suggesting that you count grams of fat every day of your life. There are a few simple ways to cut down on fat, and a number of helpful tips (see Chapters 7 and 8) that should suffice to bring you near the 30 percent mark. However, one week of gram counting can be an invaluable learning experience, paving the way for a lifetime of realistic, efficient fat-cutting.

Find out how many grams of fat equals 30 percent of your calories and try to stick to it. Use the list in Appendix 1 of this book to guide you, and try it for one whole week. You may well learn (1) how much fat you really ingest, which is probably far too much; (2) how you must begin to substitute healthier, low-fat foods if you are to cut down on fat and not starve; and (3) exactly what kinds of changes are necessary to meet the 30 percent goal.

The latter point is most crucial. Once you know from experience what you need to do, the goal will no longer be an amorphous horizon with forgettable consequences. Count grams for a week if you can; it will help crystallize your effort to lower fat in your diet, a move that will certainly lower your risk of cancer and probably prolong your life.

Here are my basic suggestions on how to reduce the fat in your diet:

1. Cut down on red meat; choose chicken and fish more often.
2. Eat more fruits; vegetables; whole-grain products, including breads and cereals; and more beans, peas, and seeds.
3. Choose *lean* meats and poultry, and trim off all visible fat before eating. Take the skin off chicken before cooking or before eating.

Add fish to your diet—even the fattier fishes have less fat than red meat, and contain oils that are beneficial.

4. Cut down on butter, margarine, and oils (especially salad dressings, creamy and/or oily sauces, oils for cooking). When possible, use olive oil for dressings and cooking instead.

5. Select low-fat or skim-milk dairy products (cut down on whole-milk products and avoid cream).

6. Broil, poach, or roast meats and drain off all fat after cooking.

Adhering to these six points is a sure bet for substantial fat-cutting. Consult Chapter 7, "The Cancer-Prevention Diet Guide," and Chapter 8, "You Can Change Your Eating Habits" for additional tips on how to achieve a low-fat diet.

NATURALLY OCCURRING CARCINOGENS

The idea that natural foods can contain carcinogens has had a curious effect on the national effort toward cancer prevention. As detailed in Chapter 3, Bruce Ames, the famed UC Berkeley biochemist, used his simple but widely applicable test (the Ames test) to discover that some chemicals occurring naturally in plant foods were mutagenic (they can cause damage to cellular DNA) and possibly carcinogenic. When he published an article in *Science* in 1983, describing the potential cancer-causing properties of foods like celery, alfalfa sprouts, and some herbal teas, the uproar shook the health-conscious community to the roots.

It was also used by industrialists and their supporters as a smoke screen against the continuing avalanche of criticism, from citizens' groups, concerning environmental carcinogens and chemical additives and pesticides in foodstuffs. Edith Efron's book *The Apocalyptics* argues against laying blame at the feet of corporations for the presence of environmental and food-related carcinogens, and for stifling regulatory action to ban or curb these carcinogens. Efron, like many others, invokes Bruce Ames's work as proof that the nation has been deluded about the impact of man-made carcinogens. The assumption is that, if carcinogens exist in natural foods, there's no telling how much of the cancer rate is due to these agents and not to industrial chemicals. According to Efron's view, the U.S. public and government are gripped by the wrong-headed notion that industrial agents are the primary cause of cancer, when in fact nature may have as much or more to do with cancer causation.

This is *not* a necessary interpretation of Bruce Ames's discoveries. First, it is very unlikely that natural plant mutagens directly cause many cancers. That does not mean we need to ignore his findings; on the contrary, they need to be examined more carefully. Second, there is no human justification (though there may be profit-related justification) for being anything *less* than vigilant about regulating the use of chemicals that are known or strongly suspected carcinogens in our air, food, or water supply.

Celery, parsley, figs, fava beans, sassafras, certain mushrooms, parsnips, potatoes, various mustards, horseradish, black pepper, and alfalfa sprouts are on Bruce Ames's list of natural foods that *may* have carcinogenic potential. This would be hard to prove in population studies, and most of them have yet to be shown to cause cancer in laboratory animals (only to damage cell structure). Primarily, the mutagens they contain are "natural pesticides," synthesized by these plants through evolution to defend themselves from insects, fungi, and other threats. According to Ames, a number of the mutagens are probably powerful carcinogens—perhaps more powerful than some man-made pesticides. *However, there is no solid evidence that these foods actually cause any human cancers.*

There is little we can do to control the levels of natural pesticides in plant foods, while there is a lot that can be done to control man-made pesticides, environmental pollutants, and harmful food additives. If the food industry is going to add harmful chemicals to the products we eat, we have a right to expect government regulation to protect us from unwittingly ingesting carcinogens. If they are suspected carcinogens, substitution should be found or safe levels determined. Such is often the case, though recent political agitation against government regulation threatens the safety net that consumers need and deserve.

In the case of natural foods, it makes sense that regulatory action would be a last resort. Before they ban celery, I hope that some pretty convincing experimental evidence of cancer risk is forthcoming. It is also unlikely that the foods Bruce Ames is concerned about are direct causes of cancer; these very foods (along with other fruits and vegetables) contain anticarcinogens that may negate the effects of the mutagens they contain. As one nutritionist remarked: "Natural foods are innocent until proven guilty."

We all tend to believe that there is a balance in nature, but for many scientists such belief is not enough. However, the sophisticated tools of modern biochemical research *are* confirming the idea that natural anticarcinogens—like beta-carotene, vitamin C, vitamin E, and selenium—exist side by side with any naturally occurring carcinogens and nullify their effects. For example, there may be enough vitamin A in parsley to counter any mutagens it may contain. Bruce Ames himself has hypothesized that natural anticarcinogens counter the natural carcinogens, although he believes that more research needs to be done and has not backed away from his position about the mutagenic power of natural pesticides.

Certainly there is no need to panic with regard to the foods cited by Ames. If you eat more foods that are allies and take the nutrients I have recommended (especially A, C, E, and selenium) you will be tipping the balance in your favor and exposure to any plant mutagens will be inconsequential. This may seem imprecise, but the data on carcinogens in these plant foods is itself imprecise.

Besides the foods mentioned by Ames, there are a number of naturally occurring carcinogens cited as cause for concern by the Committee on Diet, Nutrition, and Cancer and other sources. Most of them are not common in the American diet, but take note of those you might ingest.

1. Mushrooms: A group of chemical compounds called hydrazines are found in two different types of mushrooms: *Agaricus bisporus* and *Gyromitra esculenta*, both consumed in many parts of the world. The hydrazines they contain have caused cancers in experimental animals.
2. Coltsfoot and comfrey: Substances called "pyrrolizidine alkaloids" exist in coltsfoot and comfrey, which are sometimes used as herbal teas, and in other plant species. These alkaloids have caused tumors to develop in rats.
3. Cycad nuts: These nuts aren't very common in the U.S. but are eaten in some parts of the world. They contain cycasin, a potent carcinogen in animal tests.
4. Sassafras: Safrole is a component of sassafras tea and "natural" root beer. Some adult rats fed sassafras over a long period developed liver tumors.
5. Estragole: A derivative of plant oil, like safrole, estragole is present in two seasonings—tarragon and anise. Estragole has been found to be a mutagen and caused tumors in mice.
6. Bracken fern: Quercetin, a substance in bracken ferns, a plant food consumed in several parts of the world (especially Japan, although not in the U.S.), is believed to be carcinogenic. High levels of bracken fern in the diet have been directly linked to bladder cancer. If you go to Japan, stay away from bracken fern.

Thankfully, the above-mentioned foods are not staples in the U.S. diet (although the mushrooms are common). You probably won't have to summon up too much willpower to deny yourself these culinary delights.

NITRATES AND NITRITES

Nitrite is a food additive, used primarily in the process of salt-curing meats, such as bacon, ham, hot dogs, sausages, and luncheon meats. It is used—usually as sodium nitrite—to prevent botulism and add coloration (it gives these meats their pinkish color). Nitrite is also found in smoked and salt-pickled foods, as well as some baked goods.

There is contradictory evidence as to whether nitrites are carcinogenic in and of themselves. However, nitrites can combine with amines (by-products of protein metabolism) in the stomach to form compounds called nitrosamines. The evidence about nitrosamines *is* clear; they cause cancer. In laboratory tests, nearly all of three hundred different nitrosamine compounds caused cancer in one or more species.

Nitrosamines are implicated as a major cause of stomach cancer and cancer of the esophagus. There were an estimated 24,800 new cases of stomach cancer in 1988 and 14,400 deaths from this disease. There were about 9,800 people contracting cancer of the esophagus in 1988, and 9,100 deaths. Although scientists can't be sure exactly how many of these cases are caused by nitrite consumption, there is evidence that many are. Studies conducted in South America, Chile, Iran, China, England, and the U.S. (Hawaii) have shown a connection between higher rates of stomach and esophagus cancer and higher levels of nitrites or nitrates in the diet or drinking water.

Sometimes nitrates are used as food additives. Nitrates also occur naturally: they are a component of vegetables such as beets, radishes, celery, lettuce, spinach, and collard greens. Nitrates are generally safe and do not form nitrosamines. The problem with nitrates is that they can be converted into nitrites by bacteria in the digestive tract or by saliva in the mouth. Naturally occurring nitrates are an excellent example of the balance-in-nature concept: Vitamin C can not only prevent the formation of nitrosamines, it may also block the conversion of natural nitrates into nitrites that can become carcinogenic compounds. Vitamin C is present, to some extent, in all these vegetables.

Nitrites, however, are additives in meat products with few "balancing" nutrients built in. We should cut down on our intake of these foods as much as we can. Those of us who are addicted to bacon, hot dogs, sausages, or the like, are the ones who need to reduce our intake the most. An occasional hot dog, or bacon limited to breakfast once a week, should not be of any great consequence and is certainly preferable to constant indulgence.

Here is a list of foods that usually contain nitrites:

hot dogs
bologna

liverwurst
ham
salami
sausages
bacon
smoked chicken
smoked turkey
smoked fish (lox, smoked salmon, kippered salmon)
pickled meats or vegetables

As a simple precaution, cut down on all of these products, and find substitutes when and where you can. You might be able to find nitrite-free bacon, hot dogs, and sausage—probably in health-food stores. Remember that most of the meats high in nitrites are also high in fat and sodium content, so they have three strikes against them.

You may have heard that beer contains nitrosamines. It is true that until five years ago, the process of heat-drying barley produced nitrosamines at unsafe levels. A new process has since been instituted, and the nitrosamines in beer are now down to a very low level considered safe.

Finally, if you eat foods high in nitrites or nitrates and find it hard to cut down, it is especially important to eat foods containing vitamin C and vitamin E, and to take additional supplements I have recommended in Chapter 5, "Foods That Are Allies" (see also Chapter 7). Both C and E help block the formation of nitrosamines in the stomach.

AFLATOXINS

There are a variety of molds and fungi that are suspected of producing carcinogens. The most prominent of these substances are the aflatoxins—highly potent carcinogens produced by a fungus called *Aspergillus flavus.*

Aflatoxins most commonly develop in nuts, grains, seeds, and rice. This occurs only if such foods become moldy. Aflatoxins are very powerful carcinogens in tests with animals, and studies over the last few years have shown a direct relationship between their levels in food and rates of liver cancer in Africa, China, and Southeast Asia.

Primary liver cancer is not very common in the U.S. Still, aflatoxins can pose a threat and should be avoided. Food products that can develop aflatoxins include:

Peanuts and peanut butter
Pecans, pistachios, and almonds
Corn products, such as cornmeal and grits
Cottonseed meal

Vegetable oils and fresh corn are unlikely to contain aflatoxins. Frozen and canned corn should be O.K. The best advice on aflatoxins is to make sure that nuts, grains, and seeds—especially those mentioned—are kept sealed and in a dry place. *Avoid all molding food, but especially molding, damp, or shriveled nuts, grains, or seeds.* Nuts that don't taste fresh and "snap" when eaten should be tossed out. Refrigeration of nuts and nut butters will help prevent molding.

PESTICIDES

Pesticides are commonly present in fresh fruit and vegetables and animal-food products. Great surges of publicity have been devoted to individual chemicals deemed carcinogenic that are present in our food supply. I will clarify the possible effects of these agents and what, if anything, you can do about them.

1. PCBs: PCBs are polychlorinated biphenyls. Industrial contamination of the environment with PCBs has been widespread over the past half century. Awareness of the toxic and cancer-causing effects of PCBs grew slowly, and in 1979 the Environmental Protection Agency suspended their manufacture and use in commerce. The FDA has also established limits for levels allowed in different foods.

PCBs have assimilated easily into our food chain and have concentrated in fish, milk, eggs, and cheese. Scientists have been concerned about PCBs' possible contribution as a tumor promoter—especially in increasing risk of malignant melanoma. The good news is that levels of PCBs in the environment and in the target foods have steadily declined, and are now considered "well below the tolerance level in individual foods."

2. Organochlorine pesticides. There are two classes of very common pesticides that have been studied carefully for possible cancer-causing chemicals—organophosphates (generally found in vegetable and cereal products) and organochlorines (generally found in animal products like meat, poultry, fish, and dairy foods). Of the organophosphates, only parathion has caused cancer consistently in rats. As a class, the organochlorines appear more likely to contain carcinogens. Among the organochlorine pesticides cited by the Committee on Diet, Nutrition, and Cancer as potentially cancer-causing are DDT, kepone, toxaphene, chlordane, heptachlor, lindane, and hexachlorobenzene.

As with PCBs the organochlorine pesticides are found mainly in animal foods that are high-fat. Although these pesticides are probably not major causes of human cancer, their presence is simply another reason to cut back on high-fat foods. Because there may also be pesticide residues on fresh fruits and vegetables, it is a good idea to seek out in health-food stores organically grown natural produce, cultivated without pesticides. For information about pesticides—in your food or environment—call the EPA's pesticide hotline: 1-800-858-7378.

FOOD ADDITIVES

Food additives are usually chemical substances added to food in order to preserve freshness, improve taste, retain nutrient value, and add color or thickness. Almost three thousand different substances are now being used as food additives, but, for complex reasons, only about five hundred have been defined as such and are therefore subject to regulation.

Under the FDA's Delaney clause, known carcinogens must be banned from food or their safe levels must be determined. A few carcinogenic additives have been banned under this clause, though curiously a number of others have not. Furthermore, thousands of additives have been classified "Generally Recognized as Safe" (GRAS), and are not even subject to the Delaney clause. Some of these GRAS substances have yet to be properly tested for carcinogenicity.

According to the Committee on Diet, Nutrition, and Cancer, the FDA having recognized "the need to acquire better data and to standardize testing procedures and the criteria for acceptability . . . has recently initiated a review of direct Food Additives." The FDA commissioned a panel of scientists from the Federation of American Societies for Experimental Biology to conduct an ongoing review of food additives. The safety, or lack of it, of many GRAS substances has now been established. However, the safety of others is still unclear. Of course, this review is welcome; we can only hope for more testing, tighter regulations of potentially harmful additives, and outright barring of carcinogenic substances. But take note: nitrites and saccharin, two substances shown to be carcinogenic in animals and suspected of some potential carcinogenicity in humans, are still on the GRAS list. They're not even subject to the Delaney clause.

This means that once again it is up to us to be aware of what's in our food and avoid, if we can, questionable additives. It doesn't mean we should become worry warts, *only label readers.* I would like to note again that laboratory tests with animals involve very high levels of additives—more than most humans would typically consume. Therefore, additives that cause cancer in rats and mice may not play a direct role in human cancers. Nevertheless, many should be deemed unsafe. The following chart can be your guide to food additives which, *based on animal studies,* are (or may be) carcinogenic and should be avoided. A few have been banned, but most have not.

FOOD ADDITIVES AND CONTAMINANTS: SUSPECTED OR PROVEN CARCINOGENS

Agent	Diet Source	Tumor Site
Intentional Additives		
Cyclamates	Sweetener	Bladder
Saccharin	Sweetener	Bladder
Dulcin (p-phenethylurea)	Sweetener	Bladder, liver
Xylitol	Sweetener	Bladder
Sucrose	Sweetener	Liver
Safrole	Flavoring agent	Liver
Oil of calamus	Flavoring agent	Small intestine
Cinnamyl anthranilate	Flavoring agent	Liver, kidney, pancreas
Diethylpyrocarbonate	Preservative	Lung
8-Hydroxyquinoline	Preservative	Multiple sites
Thioacetamide	Seed grain mordant	Liver
BHT (butylated hydroxytoluene)	Preservative	Liver (promoter)
Trichloroethylene	Extractant	Liver
Carrageenin	Emulsifier	Sarcomas
Myrj 45 (polyoxyethylene monostearate)	Antistaling agent	Bladder
Tannic acid	Wine, fruits	Liver
Tween-60 (sorbitan monostearate)	Antibloom agent in chocolates	Skin (also promoter)
Carboxymethylcellulose	Ice-cream stabilizer	Subcutaneous tissue
Unintentional Additives		
Polyvinyl chloride	Packaging material	Several sites
Acrylonitrile	Packaging material	Forestomach Nervous system
DES (diethylstilbestrol)	Animal drug residue	Multiple sites
Various organochloride pesticides	Residue in diet	Liver
Parathion	Residues in diet	Adrenals
PAHs (polycyclic aromatic hydrocarbons, e.g., benzo[a]pyrene)	Air pollution, charcoal broiling	Several sites
PCBs (polychlorinated biphenyls)	Freshwater fish, packaging materials	Liver
Cycads and cycasin	Cycad nuts	Liver, kidney, intestines
Aflatoxin	Milk, mold in cereals, peanuts, and corn	Liver, stomach, kidneys
Nitrosamines	Nitrite and amines in foods	Several sites
Tannins	Tea, wine	Liver, sarcomas

Agent	Diet Source	Tumor Site
Bracken Fern	Fern species	Bladder
Pyrrolizidine alkaloids	Herbal medicine, teas, and food plants	Liver
Patulin	Mold in apple juice	Local sarcomas

Chart derived from NAS Committee on Diet, Nutrition, and Cancer report: "Diet, Nutrition, and Cancer," 1982, pp. 226–27. Most findings cited as references from the International Agency for Research on Cancer.

Over the last seventy years, a handful of dangerous food dyes have been banned, and many are no longer being produced. Nevertheless, a number of food, drug, and cosmetic dyes that are potentially toxic and/or carcinogenic have not been regulated and should be avoided. In 1984, this list included Red Nos. 3, 8, 9, 19, and 37, and Orange No. 17. The FDA dragged its feet (with pressure from the food industry) on regulating these six colorings, which are all suspected of cancer-causing capabilities. In fact, the FDA appointed a panel in 1985 to make a final decision on these particular dyes after *twenty-five years of study and twenty-seven extensions of the deadline.* Finally, within the last two years, the FDA has taken action: Red 37, Red 8, Red 9, Orange 17, and Red 19 can no longer be used in any products.

Such food colorings are most commonly found in soft drinks, candy and confections, baked goods, gelatins, ice cream, dessert powders, maraschino cherries, and many other snack foods. While we wait for final word from the FDA, consider it advisable to watch for and avoid the suspect food, drug, and cosmetic colorings (by reading labels). Once again, our knowledge of how to translate laboratory findings tells us not to worry that our children will get cancer from the cherries atop their ice-cream sundaes. Simply stated, we should try not to overindulge in additive-laden snack foods. Refrain from using over-the-counter drugs and cosmetics that list the worrisome dyes. For your guidance, here is a list of dyes still being used that are proven or suspected carcinogens, to look for and avoid:

Dye	Uses
Red No. 3	Food and drugs (candy, desserts, baked goods)
Yellow No. 5	Food, drugs, and cosmetics (pet food, beverages, baked goods)
Yellow No. 6	Predominantly food (beverages, candy, desserts)
Red No. 8*	Ingested drugs and cosmetics
Red No. 9*	Ingested drugs and cosmetics
Red No. 33	Ingested drugs and cosmetics
Orange No. 17*	Drugs and cosmetics
Red No. 19*	Drugs and cosmetics

Dye	Uses
Red No. 36	Drugs and cosmetics
Red No. 40	Beverages, candy, desserts, pet food
Blue No. 1	Beverages, candy, baked goods, drugs, cosmetics
Blue No. 2	Pet foods, candy, beverages, drugs
Green No. 3	Beverages, candy

Chart derived from "Public Citizen Health Research Group Report" to the FDA, December 17, 1984.
*Banned only for use in all products as of July, 1988.

The problem of saccharin underlines the sometimes curious regulating decisions of the FDA. A ban was proposed in 1977 after many laboratory experiments in which rats given fairly large doses of saccharin developed bladder tumors. Large population studies and studies of bladder-cancer patients have been inconclusive, though a few have demonstrated a small increased risk associated with saccharin use. A study by the NCI involving over 3,000 bladder-cancer patients and almost 6,000 population controls showed no association except among white nonsmoking women, whose risk of bladder cancer was elevated after heavy indulgence in saccharin-containing products.

Saccharin was never banned, and in 1985 the AMA's Council on Scientific Affairs announced that it is safe for humans. They did not, however, "condone" its use, and they urged careful consideration of use by pregnant women and children.

Cyclamates, on the other hand, were a class of artificial sweeteners that *were* banned in 1969. There were no adequate population studies conducted because, when cyclamates were commonly used, they were rarely consumed in products that didn't also contain saccharin. Although some laboratory studies have shown cyclamates to be carcinogenic, there is stronger experimental evidence that saccharin is carcinogenic. Why then is saccharin allowed and cyclamates banned?

All told, the risk of contracting bladder cancer from saccharin use is estimated to be extremely small. Nonetheless, I recommend that you avoid *heavy* intake of diet foods and soft drinks containing saccharin. The use of saccharin by children and adolescents is discouraged because the longer one is exposed, and the greater the exposure, the higher the risk. Pregnant women should not ingest saccharin because the risk to the fetus is unknown. Don't worry if you've eaten diet foods containing saccharin or have had a weakness for saccharin-sweetened sodas. The additional risk is minor, but try not to indulge any long-term, heavy intake from now on.

An alternative to saccharin sweetener is *aspartame*, which now has the commercial moniker Nutrasweet. Aspartame has begun to take possession of the most-used-artificial-sweetener-in-soft-drinks title.* For a period of time, combinations of saccharin and aspartame were used in soft drinks (they still are), though currently aspartame alone is more common (the labels read: "100% Nutrasweet"). Other products, including chewing gums, cereals, noncarbonated drinks, puddings, gelatins, and other desserts are using Nutrasweet. The list lengthens daily. Sugar substitutes are being marketed (brand name, Equal).

Aspartame itself is a type of compound of the amino acids, phenylalanine and aspartic acid. Many studies have been conducted testing aspartame to determine if it has carcinogenic properties. It came up clean in a range of studies except one, in which there appeared to be an increase in the number of brain tumors in rats fed large doses of aspartame. Follow-up studies have not shown these same results, so the FDA has declared that aspartame is not carcinogenic in animals. All told, experimental evidence points to aspartame (Nutrasweet) as a reasonable alternative to saccharin, for which the evidence for carcinogenicity is stronger. (However, strong evidence does not exist for the carcinogenic effects of either sweetener.) Aspartame also tastes better. Nevertheless, it is a good idea to limit your intake of aspartame, since there are still unanswered questions. An ongoing debate rages as to whether aspartame has any neurological side effects, such as headaches or seizures. The aspartame issue has yet to be completely resolved.

Preservatives are commonly used to keep boxed and canned foods fresh; you're likely familiar with them as multisyllabic chemical names on food labels. Two of the most common are antioxidants, BHA (butylated hydroxyanisole) and BHT (butylated hydroxytoluene). Some studies suggest that they can cause cancer; others indicate they inhibit cancer through their antioxidant powers. The jury is still out on these two. Propyl gallate is another preservative, which, though poorly studied, may increase cancer risk.

A SPECIAL NOTE ABOUT IRON

It has long been known that certain minerals can *cause* cancer. Arsenic, lead, nickel, and cadmium are trace minerals that may occur in foods, though at levels deemed unlikely to be carcinogenic. Exposure to these minerals occupationally or in the environment is more likely to be hazardous.

Iron, however, is a mineral we need and ingest in large quantities.

*As of this writing, a new artificial sweetener has joined the pack. The FDA has approved acesulfane K (brand name: Sunette) for use in dry foods or as powder. Once again, confusion reigns: While most studies have cleared acesulfane K of carcinogenicity, a few have not. (The FDA claims them to be defective.) Keep a media watch for more information.

In and of itself, iron is not carcinogenic. Iron is clearly required for the synthesis of hemoglobin, the substance inside red blood cells that transports oxygen. Our immune systems may suffer if we are subjected to severe iron deficiency.

On the other hand, recent studies have turned up preliminary evidence that excess iron in our bodies may be a common condition, and that this excess can seriously hinder our immune systems—perhaps leaving us more vulnerable to infection and cancer.

It has been known for years that bacteria require iron to survive. It has recently been established that cancer cells also gobble up iron in order to live and reproduce. In a recent review, Dr. Eugene Weinberg of Indiana University amassed a voluminous body of research by immunologists, all of which points to a series of cagy and complex maneuvers by the immune system to withhold iron from bacteria and cancer cells, hence starving them of their lifeline. According to Weinberg, iron seems to function as a coveted prize in the war between the host's defenses and the foreign invaders trying to stake their claim; the side that is able to retain more iron in its coffers may tip the balance in its favor.

Excess iron not only is a source of sustenance to bacteria and malignant cells; it also detracts from the smooth operation of the immune system. Dr. Maria de Sousa, in her research at the Sloan-Kettering Institute in New York, has been able to show that key immune cells— the lymphocytes—may get "stuck" in iron-rich sites in the body, taking them out of circulation. These lymphocytes are needed to eliminate bacteria or cancer cells as they appear. When the lymphocytes are out of service, the body is left more vulnerable to infections and tumor growth.

Old red blood cells are broken down in the spleen in order to have their iron recycled. In instances of iron overload, the spleen is often the first place traveling lymphocytes get trapped. Sometimes they will start to proliferate abnormally, followed by the malignant changes in splenic macrophages that lead directly to Hodgkin's disease.

Hodgkin's disease is only the most glaring example. People whose systems are overloaded with iron (a more common condition than anyone ever suspected) could be at higher risk of contracting leukemias, lymphomas, some solid tumors, and perhaps immunodeficiency diseases.

The research is still early, but it is time to reconsider our iron intake. Most of us get enough iron from the meat and vegetables we eat. Shellfish, whole-grain cereals, dried beans, apricots, prunes, and raisins are good sources of iron. Iron deficiency is far less common than we have been led to believe. If you are tired, don't simply assume that you are anemic owing to iron deficiency. Consult your doctor and find out if you really are anemic before taking any iron supplement. Menstruating women may suffer iron loss, but check with your doctor before taking iron for this or any other reason.

Iron as a supplement has been vastly oversold. Because of its possible deleterious effects, I don't recommend additional iron unless it has been prescribed by your doctor for a specific purpose. I have reported the early results of this potentially groundbreaking research not to frighten but to give you the opportunity to make an informed decision about iron.

THE COFFEE QUESTION

In the last few years, coffee has joined the company of other guilty pleasures under the harsh light of interrogation about carcinogenicity.

Studies of the possible cancer-causing effects of coffee have not been conclusive. The link between coffee consumption and bladder cancer is not strong. Several studies have linked coffee drinking to greater risk of pancreatic cancer, while some others have not. One such study indicated that there is no increased risk if you consume up to eight cups a day; more than that and your risk for pancreatic cancer goes up. In the laboratory, extremely high doses of caffeine were found to be mutagenic, which is not sufficient to call it a carcinogen.

Caffeine, which is contained in coffee, tea, chocolate, and many sodas, may or may not be a culprit in the coffee question. It certainly is hazardous to our cardiovascular and nervous systems. Caffeine also contributes to fibrocystic disease. Many women with benign breast lumps who have gone off their caffeine regimes (stopped drinking coffee, tea, sodas, and eating chocolate) have enjoyed a complete reversal of their condition. There is no known link, however, between caffeine and breast cancer.

Teas contain not only caffeine but tannins as well. Tannins are present in many plants, and they have been proven to be mutagenic. There still is no real evidence that tannins cause cancer. It is known that milk added to tea will bind tannins in such a way as to prevent their harmful effects. Add some milk as a safety precaution, if you consume large quantities of tea.

Decaffeinated coffee presents a special problem. The process for removal of caffeine may include methylene chloride, a proven carcinogen. The solution is simple: a number of major brands of coffee advertise the fact that they do not use chemicals to decaffeinate. Make sure to select those brands.

To prevent any possible increase in your risk of pancreatic or bladder cancer, I recommend that you keep your coffee intake relatively low. Don't drink more than four cups a day if you can help it, stick to one or two a day if you can, and substitute water-decaffeinated coffee,

Postum or herb tea (avoid the herbs mentioned on page 108) if you don't think you'll suffer from daytime somnambulism as a result of stopping altogether.

COOKING PRACTICES

The next chapter will detail the proper storage, preparation, and cooking of plant foods and focus on how to retain vital nutrients. However, advice on cooking methods for animal food products is appropriate here because the wrong kind of cooking can turn foods that are allies into enemies, and can turn foods that are already enemies into even worse enemies.

Charcoal broiling or barbecuing of meats—whether over a wood or charcoal broiler—often picks up polycyclic aromatic hydrocarbons (PAHs) from the smoke caused by fat dripping onto hot coals or a wood fire. Among the PAHs is benzo(a)pyrene, a very potent carcinogen akin to the tar in cigarette smoke. By one estimate, *eating a charcoal-broiled steak may expose us to the same quantity of PAHs as we would receive from smoking six hundred cigarettes.*

Smoked foods—including bacon, ham, turkey, fishes, and cheeses— also contain PAHs, picked up during the smoking process. These smoked products may also contain nitrites, and therefore should be avoided for two very compelling reasons.

Protein foods undergo "pyrolysis" when cooking. Frying, flat grilling, and broiling meats, poultry, and fish at very high temperatures produce pyrolosins that are mutagenic: they can cause damage to cellular DNA. The more burned or even browned these foods are, the more mutagens they contain.

The browning and burning of starchy foods, including french fries, baked and cereal products, and even toasted bread can produce mutagens. There is no evidence to suggest that we should stop eating these foods, but there is good reason to avoid overbrowning or burning them.

Here are my basic cancer-preventive cooking guidelines:

- Boil, poach, or steam protein foods when possible.
- Baking and roasting are better cooking methods than broiling or frying.
- Microwave cooking is an acceptable method.
- If you do broil or fry meats or other proteins, don't brown them excessively or burn them.
- Avoid charcoal broiling and barbecuing.

If you do charcoal broil or barbecue, wrap the meat in foil (though you won't get the charcoal flavor) and/or keep the grilling temperature low and the meat as far from the heat source as possible, reducing exposure of the food to flames and smoke. Barbecue sauce dripping onto coals may also increase smoke; avoid this when possible.

I have given you a great deal of information on the foods that are your allies and foods that are your enemies. For many of us, shifting the balance toward allies and away from enemies requires a monumental change in our eating habits. In the next two chapters, I will try to help you effect such a change. Below is a summary of our food enemies.

FOOD ENEMIES AND COOKING PRACTICES TO BE AVOIDED

- Lower the percentage of fats in your diet to 30 percent or less. See methods recommended in this and the next two chapters.
- Cut down on saturated and polyunsaturated fats and oils; preferably use olive oil, a monounsaturate.
- Avoid the plant foods I've listed on page 108, cited by the Committee on Diet, Nutrition, and Cancer, and other sources, as potential carcinogens.
- Reduce or eliminate smoked and pickled foods (hot dogs, bacon, luncheon meats, smoked fish and poultry, etc.) that contain nitrates or nitrites.
- Make sure that nuts, grains, and seeds are properly stored to prevent molds from forming; you'll be avoiding exposure to carcinogenic aflatoxins.
- Seek out organically grown natural foods (fruits and vegetables), from health-food stores or elsewhere, to reduce exposure to produce contaminated with pesticides.
- Be a label reader for the food additives and dyes I have listed in this chapter as carcinogenic. Avoid products that contain them to the greatest extent possible.
- Cut down on diet foods and sodas containing saccharin.
- Don't take iron supplements unless specifically recommended to do so by your doctor.
- If you drink a lot of coffee, reduce your intake to one or two cups a day. Avoid decaffeinated coffees, except those that use a nonchemical process to decaffeinate.
- Don't fry or broil as much—steaming and boiling are best; roasting and baking are better; microwaving is acceptable.
- Don't overly brown or burn meats and fish or starchy foods when you cook, regardless of the method. Stop charcoal broiling and barbecuing!

7

The Cancer-Prevention Diet Guide (CPDG)

The Cancer-Prevention Diet Guide is really quite simple. And it's more than cancer preventive—it's a way of eating that's health-promoting in every possible way. Its physical rewards span a wide range from stronger bones and teeth and better skin to heightened immunity to many diseases. The psychological rewards are a sense of well-being stemming from improved physical health and a sense of security from the knowledge that one's risk of cancer is lowered.

It's sound for children as well as adults (except for the vitamin/mineral recommendations, which are for adults only), and the sooner you can get your children used to this style of eating, the better their chances will be for a healthy and cancer-free later life. I have purposely made the diet guidelines into a short, separate chapter so that you can see them at a glance. I've also repeated the heart of the guide, the Cancer-Prevention Daily Diet, in Appendix 5 so that you can cut it out of the book and attach it to your refrigerator or bulletin board for easy reference.

Remember that these guidelines differ from heart diets in that polyunsaturated fats (mainly vegetable oils) are not encouraged. Any fats in excess of 30 percent of your daily calorie intake are to be avoided, and as much as possible, the fat in your diet should come from *monounsaturated* oils or fats.

I am referring to the Cancer-Prevention Diet as a "guide" because it is not a rigid set of rules or a highly specific regime. If you do your best to stay within the guidelines, you will receive many health benefits and be lowering significantly your risk of many types of cancer. But you need not stick to them as if they were the ten commandments, except during the first few weeks after you begin. This period of adjustment is necessary for the process of change to take hold. After that, if you slip by having bacon, fatty meats, or rich pies *on rare occasions,* just be sure you're getting enough "allies" to offset them and keep within the guidelines as a general rule.

The Cancer-Prevention Diet Guide is your ticket to freedom. By staying within its structure, you are freeing yourself from excess fear of cancer, and you are free to vary your diet so that you're not in culinary prison. I'm purposely providing clear parameters but not confining you to a limited menu that will drive you crazy and invite abandonment.

THE GENERAL RULES

Eat More of the Following

- Whole grain foods (breads, cereals, etc.)
- Fresh fruits and vegetables (especially salads that combine high A and C foods)
- Complex carbohydrates (grains and cereals, fruits and vegetables)

Low-fat foods

- Low-fat dairy or skim-milk products
    Skim or low-fat milk
    Low-fat cheeses
    Low-fat yogurts
- Chicken (without skin)
- Fish and shellfish (fresh and water-packed)
- Lean beef, veal, and lamb
- Fruits, vegetables, peas, and beans
- Grains and cereals, breads and pastas

High-fiber, low-fat foods

- Whole-grain products
    Bran cereals, whole-wheat or grain cereals, shredded wheat, oatmeal
    Whole-wheat or rye crackers
    Pumpernickel, rye, or whole-wheat breads and rolls
    Bran muffins
    Baked goods, pastas, or pancakes with whole-grain flours
    Grain foods including barley, brown rice, buckwheat, millet, oats, rye, and whole wheat.
- Vegetables
    Carrots, broccoli, corn, Brussels sprouts, potatoes (sweet and

white), cabbage, celery, green peas and beans, parsnips, kale, turnips, spinach, cauliflower
- Peas and beans
  Kidney, white, navy, lima, and black beans
  Lentils and split peas
- Fruits
  Apples, apricots, pears, bananas, berries of all kinds, grapefruit, oranges, cantaloupes, pineapples, prunes, raisins

Eat Less of the Following

- Baked goods
- Coffee and sodas
- Sugary foods, snacks
- Any foods with high salt content
- Alcohol

High-fat foods

- Whole-milk products
  Full-fat hard and soft cheeses
  Butter and butterfat
  Cream products (sweet, sour, and whipped)
  Ice creams
- Duck, goose
- Fried fish, oil-packed canned fishes (i.e., tuna, sardines)
- Pork, beef, veal, and lamb with excess visible fat (marbling)
- Nuts, peanut and other nut butters
- Pies, pastries, cakes, cookies, potato chips, crackers (refined flour), puddings, chocolate desserts

Low-fiber foods

- Baked goods, snacks, and starches from refined flours
  White breads
  Breads, biscuits, muffins, and croissants (white, refined flours)
  Most crackers, cookies, chips, cakes, pies, and pastries

Exclude Altogether if You Possibly Can

- Charcoal-broiled and barbecued meats
- Hot dogs, sausages, and bacon
- Smoked, salt-cured, or pickled meats, poultry, and fishes

• Snacks with many food additives and preservatives (see Chapter 6, "Foods That Are Enemies," for additives to avoid)

Remember the Four-Star Foods

Include at least one daily. These fruits and vegetables are high in fiber, vitamin A (often as beta-carotene), *and* vitamin C. Many of them also include vitamin E, selenium, and indoles, so you can kill many birds with one stone. Find which ones you like best and prepare them every which way you can (without much butter or margarine). Here they are:

Asparagus
Broccoli
Brussels sprouts
Cabbage
Carrots
Cauliflower
Dark-green, leafy vegetables
Cantaloupe
Green pepper
Kale
Red pepper
Spinach
Strawberries
Sweet potatoes
Tomatoes
Winter squash

THE CANCER-PREVENTION DAILY DIET

Meats, Fish, and Other Proteins

2 servings per day

Select Often	Select Occasionally	Select Rarely
Poultry	Lean Beef	Pork
Fish	Veal	Ham
Beans	Lamb	Fatty Meats
Tofu	Eggs	Hard Cheeses

Vegetables

3 servings per day
  1 from high vitamin C group
  1 from high vitamin A group
  1 from moderate/high-fiber group (between 1–4+ grams per serving)

The following checklist tells you which vegetables are from the high vitamin A, C, and fiber categories. Many that are high in one category and not checked in others may still provide those other nutrients. Brussel sprouts, for example, while high in C and not checked as high in A, do contain a fair amount of vitamin A. I am guiding you toward those foods richest in each specific anticancer nutrient to assure you of optimal intake. This also holds true for the fruit checklist that follows.

VEGETABLE	HIGH VITAMIN C	HIGH VITAMIN A	MODERATE/ HIGH FIBER
Asparagus	✓	✓	✓
Beets			✓
Broccoli	✓	✓	✓
Brussels sprouts	✓		✓
Cabbage	✓		✓
Carrots		✓	
Cauliflower	✓		
Corn			✓
Dark, leafy greens			
beets	✓	✓	
chard		✓	
collard	✓	✓	
dandelion		✓	
kale	✓	✓	✓
kohlrabi	✓		
mustard	✓	✓	
parsley		✓	
romaine lettuce		✓	
spinach	✓	✓	✓
turnip	✓	✓	✓
watercress	✓	✓	
Eggplant			✓
Endive		✓	
Green beans			✓
Green pepper	✓		
Peas	✓		✓

VEGETABLE	HIGH VITAMIN C	HIGH VITAMIN A	MODERATE/ HIGH FIBER
Red pepper	√	√	
Sweet potatoes	√	√	
Tomatoes	√	√	
Winter squash		√	√

Note: You can substitute one portion of high-fiber beans, either fresh or dried (green, lima, kidney, soybeans, or white beans; chick peas or lentils) for the one high-fiber vegetable.

Fruits

2 servings per day
   1 from high vitamin C group
   1 from moderate/high fiber group (1–4+ grams per serving)

FRUIT	HIGH VITAMIN C	MODERATE/HIGH FIBER
Apples		√
Apricots (fresh or dried)		√
Avocados	√	
Blackberries		√
Cantaloupe	√	√
Cranberries		√
Grapefruit	√	
Honeydew		√
Lemons	√	
Limes	√	
Oranges	√	
Papayas	√	
Pears		√
Pineapple	√	
Prunes, dried		√
Raspberries	√	√
Strawberries	√	√
Tangerines	√	
Watermelon		√

Whole Grain Foods*

2 servings per day (or as many as needed to reach 30–40 grams of fiber per day)

Choose from the following groups.

CEREALS†:
Bran cereals
Whole wheat or grain cereals
Shredded wheat
Oatmeal

GRAIN FOODS:
Barley
Brown rice
Buckwheat
Millet
Oats
Rye
Whole wheat

WHOLE GRAIN BAKED GOODS:
Whole wheat or rye crackers
Brown, rye, or whole wheat breads
Bran muffins

*See p. 87 for fiber content of various foods.
†See p. 84 for fiber content of breakfast cereals.

Dairy

1–2 servings per day
Any low-fat or skim-milk product, cheese, or yogurt

DAILY SUPPLEMENT LIST

System 1: Ideal

Take in the A.M.:

Vitamin A	10,000 IU and 15 mg. beta-carotene
Vitamin B	B-complex pill (high B50 or B100)
Vitamin C	2–5 grams (2,000–5,000 mg.)*
Vitamin E	200–600 IU
Selenium	100–200 mcg.
Calcium	800–1200 mg.
Magnesium	400–600 mg.
Zinc	25 mg.
Copper	3 mg.

Use a multivitamin/multimineral pill, or antioxidant combination, if you prefer to take fewer pills. Try to avoid those that contain iron. (See section on iron in Chapter 6, "Foods That Are Enemies.")

*Divide doses of C as needed and take additional quantities in the P.M.

System 2: Good

In the A.M.: Take an antioxidant combination that includes beta-carotene, C, E, selenium, and zinc. Back this up with a super B-complex, one or more grams of C, and additional E. (That brings you down to 4+ pills in the morning, depending on how much extra C you take.)

In the P.M.: Take the additional C you need to meet your daily requirement. Divided doses can be taken at noon and after dinner.

System 3: Okay

In the A.M.: Take an antioxidant combination with a B-complex pill and a gram of C. This keeps you down to 3 pills in the morning.

In the P.M.: Take the additional C you need to meet your daily requirement in one or more additional doses when most convenient.

For all three systems, let the contents of your antioxidant pill be your guide. Check the values of A, C, E, selenium, and zinc it contains against my ideal recommendations and see how well it fares. Shore up this pill with B, C, or E according to Systems 2 or 3. Try to include calcium and magnesium, zinc and copper. *Watch that your total values don't exceed my recommendations in System 1.* Of course, if you can hack it, System 1 is ideal; come as close to it as you can within your pill-taking capabilities.

SPECIAL RECOMMENDATIONS FOR:

Smokers and Drinkers

Extra vitamin A and C-rich foods
Add another 15 mg. beta-carotene supplements
Choose amount of vitamin C from high end of recommendation: 4–5
  grams

Suntanners

(Whenever you tan, or as a rule if you tan regularly.)

Extra beta-carotene rich foods
Add 15 mg. more beta-carotene
Take vitamin E from high end of recommendation (600 IU)

When You Eat Foods with Nitrites

Extra vitamin C and E-rich foods
Choose amount of vitamin C from high end of recommendation: 4–5
   grams
Take vitamin E from high end of recommedation (600 IU)

When You Are Exposed to Chemical Carcinogens

(In industrial or home settings—see Chapters 15 and 16 for
   examples)

Extra vitamin A, C, and E-rich foods
Add 15 mg. more beta-carotene supplements
Choose amount of vitamin C from high end of recommendations:
   4–5 grams
Take vitamin E from high end of recommendation (600 IU)

MORE TIPS ON FAT-CUTTING

A food with 2.5 grams of fat per serving is considered low; more than
10 grams is considered high.
   To figure your daily fat intake:

1. Estimate your average daily calorie intake; use a calorie counter.
2. Add together the grams of fat from each food you eat in a day (see
    Appendix 1 for grams of fat per serving for many foods; for others,
    check labels).
3. Multiply the number of fat grams by 9 and then divide by your total
    calorie intake. This will tell you the percentage of daily calories
    coming from fat. This will tell you how many grams of fat you must
    eliminate—to reach 30 percent or less.

Dairy Products

Skim-milk products are preferable to low-fat milk products, and low-fat products are preferable to whole-milk products. Items marked "low-fat" are therefore the viable middle ground for those who don't like skim-milk foods.

Most hard and many soft cheeses are high in fat content. Cottage cheese isn't bad (low-fat cottage cheese is better). Part-skim cheeses are often very good—especially part-skim mozzarella.

Even skim or part-skim cheeses have a fairly high percentage of their calories coming from fat. Cottage cheese, both large curd and small curd, may be low in calories but it does have a moderate fat content. Low-fat cottage cheese is best. Here are some high-fat cheeses to worry about, and some alternative brand-name low-fat cheeses, for those of you who love cheese and don't want to give it up:

High-Fat Cheeses
American cheese
Blue cheese
Brie
Camembert
Cheddar
Cream cheese
Jack
Mozzarella (whole milk)
Provolone
Swiss

*Brand-Name, Low-Fat Alternatives**

CHEDDARS
Olympia low fat
Kiel Kase
Heidi Amm low-fat Cheddar
Green River part skim

CREAM CHEESES
Lite cream cheese
Neufchatel

*Low-fat cheese list derived from suggestions by William E. Connor and Sonja Connor, in *Medical Self-Care*, January–February 1987.

MOZZARELLAS
Mini Chol imitation mozzarella
Hickory Farms Lite
Part-skim mozzarella (check package: some are not very low-fat)

SOY-BASED CHEESES
Soyarella
Tofu mozzarella
Soya Kaas

PROCESSED CHEESES
Lite Line
Lite n' Lively Cheese Slices

ALL VARIETIES LOW-FAT OR SKIM COTTAGE CHEESE

Low-fat yogurt has about one-half the fat of regular (whole-milk) yogurt. The low-fat variety comes in all sorts of flavors and brands and can be used creatively. Some brands have no-fat yogurt, which are the best of all.

Spreads and Salad Dressings

Use as little of the saturated fats (butter, animal fats, lard, shortenings, palm and coconut oil), and polyunsaturated oils (vegetable oils like corn, safflower, etc.) as possible. When you need to use oil, choose the monounsaturated variety. Olive oil is the most monounsaturated, and peanut oil is second. Remember that low-fat yogurt goes a long way—with spices and a bit of lemon juice—toward making excellent salad dressings and dips. Try to stay away from regular mayonnaise. Reserve butter for a small dab on bread, potatoes, pasta, and vegetables. And even here yogurt or olive oil can often be substituted.

Chicken and Fish

Chicken and fish are less fatty than red meat (beef, lamb, and pork). Fish is perhaps the best low-fat animal source of protein (with lots of additional nutrient factors). Even the fattier fishes are O.K.; studies show that fish oils can help prevent heart disease. The white meat of chicken is less fatty than the dark, but you should remove the skin, the fattiest part of the chicken. Veal has less fat than beef and pork and is therefore the meat of choice.

Beans (lima, kidney, navy, white, garbanzo, etc.), and tofu (soybean curd) are good sources of protein and alternatives to meat, fish, and poultry. Most of them have a low to moderate fat content, and are high in fiber to boot. Nuts are high in unsaturated fats; but they are still a good source of protein and other nutrients. Although they shouldn't be overeaten, owing to their fat content, they are recommended in moderate amounts; only fresh, sweet-tasting, unsalted nuts should be selected.

The best (low-fat) fishes are:

Shellfish: lobster, crabs, scallops, clams, and oysters. Shrimp is also low in fat. (Like many shellfish, shrimp was once considered high in cholesterol. Recent studies have changed this view, and shellfish probably contain factors that inhibit cholesterol absorption.)
Bass, cod, flounder, fillet of sole, haddock, perch, halibut.

Higher-fat fishes (though still not as high as the fattier red meats) are:

bluefish, salmon, sardines (canned in water, not oil), herring, anchovies, whitefish, mackerel.

You needn't avoid the fattier fishes as you should avoid red meats. Fish oils have health-giving properties and play a role in preventing heart disease.* Moderation is the key. But don't fry fish. Oils or heavy batter turns your low-fat meal into a greasy high-fat meal. Bake, broil, or sauté in very little oil.

SHOPPING FOR MEATS

When you do buy red meats, choose those with the least fat, and look for excess "marbling"—the fat layers tucked between the muscles. Veal is the least-fatty red meat. As cuts, London broil, flank steak, and round roasts are less fatty than T-bone steaks, ribs, and rib roasts. Buy hamburger or other meats marked "lean" or "select." Before cooking, trim any chunks of fat off the steaks, chops, or roasts. Bypass altogether the supermarket aisle that has bacon, sausage, salami, hot dogs, and salt-cured luncheon meats, which are not only high in fat but high in salt and nitrites as well. Most sliced ham has slightly less fat. If you need a lunch-meat substitute use sliced turkey, chicken, lean roast beef, and water-packed tuna as much as you can.

---

*A recent Harvard Medical School study showed that in rats fish oils may slow the spread of tumor and growth. More research is needed to find out whether such effects occur in humans.

STARCHES

Starches are complex carbohydrates derived from plant foods like grains, beans, and peas. They can be one of the pleasures of a low-fat diet. Potatoes, whole-grain breads and cereals, brown rice, and pastas are complex carbohydrates that are reasonable sources of fiber and vitamins. *They are excellent foods unless soaked with butter or rich gravies.* The more-refined starches (i.e., white bread as opposed to whole wheat, white rice as opposed to brown) have less protein, vitamins, minerals, and fiber than whole-grain products. Remember this as you shop for complex carbohydrates.

LOW-FAT DESSERTS

Store-bought low-fat sweets, cakes, puddings, and frozen treats are now fairly easy to come by. Check your labels. When baking your own, use low-fat milk products, and as little butter and shortening as possible. Avoid products that list hydrogenated fats.

Low-fat ice-cream substitutes can fulfill that craving for sweet-cold. Sherbets and ices are no-fat alternatives. Still high in calories from sugar, ice milk is usually low-fat and moderate in calories and there are many excellent brands now on the market. Frozen low-fat yogurt is tasty and preferable to ice cream. Some of the best low-fat icy treats are the wide variety of "fruit bars" now being marketed. They usually have little or no fat content, are reasonable in calories, and taste great. Watch out for Tofutti—some of these products are actually high fat, while others, marketed as "extra-light," are very low fat. After cultivating a taste for one or many of these ice-cream alternatives, you may find that they digest more easily and are more truly refreshing (especially on a hot day) than thick scoops of heavy ice cream.

TIPS ON FIBER

Whole-grain cereals are among the best sources of fiber, but you can't always tell from the advertising on the box which ones actually have a high-fiber content. Refer to page 84 in "Foods That Are Allies" for a complete list of breakfast cereals and their fiber content. For quick reference, here is a list of the high-fiber cereals (4 grams or more):

High-Fiber Breakfast Cereals

Cereal and Grams of Fiber per 1-Oz. Serving

12 GRAMS
Fiber One (General Mills)

9 GRAMS
All-Bran (Kellogg)

5 GRAMS
Post Natural Bran Flakes
Quaker Corn Bran
Bran Chex (Ralston Purina)

4 GRAMS
Nabisco Shredded Wheat 'N Bran
Familia Swiss Birchermuesli (Biofamilia)
Kellogg's Bran Flakes
Fruit & Fibre Harvest Medley (Post)
Fruit & Fibre Mountain Trail (Post)
Fruit & Fibre Tropical Fruit (Post)
Fruitful Bran (Kellogg)
Post Natural Raisin Bran
Kellogg's Raisin Bran
Cracklin' Oat Bran (Kellogg)

Don't feel that you must choose from the "very high" category only. If you don't like the cereals in this category, find one or more in the high or moderately-high category that you'll enjoy on a regular basis. Eating fiber regularly is the key.

You will have to do more than eat breakfast cereals to achieve a level of 30–40 grams of fiber every day. Think creatively about using other forms of unprocessed bran in appetizers, muffins, breads, salads, meatloafs, etc. *Most important, eat more of the high-fiber foods listed earlier in the section on requirements for fruits, vegetables, and beans. These high-fiber foods also contain many of the valuable anticancer vitamins and minerals as well.*

Breads, Crackers, and Rice

Foods made with whole-wheat flour—as opposed to bran—generally have good but not great fiber content. The coarser the form of grain, the more fiber and the greater the bulk-producing effect in our diet. Some moderate-high fiber foods of choice in this category include:

bran muffins
cat bran
brown rice
buckwheat
whole-wheat breads
whole-wheat crackers, thins, and wafers
rye crackers, thins, and wafers
graham crackers

Can we get too much fiber? The answer is yes, but a non-adamant yes. Too much fiber makes it difficult for us to absorb the zinc, iron, and copper in our diets. Fiber can bind to these minerals. If our diets don't exceed 50 grams of fiber per day, and we get enough of these minerals (especially zinc, through zinc-rich foods and/or supplements), we should not experience any deficiency of these minerals.

By increasing fiber in your diet, you're not only going a long way toward preventing colorectal cancer, but also improving the functioning of your digestive tract. You are blocking some of the deleterious effects of fat, contributing much-needed bulk, and possibly lowering blood cholesterol levels.

TIPS ON FOOD PREPARATION AND COOKING

How you store and cook fresh fruits, vegetables, and grains is an important factor in whether you lose some of their critical nutrients. How you cook meat, fish, and vegetables is crucial to whether or not you create dangerous carcinogenic agents in these foods.

Very little vitamin A and E is lost in the storage or cooking of fruits and vegetables. They are both fat-soluble vitamins, and are not easily destroyed. Vitamin C, however, a water-soluble vitamin, is easily lost when exposed to oxygen, heat, or light for long. Using fresh produce, selected when seasonal, and eaten soon after purchase, is the best way to retain the vitamin C. Vegetables frozen while fresh are the next-best alternative, while canned and dried fruits and vegetables tend to lose far too much vitamin C and other vitamins. (Dried fruits do retain vitamin A.)

Produce containing vitamin C should be cooked as little as possible because the longer you cook these foods the more C is lost. The same goes for the B vitamins, which are also water soluble. Steaming vegetables is by far the best cooking method. Eating them raw is even better. Brisk stir-frying (with little oil) or quick boiling is fine, too. Undercooking is the watchword. Gone are the days (or if they're not, they should be) when eating vegetables meant staring at a plate of depressingly limp or mushy stalks, stems, pods, or leaves.

Basic Rules for Storing and Cooking

- Keep fruits and vegetables refrigerated. Eat them as fresh as possible and cook them as little as possible.
- Make sure to properly store and seal grains, nuts, and seeds in a cool, dark, dry place (to avoid spoilage and contamination with molds such as those that produce aflatoxin).
- Bake, boil, or broil (but *don't* overly brown) whenever you can, using little or no oil or butter.
- When sautéing, stir-frying, or roasting, cook with as little oil as possible, preferably no more than one tablespoon per two servings. If oil becomes brown, throw it out. If food becomes brown, charred, or covered with browned oil, throw both out. If you should deep-fry, don't use the oil twice. *Heating and reheating fats may cause the formation of free radicals and other harmful substances.*
- Don't order deep-fried foods in fast-food joints or other restaurants, since many of these establishments reuse their frying oil from day to day. Some places have been known to reuse oil daily for over a month!
- Use olive oil or peanut oil for cooking. These high-in-monounsaturated-oils may have less harmful effects than the saturated or polyunsaturated variety.
- Avoid barbecuing, charcoal broiling, burning, or overly browning meats, chicken, and fish to avoid formation of dangerous mutagens (see Chapter 6, "Foods That Are Enemies," p. 119, on Cooking Practices).

8

You Can Change
Your Eating Habits

Some people are lucky—or just plain smart—and have been eating a sound, balanced diet since childhood, one not too far from the CPDG. The main problem with the diets many of us were led to believe were healthy was the preponderance of red meat and high-fat dairy products like whole milk. Otherwise, the balanced diet of yesteryear is not too far from the cancer-prevention diet guidelines herein. The primary difference is the emphasis on low fat and high fiber, and the focus on particular vitamins and minerals.

In our newly health-conscious society, many who didn't eat well to begin with have changed their ways down the line. You may know them: people who have suddenly developed a passion for vegetables: they eat lots of them raw, steamed, baked, or stir-fried, with little butter or oil. They are the ones who, at lunch, blithely order a smidgen of low-fat cottage cheese, surrounded by slices of carrots, broccoli, cauli-flower, and then top it all off with half a grapefruit for dessert. The drink: seltzer water with a twist of lemon or lime. In the early morning, they jog for an hour or work out at the local health club/spa. Surely an admirable routine.

If you are one of those blessed souls, you can skip this chapter. It's meant for types like me who, from an early age, have been hooked—really hooked—on pizza, spareribs, oily Chinese and Indian foods, cake and ice cream with whipped-cream toppings.

I had a very tough time changing my eating habits. By the time I was twenty, I was perennially ten to fifteen pounds overweight. I would try, from time to time, a crash or fad diet, or develop my own self-styled regime. Like most dieters, I would drop a few pounds then just as quickly put them back on, until one day I woke up and found myself

137

forty pounds overweight. I knew then that a serious change was required and that I could no longer go it alone.

I joined a local diet center, where counseling was offered to stay on a reasonably strict but nutritionally sound program. I joined because I knew I needed the structure, the moral support, and the routine of weighing in. The problem had become so serious that I knew I had to devote a great deal of energy and conscious awareness to what I was eating and why.

After three weeks of strict adherence—and fidgety anxiety—I discovered several things: that I had been ruled behaviorally by food; I had lost the real pleasures of eating; I had become unaware of how I felt physically when eating loads of fattening and unhealthy food; nor was I any longer aware of how it felt to be forty pounds overweight.

You don't have to be obese to suffer from these problems. Many people who aren't obese—perhaps by virtue of metabolism or because they don't eat large quantities—are still ruled by eating in some way. Being obsessive about food—whether one is overweight or not—will require a major shift in habits and attitudes.

Those of us who become addicted to pizza, oily Chinese or Mexican or Indian foods; hamburgers, hot dogs, french fries; cakes, candy, sodas, etc., lose touch with the real pleasures of eating, and with the bodily sensations connected to eating. That's not to say these foods aren't fun—they are. They were fun when we were all children and wanted every day to be our birthdays, which is often where the problem begins. Few of us shed easily the childhood associations with "fun" foods that we chose—or were fed—to reduce unhappiness, anxiety, or anger. Many of us were "forced" to eat vegetables (often of the overcooked frozen variety) and "rewarded" when we did, with ice cream or other sugary desserts and cookies. Who can blame us as adults for turning our diets into one never-ending birthday party—especially when our adult anxieties often mirror childhood disappointments we may never have resolved?

My experience is unhappily common. It isn't until the inevitable girth appears, and our adult status or attractiveness is threatened, that we take matters in hand and begin dieting, which sometimes means eating sensibly for the first time in our lives.

Then something almost shocking occurs. We discover what it feels like to eat healthy foods. How it tastes. How it feels physically. The positive effects it has on mind and body.

Once we have sloughed off the old addictions, lost a few pounds, and begun to feel better, we suddenly realize the contrast. When we remember that we used to eat tons of greasy, salty meats; creamy sauces; ice cream; absurdly sweet pastries, pies, and cakes, the memories begin to become mildly nauseating. No longer do we salivate reflexively like Pavlov's dogs, huffing and puffing with an anxious urge to gobble down goodies. One moment's reflection, a few deep breaths, and we know we couldn't swallow much more than a few bites of some of the foods we once craved. We don't realize this until we're out of the woods, because the body's nutritional requirements—which are fully in line with the Cancer-Prevention Diet Guide—are felt physically and psychologically. In order to ignore the body's nutritional needs, we have to lose touch with a range of physical sensations.

On my diet, water was a major requirement—eight glasses a day. I recommend drinking a lot of water each day, for two reasons: (1) because our bodies require a great deal of fluid for their biochemical processes, and (2) because it has a detoxifying effect, flushing metabolic wastes quickly and efficiently out of the body.

Drinking the eight glasses hastened my weight loss, made me feel full and therefore less hungry, and produced a feeling of well-being, owing in part to the continuous and efficient removal of toxins and waste products from the body.

The sensations associated with my own dietary change—eating more chicken and fish and less red meat, more fruits, vegetables, whole grains, and water, and less of all the fatty, sugary foods that were once my wont—were sublimely pleasurable. I lost the forty pounds in just over one year (a long period owing to a gradual but deep-set change) but I have kept it off five years later.

It's been relatively easy to keep the pounds off, because I can no longer eat what I used to. It's physically impossible. However, today I don't eat as healthfully as I did while on the strict diet. I indulge in an occasional slice of pizza. Once in a while my craving for Häagen Dazs overwhelms all my diet and cancer-prevention sensibilities. And Chinese food—I must have it every so often, even if they do use a lot of (polyunsaturated) oils.

I have not, however, gone back to any of these foods on a regular basis, and I don't believe I could. Having been to culinary hell and back, my body won't stand for it.

It should come as no surprise that the CPDG dictates a pattern of eating that many nutritionists have for years advocated as healthful. Today, we know much more about the powers of specific vitamins and minerals, the importance of fiber, and the real dangers of high fat, but the basic prescriptions are not far afield from the "balanced diet" of yesteryear.

However, with new knowledge of the diet-cancer connection, we have one more—and very critical—motive to change our eating habits. A dietary shift will provide multiple benefits, *including* cancer prevention.

HOW TO START WITH THE CPDG

Start with as much discipline as you can muster. The closer you can stay with the CPDG guidelines, the easier it will be for you to change. For two weeks, be a disciplinarian with yourself. Force yourself to cut out fatty meats; eat all the fruits, vegetables, and fiber called for. Drink a lot of water. Carefully count your grams of fat and don't go over the limit.

If you stick to this for just two weeks (a few people need three or four), you will feel a difference. If you have been overweight, you will drop a few pounds. But, even if you weren't overweight, you will feel lighter, cleaner, and more alert. In the beginning, you'll miss the foods you've cut out—they may even haunt you in your dreams! After about two weeks, though, you'll feel different. Cravings will begin to cease, and you will feel your first pangs of disgust at the thought of some of your old (two-faced!) friends.

Once these feelings surface, the shift has occurred. The groundwork for a lifelong change in your eating habits has been set in place. If you recognize these early sensations at this crucial point—and you want them to grow and continue—then you're on the path. Less will power will be required. From that point on, discipline will be born of desire, not obligation. You'll feel better and want that feeling to expand.

STICKING WITH THE CPDG

The best advice I can give: if you stray from the diet guidelines, don't worry about it. Just get back on the track.

Many dieters feel guilt-ridden when they cheat or fall off the wagon. This guilt can register unconsciously, leading directly to a nihilistic "what the hell?" attitude. That leads, in turn, to abandoning the diet completely. Beware of this trap.

Although it is not as stringent as most weight-loss diets, you are bound to stray occasionally from the CPDG. If you begin eating a few fatty foods, or forget your fiber, fruits, or vegetables, you're not going to get cancer as a result. If, however, you do stray considerably—and, as a result, throw in the towel—then you will lose the cancer-preventive benefits of the diet. Dieters of all kinds often think they need the guilt or fear to keep them straight, but they don't. These are counterproductive feelings, and not good motivators. Try to keep your focus the positive desire for health.

The CPDG is designed to give you enough leeway to continue to enjoy some of your favorite foods—even the ballyhooed birthday delights. Whether your weakness is ice cream, or hot dogs, or T-bone steaks, make a concerted effort to cut down on your intake but don't worry that you'll never be able to eat them again.

If a food you love is really on the hot list—like barbecued spare ribs (fatty food, full of nitrites, *and* grilled!)—and you know you really can't live without it, let yourself have it, *but very rarely!* You're better off having it once every few months than once a week.

Remember, too, that by taking the cancer-preventive supplements I have recommended you are affording yourself an extra edge of protection. This does not mean that taking them will undo any damage caused by bad eating habits. It does mean that occasional indulgences are less likely to be harmful. For example, the vitamin C and E you take will help block the nitrosamines formed after you eat a hot dog or bacon. This is another good reason to take the supplements every day. That should be the easiest part of the CPDG.

GETTING BACK AT FOOD

As you change your eating patterns, you will try to deny yourself certain foods you ate to make yourself "feel better." I used a trick when I was dieting that was very successful. Occasionally, I would feel an irresistible craving for one such food—an ice-cream bar, for example. I would let myself go out and buy the bar and take just a few bites. Then I'd stop, take a breath, and ask myself: "Am I really feeling better?" One time in five the answer was "yes" and I would devour the rest of it, with zest. Four of the five times, however, my answer was "no"—a resounding "NO." Then I went to the nearest street-corner trash can and got rid of it. I don't mean I simply tossed it into the can. I would spot a place in the can where I could hurl it full speed to produce full splattering effect.

I did this often—with ice cream, pizza, french fries, cakes. I'd spend a dollar on them, have my few bites, ask my question, well up with frustration, then take my anger out on the junk food. It always felt good. For me, these foods had been real enemies.

You can use this technique for sticking to the CPDG as well. People addicted to salty and sugary foods especially—whether they are obese or not—are usually seeking comfort of some kind. These foods offer only the most limited, short-lived kinds of comfort. When you realize in a flash that your "crutch food" is not really helping, but is adding to your risk of cancer, it's time to heave it, full force, into the trash.

After a while, my anger abated but I realized I still might need an occasional benign bite of the once-loved, once-hated morsel. Then nibble and throw became my watchword. It may seem wasteful, but it's better to satisfy a small craving with a nibble than feel impelled to eat an entire serving of unhealthy food.

VISUALIZATIONS CAN HELP

Information is all well and good, but it also helps to talk more directly to your unconscious mind. And visualizations can work on the unconscious very successfully. They can help you relate more instinctively to the diet-cancer connection. If the connection becomes meaningful for you, changing your eating habits will follow naturally.

The sample visualizations are based on fact, not fantasy. Nutrients do help fight cancer along the lines these images follow. The "symbols" are imagined, but the metaphors and meanings are grounded in biological reality. The visualizations here are merely examples. Use them to create images of your own. Do what works best for you. Begin any visualization with a few moments of relaxation, deep breathing, and inner focusing. (For additional information on relaxation techniques, see Chapter 21, "New Ways to Mind-Body Health.")

For Fiber

Practice this visualization during or after eating a fiber-rich food. You will understand and appreciate more deeply why fiber is helpful to your body, you'll enjoy the food more, and you may soon begin to want more and more of it.

You're out in the country, at a farmhouse, with a barn. An aluminum chute runs from the open window of the barn's upper loft down to the ground. The chute is shiny, heavily greased with a thick layer of oil. The farmer tosses a huge bucket of fiber-filled whole-wheat grains down the chute. You hear the rushing sound of grain on metal. After all the grain is down, the chute is left miraculously cleared of grease; only a fresh, fine veneer of wheat dust remains. Then smell the fresh aroma of whole wheat and taste the flavor. It's like the best bowl of whole-grain cereal—hot or cold—you ever remember tasting.

You're on your way to protection from colon cancer.

Vitamins A, C, and E (ACE)

See your immune cells—the T- and B-cells that pick up bacteria and cancer cells—as an endless stream of little compact European cars hurtling down a broad avenue of a big city and branching off onto side streets. These cars are driven by people who perform vital services for the city—cops who stop criminals in the trucks, detectives on the lookout for terrorists, sanitation men who clean up the streets. The faster and more vibrant these little cars are, the more efficient and safer the city will be.

Now imagine that it's morning. The sun shines bright and everything runs smoothly, perfectly, and in fast motion. The little cars spurt gingerly from place to place, make tight curves around sharp corners. Traffic moves smoothly and energetically. The little men pop in and out of the cars, with briefcases and tool kits, wearing their proper uniforms and looking purposeful. Their movements are crisp, economical, determined.

Now flash forward. It's later in the day and everything is winding down. The cars aren't moving quickly anymore. As a result, there are traffic jams everywhere. Horns are honking. Cars are stalling out. The little men stuck inside the cars are anxious. They're late reaching their destinations. They're angry, tired, and most of all, trapped.

Now pull back, for an aerial viewpoint. With a broader view, you discover the reason for all the congestion. There are many side streets off the main avenue. You focus in on three of them. Half a block down each one is a gas station, each with the sign "ACE." Two of them are closed, and marked "No Fuel." One is still open, trying to serve an endless line of customers. Traffic is hopelessly clogged down the two streets where cars have gone, only to discover there's no more fuel.

You can solve the problem. You can restore order and vibrancy to the whole city. You send a huge tanker marked ACE through a back route to the side streets. The tanker quickly refills pumps in the two empty stations and replenishes the overtaxed one. Cars begin having their tanks filled and swing back onto the avenue. The congestion slowly unfurls, the cars start moving briskly again, the men heave sighs of relief, and begin popping in and out of their cars with energy and purpose again.

Using visualizations is but one way to get in touch with the physical part of our being, which responds to the nutrients we ingest. A low-fat, high-fiber, vitamin-mineral-rich diet meets our nutritional needs, and eventually makes us feel good. It harmonizes our food urges with our requirements for health and disease prevention. After you have been on the CPDG for a period of time, the subtle benefits become more obvious, and you receive a kind of biofeedback of new sensations that tell you you're on the right track. That's the best kind of positive reinforcement.

IV
THE
LIFESTYLE FACTOR

9

Smoking: The Most Dangerous Habit

Some of the greatest cancer hazards come from voluntary behaviors that most of us know all too well increase our risk. At the top of this list—well above everything else—comes smoking. Next are alcohol and suntanning. The challenge is how to conquer the habit/addiction of smoking, how to reduce the intake of alcohol, and how to get it through our heads that suntanning really is a serious, significant risk factor, and that we must respond by protecting ourselves.

Education—though a necessary first step with addictive habits—is not usually sufficient to bring about change. We need, as well, supportive systems for motivation and behavioral change, including support groups made up of people in the same predicament. This is especially true with nicotine, *one of the most addictive drugs* we know of.

Smoking is such a big hazard—accounting for 30 percent of all cancers—that I will devote this entire chapter to it. Those of you who don't smoke, and are not trying to help someone else give up smoking, can skip this chapter. However, if you are a nonsmoker but are interested in helping others give it up, I suggest you glance through it. If you've never been addicted to smoking or are a convert to nonsmoking, you need to be aware of some of the causes and manifestations of this habit—in order to be of any help to someone trying to relinquish it. The situation with smoking is analogous to that with alcohol: few people who have not been addicted can understand the compulsion, which is why the best alcoholic counselors are recovering alcoholics themselves. Many smokers have quit on their own without help. But they may not have been addicted, or as severely addicted as others. Those people who found it "no sweat" to give it up are often not much help to those who have to struggle.

YOU CAN QUIT

If you're a smoker, the first thing to realize and *believe deeply* is that you *can stop.* Millions of Americans have: in the twenty-three years between 1959 and 1982, the percentage of men who stopped smoking rose from 7 percent to 40 percent; the percentage of women rose from 6 percent to 23 percent. There are 37 million ex-smokers in the U.S. today.

That's a lot of people. Why not join the ranks?

DON'T BELITTLE SMOKERS

If you're a nonsmoker, remember that smoking is one of the toughest addictions—both physically and psychologically—to relinquish and that your friends and relatives who are trying to stop need all the support they can get. Constant badgering doesn't work. Ridicule is counterproductive. If you see a friend who's said he's quitting light up, don't say, "I thought you were giving up the cigarettes. It doesn't seem to work, does it? Where's your will power?" Such remarks make him feel guilty and defeated and often send him back to smoking full-time. One cigarette does not necessarily mean an inevitable reentrapment. A more effective response is: "Okay—have one. But don't give up the fight. I know you can make it."

KNOW THE FACTS

Knowing what the health hazards are is an important first step, but often it is not the decisive factor in the final decision to quit. For those with real addictions, many of the facts can be rationalized away in one way or another. Motivations other than fear of health damage work as well or better. I know one man who quit because he had laryngitis and couldn't be heard in an amateur theatrical production that was going into final dress rehearsal. For years, he had been warned about smoking by his doctor and friends, but it was his wish to perform well that clinched the change. A woman I know gave up smoking because she couldn't bear the burn holes that cigarettes made in her new clothes. What motivates motivates. And it is frequently *not* fear of ill-health— especially if the projected health damages may occur twenty years in the future. ("I'll stop tomorrow," goes the litany.)

Nevertheless, the raw facts are important and must be understood fully—and absorbed. Even if they're not the final trigger for stopping, the health facts have their cumulative effects over time. Most people would say they stopped "for health reasons." Here are the facts:

- Nicotine is a powerful drug and *the* addictive agent in tobacco, although it accounts for only 1 percent to 5 percent of tobacco's total content. Nicotine is both addictive and psychoactive, and causes chemical changes in the cells of the brain and muscles throughout the body. In reality it is a poison; a dosage of only 60 mg. can kill as effectively as cyanide.

- In small doses, nicotine is a powerful stimulant of the central nervous system and can cause an immediate rise in blood pressure and an increase in heart rate of as many as thirty-three beats per minute. It is the pleasure of this stimulation that becomes its physiological hook. Many doctors compare the addictive qualities of nicotine to those of heroin and barbiturates. Nicotine addiction may be even harder to break than that of heroin or cocaine.

- Nicotine also directly affects hormone production, muscle tension, pain sensitivity, and skin temperature, the latter making smokers prone to frostbite. A recent study indicates that the biochemical action of nicotine makes it easier for metastases to develop in people with all types of cancer.

- Smoking and smokeless tobacco combine to kill more adults worldwide than any other preventable cause of death, including war, famine, and terrorist attacks, according to the Worldwatch Institute. Senior researcher William Chandler estimated that cigarette smoking causes between 2 and 2.8 million deaths throughout the world each year.

- About 32 percent of the U.S. population is still smoking, and 320,000 deaths a year are directly attributable to this habit. About 600 billion cigarettes were smoked in the U.S.A. last year.

- Smoking is the single major cause of cancer mortality—accounting for 30 percent of all deaths. Although diet accounts for 35 percent of all cancers, remember that diet covers a lot of territory and a lot of variations. Smoking is a single factor.

- The death rate from cancer for male smokers is double that of non-smokers. Women smokers have a 67 percent higher rate than non-smokers.

- Lung cancer causes more deaths each year than any other type of cancer. For 1988 alone, there will be an estimated 152,000 new cases in the U.S. and 139,000 deaths.

- Lung cancer is one of the most difficult cancers to treat. It's difficult to detect in its early stages, so that it often has a death grip before treatment is begun. Only 13 percent of lung-cancer patients live five years or more after diagnosis. Some 85 percent of lung cancer in men is due to smoking; 75 percent of lung cancer in women is due to smoking.

- Smoking increases the risk not only of lung cancer but also of cancers of the lip, mouth, throat, larynx, esophagus, bladder, pancreas, and kidney. It may be associated with cancers of the stomach and cervix.
- Seventy-five percent of all oral cancers are caused by the smoking-alcohol connection.
- Smoking is a major cause of heart disease, and is strongly associated with chronic bronchitis and emphysema. It has been linked to conditions ranging from colds to gastric ulcers.
- Smokers are two to three times more likely to suffer strokes than nonsmokers.
- The earlier one smokes, and the more and longer one smokes, the greater the risk. The Department of Health and Human Services reports that those who smoke more than one pack a day have three times the cancer rate of nonsmokers. Those who smoke two or more packs per day have lung cancer death rates fifteen to twenty-five times higher than nonsmokers.
- The cost of smoking to the economy ranges from $38 to $95 billion, with a middle estimate of $65 billion, according to the U.S. Congress's Office of Technology Assessment.
- Cigar and pipe smokers have a greater risk of developing cancer than nonsmokers, though the risk is less than that of cigarette smokers. This is so because they usually inhale less and smoke less.
- A pipe/cigar smoker's risk of oral, esophageal, and laryngeal cancer is about the same as that of cigarette smokers. Moreover, there has been some data showing that cigar and pipe smokers are even more likely to contract bladder, kidney, and pancreatic cancer.
- Chewing tobacco has been shown to increase the risk of cancer of the oral cavity. Dipping snuff isn't any safer. Snuff that is rolled and placed between the gum and cheek results in a much greater likelihood of cancers of the mouth, cheek, gums, or larynx. Very often, tobacco chewers and snuff dippers become strongly addicted to the nicotine in these products, and soon switch to cigarettes to have larger and quicker doses of their drug.
- There is no such thing as a safe cigarette or cigar or chewing tobacco. Even the low-tar and low-nicotine brands—though preferable—are smokestacks of poisonous gases and carcinogenic chemicals.

With all these facts, it's rather amazing that cigarettes have not been made illegal. However, illegality—as in Prohibition of the 1920s or with the current drug scene—might not be an effective answer.

WHAT'S IN A "GOOD SMOKE"?

Cigarettes can contain well over five thousand chemicals along with a number of unknown products and additives that are not regulated by agencies outside the tobacco industry (nor, obviously, by anyone within it). They may include pesticides (used to protect the tobacco plants from bugs), some of which have not been tested for safety.

Nicotine, as mentioned before, is *the* addictive agent in cigarettes, but accounts for only 1–5 percent of a cigarette's contents. Without question, it alters mood as well as the body's chemistry and it's no myth that you can get a "lift" from a cigarette. Yet the tense, uptight feeling that a cigarette supposedly relieves can itself be caused by nicotine. It's a vicious circle.

When tobacco is smoked, tar results, which is not that different from the black sticky stuff used to pave roads. Cigarette smoke involves both "a toxic gas phase" and a "particulate" phase. Most carcinogens come from particles in tar, though a few come from gases. Tar contains agents that both *initiate* and *promote* cancerous changes, and co-carcinogens that, together with other agents, form cancer-producing chemicals. There are nitrosamines, polycyclic aromatic hydrocarbons (PAHs) such as benzo(a)pyrene, and various metals (including arsenic!), which cause or promote tumor growth.

As if this cornucopia of carcinogens was not enough, cigarette smoke also contains other poisonous chemicals and gases. The chemicals include acids, glycerol, glycol, alcohols, ketones and phenols; the gases include hydrogen, cyanide, nitrogen oxide, and a hefty amount of carbon monoxide. A number of these substances have been linked in animal and human experiments to lung and other cancers, heart and circulatory diseases, bronchitis and emphysema.

Using filters does help. They reduce the amount of tar, nicotine, and poisonous gases that reach your lungs. Smokers of filter-tip cigarettes have a lower risk of lung cancer than those who smoke "regular cigarettes," though their risk is still six and one half times that of non-smokers.

Low-tar, low-nicotine cigarettes may help a little. As yet, the data is imprecise, because low-tar/nicotine (T/N) cigarettes have not been marketed long enough for the long-term studies to give results. Some early studies have shown a decrease in death rates from cancer among those who smoke the low T/N brands. But remember, low T/N brands are primarily the tobacco industry's way of deflecting criticism and trying to make their product appear safe. Ads that promote low-tar cigarettes as "healthier" are an out-and-out contradiction because the danger is still so much greater than the safety factor.

"Low-tar" has been defined as less than 17 milligrams and "low nicotine" as less than 1.2 milligrams. If you smoke, check your pack.

Being told that you are a little *less likely* to die of heart disease or lung cancer should not be very reassuring. Let me repeat: the consensus of everyone from the Surgeon General and the National Academy of Sciences to the American Cancer Society is that *there is* NO SAFE *cigarette.*

WHAT HAPPENS WHEN SMOKERS SMOKE?

A long drag on a cigarette is followed by a deep inhaling that pulls the smoke down into the air passages of the lung. Black, sticky tar, with its carcinogenic chemical constituents, is deposited on the membranes of the whole bronchial system. Chemicals and gases irritate the mucous membranes and damage the cilia that catch foreign matter in the passages. After years of being exposed to smoke, the cilia are destroyed and the entire lung is partially or completely blackened—depending on how much and how long one has smoked.

Sooner or later, the cells lining the air passages may begin to transform, because of continuous exposure to chemical carcinogens. These cells then become irregular, clump together, and over a period of years may form a growing tumor. In later stages, cancer cells break away from the lung and travel through the lymphatic system to other organs. Metastatic tumors develop, and the cancer is then usually beyond treatment.

Pretty scary, isn't it? But that's a common scenario—tragically common.

ADVERTISING THE "SOPHISTICATED CIGARETTE"

In the early 1900s, lung cancer was comparatively rare. Then, in 1912, a lighter, milder cigarette was introduced—one whose smoke could be deeply inhaled. Soon after, cigarette consumption in the U.S. skyrocketed.

As you might expect, lung-cancer rates have risen at a commensurate rate. In 1950, there were 18,300 lung-cancer deaths. By 1977, the figure had risen to 75,000 and for 1988, the estimated deaths are 139,000.

What powerful forces have been at work to hook people on tobacco? They are manifold: physical, cultural, behavioral, and psychological.

Advertising picks up on cultural and psychological needs, dresses them up, and then presents them to the public. The tobacco industry spends more than $1¼ billion each year on advertising. Since 1971, television and radio ads for cigarettes have been banned. But print ads in magazines and newspapers and on outdoor billboards still flood us with images that connect smoking to power, sex, and sophistication. And the ads do more than associate smoking with qualities and values we yearn for: they also lure us into forgetting the horrendous dangers of tobacco.

Women have been a prime target of advertising ploys. An infamous example is Virginia Slims' tag line, "You've come a long way, baby. . . ." Yes, indeed, women have come a long way: in 1950 women represented only 9 percent of the deaths from lung cancer. In 1988, they represent over 33 percent! In the last two years, lung cancer has surpassed breast cancer as the primary cancer killer of women.

Teenagers, too, are a special target. The tobacco industry has a vested interest in snaring new customers at the earliest possible age, especially in the face of the continuous decrease in the smoking population from those who quit. The ads focus on luring images of maturity, sophistication, derring-do, and sexual attractiveness.

But young males have been the group most conspicuously appealed to for years. Machismo and smoking go hand in hand. We are presented with romantic images of cowboys, outdoor adventurers, great sportsmen, corporate power brokers—and almost every other male archetype—lighting up and loving it.

These images have created a smoke screen around us to which we are all susceptible. There are, however, more basic reasons why we smoke, which are sometimes exploited in ads but aren't directly addressed.

A SUBSTITUTE FOR BASIC NEEDS

If you ask veteran smokers what they get from smoking, much of the time they will say it "relaxes" and "reduces tension" in a difficult situation. We all know people who wouldn't think of making a touchy phone call without having a full pack of cigarettes, plenty of matches, and an ashtray next to the telephone. They wouldn't think of going to a party or a business lunch without being sure they're well prepared in the nicotine department, even though smoking is becoming more difficult as increasing numbers of people become intolerant of being engulfed by smoke. The cigarette is a friend, and one who's always available to give comfort in tense situations, regardless of the tension it causes others.

Psychologically the comfort comes from satisfying some of the oral needs left over from early infancy and childhood. We all have them, in greater or lesser degrees. Feeding at the breast (or bottle) was the most gratifying of our infantile experiences, meeting primal needs for warmth and oral stimulation. Denial of these needs leaves a long-lasting psychophysical imprint. The sucking and inhaling of a cigarette hundreds of times a day is as integral to the addiction as the chemical action of nicotine. In the process of quitting, it is important to address both the psychological and physiological issues and then provide ourselves with some nonfattening oral substitutes—such as chewing gum or incessant chomping on carrot sticks.

Obviously smoking is a false friend. It appears to calm us but it does so only transiently; in reality, it is a stimulant, which revs us up further, causing us to smoke more—another vicious circle. It seems to bolster self-esteem but only does so flimsily and temporarily. It helps us project images of sexuality, power, or sophistication—but in a meaningless and superficial way. When we quit, one of the false images we must give up is that a cigarette is an ever-present, reassuring friend.

HOW TO BECOME A NONSMOKER

Some people just wake up one morning and decide "that's it" and never smoke again. In the process of their withdrawal, they suffer greater or lesser miseries but never look back. My uncle, a chain smoker of unfiltered Camels, did just that. He didn't tell anyone, and no one noticed what he was up to (people often don't), even though he was as cross and jumpy as a wet monkey. On the third day, his wife said, "Henry, why are you so scratchy lately? You're dreadful."

He snapped back, "Didn't you know? I've quit smoking."

"Oh, my God," replied my aunt. "I never noticed. That's great. Be as cross as you like."

"I will," he said. And stomped off.

He was back to his jolly old self in two weeks. In the meantime, my aunt gave him a wide berth.

My California friend Bill went alone to Yosemite for the weekend. He chose a two-day hike far from civilization—and any cigarette machines—and from other hikers who might have packs. At the bottom of the trail, he burned his last pack of Merits, shed a tear or two, and set out. When he returned on Sunday, he had convinced himself he would never smoke again. He doesn't claim this hike was the most pleasant one of his career but says it was, perhaps, the most rewarding.

Most of us can't do it that way. And I can't recommend that everyone try such heroics. There are many less-disruptive ways to ease the transition. And there are many good ways to prepare for it. Whatever works for you should be the path you choose and stick to.

PREPARING TO QUIT

Step One: Face the Facts and Master the Fears

There is little question that my uncle and my friend Bill had done a good deal of mental preparation before they quit—whether they spoke about it or not. At the very least, they were aware of the health hazards of smoking. It's good to start your preparation with a full understanding of the facts. Read again the list on pages 149–150. Such a listing raises fears, but fear is not an inappropriate response, if used constructively. Smoking *is* a direct cause of cancer (and other diseases). The fear of contracting cancer from smoking is not irrational unless the fear becomes so great that our minds block out the reality. As Lord Conesford of Britain once quipped, "I have every sympathy with the American who was so horrified by what he read about the effects of smoking that he gave up reading."

We can all fall back on clever rationalizations like "Uncle Andy smoked three packs a day and he lived to be ninety-six!" What about Aunt Emily and Cousin Jake? Did they fare as well? Do we really want to play Russian roulette?

If the fear remains unconscious—and our behavior rationalized—it not only has an insidious effect on our psyches but also allows us to continue a horrendously destructive habit. It's best to know and absorb the facts and be fully aware of our fears. The best way to reduce those fears is to QUIT.

Step Two: Think Positive

Focus not on what you'll be giving up but on what you'll be gaining.

As for the health benefits, they are phenomenal! The lungs are among the most resilient and self-repairing organs we have. As soon as you stop, the levels of carbon monoxide and nicotine begin to go down. The damaged lung tissues immediately begin to repair themselves, and your circulatory system begins to function more efficiently. Within weeks, your breathing will improve, and your head will become clearer. You will feel more alive. After a year, your risks of cancer and heart disease will drop appreciably. After a few years, the cells in your lungs will have regenerated so that, in about ten years, they will be in as tiptop condition as those of someone who has never smoked.

Add to this the many other gains you'll be reaping: No more going out in the middle of a cold rainy night because you've run out of cigarettes. No more burn holes in your furniture or clothes. No more slipping outside at the office, or a party, to take a "nicotine fix" away from the nonsmokers. No more being annoyed in a restaurant by the lady at the next table who ostentatiously waves her hands in the air to get rid of the smoke. You'll be saving money. You'll have fresher breath, more wind for tennis, hiking, or climbing upstairs. No more ashtrays stuffed with butts to clean up in the morning. Your clothes won't smell of smoke. Your senses of taste and smell will improve. Make a full list of the reasons why you want to quit and the benefits that will come. Post it on your refrigerator door or on your bathroom mirror. Take a copy to work with you. Keep referring to it. Over and over again.

Begin to think of yourself as a nonsmoker—a nonsmoker who is smoking temporarily. Call yourself a nonsmoker (not out loud yet; you'll get into trouble with some skeptics!). See how it feels.

Step Three: Find Out Why You Smoke

Here is a test, taken from the *University of California, Berkeley, Wellness Letter,* based on material from the U.S. Department of Health and Human Services. It will help you determine why *you* smoke. Jot down the answers as you go.

True or False: I Smoke . . .

1. because I light up automatically and don't know I'm doing it.
2. because it's relaxing.
3. because I like handling cigarettes, matches, lighters.
4. to help deal with anger.
5. to keep from slowing down.
6. because it's unbearable not to.
7. because I enjoy watching the smoke as I exhale it.
8. to take my mind off my troubles.
9. because I really enjoy it.
10. because I feel uncomfortable without a cigarette in my hand.
11. to give myself a lift.
12. without planning to—it's just part of my routine.

RESULTS: "True" answers to 5 and 11 indicate that you smoke for stimulation; to 3 and 7, that pleasure of handling is important; to 2 and 9, that you seek relaxation; to 4 and 8, that you need a tension-reducing crutch; to 6 and 10, that you have a physiological addiction; to 1 and 12, that you smoke from habit. No doubt you smoke for a combination of these reasons.

Choosing your way to quit smoking and providing yourself with substitutes depends on what kind of smoker you are, what you think you get out of smoking, and what it seems to do for you.

Step Four: Plan Substitutes That Help You

After you've completed the questionnaire above, think up things you can do to meet the needs cigarettes fulfilled. Here are the U.C. Berkeley *Wellness Letter*'s suggestions (with some additions of my own):

- If you smoke for stimulation or a lift, find a healthy substitute like exercise. Even a quick walk around the block will do fine. Plan to exercise a lot during your first two weeks.
- If you smoke because you like something in your mouth, try sugarless chewing gum, or chew on plastic straws or toothpicks until you get over the withdrawal period. Vegetable munchies are good, too. Keep carrot, green pepper, or celery sticks handy. But stay away from sugary or fatty foods.
- If you smoke because of physiological addiction ("it's unbearable not to"), talk to your doctor about prescribing nicotine chewing gum (see page 166). It helped millions of Europeans before it was allowed in the U.S., and is one approach to handling withdrawal. Eventually you'll need to give up the gum, but most people find that comparatively easy. The other habits around smoking have already been given up.
- If the habitual factor is strongest, plan to alter your daily habits. Don't sit in the same place at meals. Talk on the telephone when standing or sitting—whichever is not habitual. Cut down gradually, in steps: first, give up smoking in the car, for instance; then on the phone; then for fifteen minutes after meals; etc.
- If handling cigarettes is important, try doodling, knitting, needlework, or some Greek worry beads that you can finger.
- If you smoke for relaxation or to relieve tension (sometimes it's hard to tell which is which), plan to practice some meditation or other relaxation techniques (see page 165) or deep breathing or physical exertion. Or plan to have a series of massage sessions after Q-Day, the day you plan to Quit.

Step Five: Choose Your Own Method of Quitting

Like my uncle and my friend Bill, many people prefer to quit by themselves—but usually not as abruptly as they did. By one researcher's estimate, over 90 percent of those who stop successfully do so with no apparent assistance. Others do better with a support group and a systematic schedule laid out for them. Do what you feel most comfortable with.

There are other choices.

"You can't quit unless you go cold turkey" is an old saw with no validity. For some who are frightened about giving everything up boom! a gradual tapering-off is not only preferable but the *only* way they can stop. For others, bit-by-bit withdrawal is agonizing and almost impossible. Whether you stop by yourself or find a group, choose the time frame that suits you best. Some groups stop immediately, others in five days, others over a period of six weeks or more.

If the way you've chosen seems intolerable, try an alternative. Keep trying. Many smokers have quit on their third, fourth—or fourteenth—try.

Step Six: Pick a Q-Day

Almost all systems—in planned groups or solo—suggest you pick a day (the American Cancer Society calls it "Q-Day") on which you plan to stop. And then stick to it. It doesn't much matter how far off it is; you may need a week, several weeks, or more than a month to "psych yourself up" or taper off. The central issue is to choose some date, and to choose one that is not apt to be stressful. Don't give yourself the chance to rationalize that you have a major report due or that you have a stressful appointment and therefore need buttressing with a cigarette.

If you plan to join a group, sign up for a specific date. The group will set Q-Day for you.

If you decide to cut down gradually, it's still important to set very specific goals. Make them simple: If you smoke three packs a day, start with cutting down to two. If you smoke two, cut back to one. Give yourself a reasonable period of adjustment to a plateau, then move on to your next goal. You can also try the "little steps" approach—even less threatening—by cutting back by very small numbers. If you smoke, say, thirty-five cigarettes a day, try cutting down by five each day for a week (to thirty, then to twenty-five, etc.).

Your eventual goal should be to cut back until you stop completely. If this is unthinkable, select a goal of a nominal figure—say, five to fifteen cigarettes a day, depending on how much you smoked to begin with (light smokers can go down lower than heavy smokers). Very often, achieving a median goal is the beginning of the end of all smoking.

Step Seven: Alter Your Smoking Habits

The American Health Foundation suggests a number of useful tips to make you aware of your unconscious smoking-behavior patterns:

- Buy cigarettes one pack at a time and keep it out of sight.
- Switch to a different brand.
- Stop using all smoking paraphernalia, such as cigarette cases, holders, and lighters.
- Remove ashtrays from tables and desks at home and at work. Just seeing an ashtray can trigger an urge to smoke.
- Eliminate "unnecessary" cigarettes. Smoke only when a cigarette is craved strongly. Don't struggle with yourself over a craved cigarette but simply refrain from those that are not "important."
- When the urge to smoke comes, take a very deep breath and let it out very slowly through your mouth. Relax and try to wait *five full minutes* before lighting up. Often, the urge to smoke passes quickly.

These tips will give you an awareness of your habit, what triggers your urge to smoke, and what smoking seems to do for you. Your habit goes from an unconscious to a conscious level, where it can be changed and eliminated.

Step Eight: Keep a Record

The advantage of recording each cigarette you smoke is that it really draws your attention to when, how, and why you smoke. And, for some, being conscious of this is enough to make them stop altogether or cut down drastically. Almost all behavioral experts agree that keeping a record really helps.

An extraordinary physician and acupuncturist in Mill Valley, California, Dr. Martin Rossman, who had conducted many successful stop-smoking workshops, suggests you keep a daily smoking diary something like this:

SMOKING DIARY   DATE_____

	Situation	Emotion	Craving*	Cues	Expected gratification†	Experienced gratification†
TIME						
6 A.M.						
7 A.M.						
8 A.M.						

SMOKING DIARY   DATE_____

	Situation	Emotion	Craving*	Cues	Expected gratification†	Experienced gratification†
9 A.M.						
10 A.M.						
11 A.M.						
NOON						
1 P.M.						
2 P.M.						
3 P.M.						
4 P.M.						
5 P.M.						
6 P.M.						
7 P.M.						
8 P.M.						
9 P.M.						
10 P.M.						
11 P.M.						
MIDNIGHT						
1 A.M.						
2 A.M.						
3 A.M.						
4 A.M.						
5 A.M.						

Situation code:
M = after a meal
D = driving
A = anxiety/tension
C = coffee
S = social (seeing or being with another smoker)
AA = alcohol
B = bored
T = telephone

*Rate intensity of craving from 1 to 5, with 5 indicating strongest craving.
†Rate expected gratification and experienced gratification from 1 to 5, with 5 indicating strongest gratification.

Step Nine: Set Up a Support System

If you are quitting without a group, find a relative or friend who's empathic to your desire to quit—one whom you can check in with frequently and who will bolster your morale and resolve. (*Don't* choose someone who'll be preachy or sarcastic if you backslide.) Smokers benefit greatly from the empathy of others who understand the agony and the humor involved in the struggle with their wretched butts. Seek out and enjoy the understanding of someone who's been through it, is going through it now, or can identify with your plight because of some other personal experience with addiction.

Best of all, of course, is a friend who wants to quit at the same time you do. The "buddy system" works well.

Step Ten: Be Prepared for Some Withdrawal Symptoms

Whether you choose to quit alone or with a group, or do it cold turkey or gradually, be prepared for a few withdrawal symptoms. Although some people experience almost none, more likely than not you will have one or more of these symptoms:

- Craving for tobacco (obviously)
- Increased appetite
- Drowsiness or difficulty sleeping
- Restlessness and impaired concentration
- Irritability
- Anxiety
- Constipation
- Stomach ache
- Coughing (getting rid of the poisons)

Be ready for these symptoms and plan to indulge yourself in other ways: frequent naps, movies (where no smoking is allowed), a good massage—anything that relaxes and pleases except overeating. Keep reminding yourself that the symptoms will pass quickly—usually lasting from a few days to three weeks—and that they are simply signs that your body is busy cleaning itself, throwing off the poisons and readjusting to a healthier balance. The possibility of experiencing these symptoms are a good reason why you should quit on a weekend or holiday when you can coddle yourself without having to finish a body of work or face your boss.

The small pains you may suffer are the "new birth" signals—the genesis of a healthier self. It won't be long before you see the light at the end of the tunnel and wonder why you ever smoked.

Step Eleven: Changing Your Diet Helps a Lot

An acid stomach craves nicotine, so if you keep your system on the alkaline side, you'll have fewer urges to smoke. Blood-sugar swings also create cravings. Follow these tips suggested by Dr. Martin Rossman:

- Avoid coffee, tea, alcohol, citrus juices and citrus fruits, tomatoes, and vinegar. All these create acidity.
- Eat dark-green leafy vegetables, like spinach and beet greens. Make a large soup of dark greens. Keep it on hand to be used as a snack.
- If you're taking vitamin C as a supplement, switch from ascorbic acid to calcium ascorbate or ph vitamin C. The latter are nonacidic.
- Avoid refined sugars.
- Drink 6 to 8 glasses of water a day. This not only helps with acidity but also with flushing cigarette poisons from the system faster.
- Eat regularly, and avoid skipping meals. Have fruit (nonacidic), whole-grain snacks, nuts, or seeds between meals to keep blood-sugar levels stable.
- Experiment with herb teas and find one that is calming for you. Those with chamomile, valerian, and passionflower are good relaxers. They will be helpful in the first days of quitting.

What About Weight Gain?

Many people fear they'll balloon to immense size if they quit smoking, but many have stopped without gaining any weight at all. However, you do need to watch your food consumption carefully.

- Try not to substitute food for cigarettes, except for very low-calorie raw fruits and vegetables—carrot sticks and the like.
- Water helps. It keeps you feeling full and adds no calories. Drink 8 glasses a day.
- Cut down slightly on your daily caloric intake. Quite apart from the temptation to eat instead of smoking, studies prove that smokers have a higher metabolic rate than nonsmokers. For instance, someone who burns 2,200 calories on a day that he smokes 24 cigarettes will burn up only 2,000 calories on a day that he doesn't smoke. Reduce your daily intake accordingly.
- Don't use weight gain as an excuse not to quit. Smoking is far worse for your health than a few excess pounds. Moreover, most people who gain weight when they quit do so only temporarily. They are apt to shed it rather quickly later.

Step Twelve: Consider Using Other Aids and Techniques

If you are quitting on your own, you might want to investigate some additional supports or alternative methods that have proved their effectiveness. There are a wide variety of them. Some, like behavior therapy, are directly focused on smoking behavior. Others, like relaxation training, are stress-reduction techniques that make your efforts easier.

Quit Kits

Both the American Cancer Society and the American Lung Association offer these, and they are replete with information and self-starting program materials. The American Lung Association offers a "Freedom from Smoking" package and the ACS has a "7-Day Quit Plan" (see Appendix 3 for phone numbers and addresses).

Cassettes and Videotapes

In the stores, there is a cornucopia of audio and video cassettes to help you do everything from managing stress to cooking chicken cordon bleu. Stop-smoking tapes are available too. If you want vocal or visual guidance but haven't the time, patience, or temperament for a group, seek out the tape that suits you. One video I recommend is the American Cancer Society's *Freshstart: 21 Days to Stop Smoking ($29.95)*. It is especially designed to help you stay off cigarettes once you've stopped, often the most difficult aspect of quitting. Twenty-one daily segments of about three to four minutes each see you through the toughest hours. Comedian Robert Klein is host. He's empathic during the end of week four: "You can become as nervous as a long-tailed cat in a roomful of rocking chairs." He also suggests you write your motives and carry the list around with you. One of Klein's was "I want to see my children grow up."

Audio cassettes, which are less expensive, are often as helpful as video—if not more so. They allow you to close your eyes for meditation and your own imagery. Ask your local bookstore or record or video retailer for information about the stop-smoking audio and video cassettes available. Popular health magazines often advertise such cassettes.

Hypnosis

Hypnosis has proved very effective for some people. An editor at Harper & Row was persuaded by an author friend to fly to Cincinnati for the weekend to see her hypnotist at the author's expense. He had one session, a semi-agonizing weekend, and that was it. Whether it was the hypnosis, the free flight, or the potential embarrassment of not quitting after all that effort is hard to say. But hypnosis *does* work and self-hypnosis repeated for a few minutes two or three times a day seems to be even more effective.

In the hands of an experienced clinical hypnotist, you are absolutely safe. There is no magic or mumbo-jumbo. Hypnosis is simply a form of intense concentration, and a way of speaking to your unconscious. A hypnotist can either hypnotize you or give you systems for hypnotizing yourself, or both. The best results seem to be achieved with a combination of daily self-hypnosis and several therapist-run hypnotherapy sessions spread over a number of weeks. The sessions should begin before you stop smoking and continue afterward for reinforcement. Learning self-hypnosis can be valuable for solving other behavioral problems as well.

Studies from around the country report hypnosis success rates from 5 to 85 percent, so the effectiveness is still uncertain on a nationwide scale. However, one report indicated a reduction in withdrawal symptoms for 85 percent of those treated. And ameliorating withdrawal greatly enhances anyone's attempt to quit.

To find a hypnotherapist, contact your nearest hospital, university medical center, or mental-health clinic. Or call or write one of the hypnosis organizations listed in Appendix 3.

Acupuncture

Acupuncture is being accepted more and more in the Western world as a valid approach to many addictions and illnesses. New York's Lincoln Medical and Mental Health Center in the Bronx, which has a famous treatment center for addictions, now uses acupuncture with counseling as its treatment of choice for all addictions, including smoking, alcohol, drugs. They've had remarkable success.

Acupuncture is an ancient Chinese healing practice. In Chinese medicine, all mental and physical disorders and addictions are thought to result from an energy imbalance in the body. To restore balance and to redistribute the energy along the energy pathways (meridians), hair-thin needles are inserted in various parts of the body. The insertion is painless. Documented results include healing of stress-related illnesses and relief from pain, depression, addictive cravings, and withdrawal symptoms.

For smoking, needles are usually placed in two points in the external ear (points on the lung meridian), points near the knees, and at various other lung meridian points on the body. Many acupuncturists recommend, in addition, a staple puncture, which stays in the external ear for a week at a time and can be pressed by the patient to decrease cravings whenever they occur.

A friend of mine, who quit on her own, used these "needle staples" and found them enormously helpful in reducing cravings. "When an urge to smoke comes, you just press the staple, which looks like a gold earring stud, and voilà! the urge magically diminishes. And it doesn't hurt at all."

Acupuncture can be an excellent support, particularly for those who are impatient with making lists and who don't want to analyze, but just want to *quit*. Visits to the acupuncturist or treatment center are usually limited to anywhere between two and five sessions of only a few minutes.

To find an acupuncture practitioner or clinic, write or call the acupuncture reference listed in Appendix 3 and ask for information about referrals.

The Relaxation Response

The "relaxation response" is a term coined by the famous Harvard cardiologist Dr. Herbert Benson. It covers a variety of stress-reduction techniques, all of which involve sitting in a quiet place, progressive muscular relaxation, deep breathing, and inner focusing. There are a thousand approaches to meditation and relaxation—most of them built on Eastern medical or religious practices. Some, like transcendental meditation, involve a mantra, a word or phrase that is repeated over and over again, particular positions (such as the yoga lotus position), and even prayer. Dr. Benson's system is deceptively simple: In a relaxed position, you clear your mind of its usual "busyness," and become aware of your breathing while simply repeating the word "One" silently to yourself. Try it. (For a fuller description, see page 301 in Chapter 21, "New Ways to Mind-Body Health.") Getting the full benefits of the relaxation response, however, is not that easy. Discipline and consistency are required, but it's worth the effort. With practice comes greater proficiency, deeper relaxation, and more health benefits.

The common denominator of all relaxation techniques is a lowering of various physiological functions, including blood pressure, heart rate, and oxygen consumption. Relaxation training is a proven stress-management technique and, as such, can help eliminate the need for smoking and relax the anxious craving for cigarettes. Relaxation techniques may not be all you will need to quit smoking, but they are an excellent way to bolster any plan you may choose. If you can reduce your generalized pool of anxiety and respond more healthfully to stress, you have a better chance of stopping and staying off tobacco. Practicing the relaxation response techniques also brings a host of other health benefits. To learn more, read *The Relaxation Response* by Herbert Benson, M.D. (published in paperback by Avon).

Nicotine Chewing Gum

I've already suggested nicotine chewing gum as a good withdrawal aid. Many ex-smokers swear by it. Only approved a few years ago in the U.S., it has been used for years in Europe and Scandinavia, where it has proved to be moderately successful. In the U.S., it is only available with a doctor's prescription (one brand name: "Nicorette"). Nicotine chewing gum seems best suited for those who are particularly "physically" addicted, though most people who can bear chewing gum find it very helpful indeed. The nicotine in the gum helps satisfy the craving and slowly—after many months—one is encouraged to cut down and stop chewing the gum as well. This second step is made easier by the fact that the gum doesn't taste all that great; it is slightly irritating to the mucous membranes of the throat and mouth.

If you feel that physical addiction to tobacco is one of your biggest obstacles, you may want to try this new approach. *However, people with cancer should not use these products, because nicotine can increase the risk of metastases.* Furthermore, those who choose this method should decide to get off the gum as soon as possible. Talk to your doctor about nicotine chewing gum and whether it's an appropriate choice for you.

Behavior Modification

Behavior therapists are psychologists who use positive or negative (aversive) reinforcement for nonsmoking. You may be taught a host of skills for self-control, or learn to reduce by altering the "trigger" that causes you to smoke. Many of the suggestions I've made in the preceding pages come from behavioral medicine and the behavioral therapists. Most stop-smoking group courses borrow heavily from the behavioral therapists for their techniques. And these techniques work.

If you are giving up outside a group, you might like a session or two with a behavior psychologist to reinforce your resolve and give you additional "tricks" not included in this book. To find such, call the behavioral-science department of a nearby university or medical center, or contact The Association for Advancement of Behavioral Therapy (see Appendix 3).

Some behavior-change techniques are what is known as "aversive," and they are significantly different from the positive reinforcement methods mentioned above and in the preceding pages.

I don't recommend them. They teach by negative reinforcement, and who needs it? The most common technique involves the delivery of mild shocks (electrical impulses) while you're smoking in a clinic. The Schick Institute has Smoking Control Centers throughout the U.S., which provide such shock or "impulse" therapy. Associating smoking behavior with the painful impulses sets up a "counter-conditioning," which, they claim, causes the behavior to cease.

Other aversive therapists use "rapid smoking," a form of forced chain smoking that you must do in a small chamber. In this way, you are forced to experience the full force of the smoke gases, resulting in stifling and stinging sensations, speeded heart rate and blood pressure, coughing, nausea, etc. The method is supposed to help you get the message about how disgusting smoking really is and associate any later smoking with this negative experience. People with known or suspected heart disease, pregnant women, and those with respiratory disorders should not participate in such methods.

There are also drugs and deterrents, such as antismoking lozenges or mouthwashes that have a horrible taste and odor. They are meant to be used after smoking as a form of aversive stimulus.

I can't recommend any of these techniques. They all involve a form of self-punishment that is tantamount to masochism. The intentions of the practitioners may be positive, but the methods range from questionable to deplorable. Although some of the aversive methods claim a rate of success comparable to the other techniques, why choose a punitive approach when you're just as likely to succeed without subjecting yourself to *more* pain and discomfort? You are teaching yourself avoidance of pain instead of searching for maximum health and happiness.

Step Thirteen: You've Done It. Congratulations!

If you've followed all the earlier steps, you will have arrived at Q-Day fully prepared, and now all you have to do is stop on the day you've chosen.

Remember all the tips and keep all the appropriate ones in full operation for at least a month. Eat right. Get lots of sleep. Exercise. Enjoy yourself. And, if you get itchy or depressed, put your work aside and meditate or call a friend or go to the movies—three a day if necessary. Your priority at this time is to stop smoking. You can get back to other duties later. Kissing may be the best oral substitute imaginable—a highly recommended activity.

If you've decided to quit with a group, below are some national organizations that offer quit programs that have proved effective over time. There are undoubtedly other groups that are just as good, but be sure to check them out to see if their particular system fits you. There are live-in programs and five-day plans. Check your yellow pages under

"Smoker's Information and Treatment Centers." Ask in advance what the costs will be, what the dropout rate is, what percentage of people succeed in quitting for an entire year, and whether there is a follow-up program.

The great advantage to a group is that there is a built-in social support system; everyone is in the same boat, and they help each other beat the smoking rap. A group also provides structure, telling you what to do each day or week, so you don't have to build that structure for yourself. There's a lot to be said for quitting this way—especially if you're too busy or disinclined to keep charts, etc.

Stop-Smoking Groups

- *American Cancer Society.* The ACS offers the "Fresh Start Program" in many of its local chapters. The groups usually range between eight and twenty-five people and are led by doctors or trained ex-smokers. There is no charge, and groups meet twice a week for four or five weeks. Group support, behavior modification (*positive* reinforcement), and strategies for dealing with stress and weight control are features of the ACS program. Some ACS quitters' groups use a buddy system, in which you are matched with someone for moral support, and some have a Stay-Off-Smoking hotline you can call seven days a week, twenty-four hours a day. An ACS flyer for the Group Action Method stresses "No fear tactics, no aversion therapy, no cold turkey!" An ex-smoker's club and a Fresh Start kit help with measuring your goals after you've quit. For further information, contact your local chapter of the ACS (see Appendix 3 for the national number and address).
- *Smokenders.* This is a for-profit corporation that offers a comprehensive group program at moderately expensive rates. Six once-a-week, two-hour sessions run individuals $295 per person; special corporate programs charge $225 per person. Introductory seminars and the group sessions take place at hotels, schools, community centers, churches, and some corporations that have accepted the Smokenders corporate program. Despite the cost, Smokenders has some real selling points. For smokers who are threatened by cold turkey, Smokenders offers a gradual, comforting approach. The emphasis is on positive motivation—not fear tactics or pushy group dynamics. You are not expected or encouraged to quit entirely until after the fifth week. The meetings that follow are for all-important reinforcement. For further information, see Appendix 3 for Smokenders.
- *The American Health Foundation.* This health organization sponsors a streamlined, moderately inexpensive five-day course to help you

stop smoking (The Stop Smoking System). You attend lectures, demonstrations, and groups to learn a variety of sophisticated techniques to enable you to stop smoking. These are very careful behavioral methods, including stimulus control (how to change your environment to lessen smoking "trigger" situations), relaxation, imagery, deep breathing, coping skills, and positive reinforcement. Taken together, this program offers a comprehensive yet concentrated stop-smoking plan. (See Appendix 3 for national address and telephone number.)

- *The Seventh-Day Adventist Five-day Plan.* This nonprofit group has sponsored the by-now-famous five-day plan for over twenty-five years. A modest fee pays for five consecutive evening sessions (usually one and a half hours), run by health workers with medical advisors in attendance, and usually occurring in hospital conference rooms or auditoriums. The five-day plan is a cold-turkey approach: you hand in your cigarettes after the first meeting. Lectures on the psychological and physiological aspects of smoking are delivered, films are shown, experiences shared, and stop-smoking procedures are demonstrated. Their emphasis on fear tactics seems to have waned over the years, replaced by positive techniques, focusing on ways to handle the physical urge to smoke with substitutions. A buddy system is sometimes used for support. The five-day plan is well structured and has a documented high rate of success (often well over 50 percent). But be prepared to stop abruptly. (See Appendix 3 for the Seventh-Day Adventist address. Contact them to get information on the five-day plan, given throughout the country.)

- *The American Lung Association.* Their Freedom from Smoking Clinics offer a seven-week course that includes class instruction, written and audio-tape materials, and in some locations a follow-up maintenance group for ex-smokers. Cost varies according to locality. (For further information, see Appendix 3 for address and phone of the ALA.)

No Matter What, Keep Trying

Whatever method you choose, I am passionate on one point: if you fall off the wagon and smoke a cigarette, don't blame yourself or your approach. It's true that often smokers who have gone cold turkey are fine for months until they succumb just once—and then they're back full tilt. The physical craving for nicotine does return, but not all in one instant; more often it's the feeling of guilt and futility that causes one to throw in the towel. Once you've quit, do everything you can to abstain. If you break down and smoke once, don't let demoralization get the best of you; get right back on track. That's how you'll stay off cigarettes for good.

THE SMOKE-FILLED ROOM

With more and more research pointing to the fact that tobacco smoke may cause cancer in nonsmokers, tougher regulations and legislation are popping up throughout the country. The national debate on this question is heating up every day.

Airlines separated smoking and nonsmoking sections some years ago. Smoking is banned altogether in most city buses, subways, and elevators. Many states now restrict smoking to specific areas in public buildings, government offices, restaurants, and hospitals. Some private corporations have followed suit. And undoubtedly many more restrictions will soon follow, as legislation catches up with research findings and the antismoking organizations grow in size and influence.

A three-year study by the EPA estimates that five hundred to five thousand nonsmokers die of lung cancer caused by "sidestream" smoke from others' cigarettes. Tobacco smoke is a major indoor pollutant in homes and especially in sealed ("sick") buildings. A 1980 report in the *New England Journal of Medicine* indicated that nonsmokers who work near smokers suffer as much loss of lung function as those who smoke about half a pack a day.

Much of the political action for smoke-free inside air has come from two citizen groups: ASH (Action on Smoking and Health) and GASP (Group Against Smoking Pollution). ASH is a national nonprofit organization dedicated to the health consequences of smoking in the environment. It lobbies for the rights of nonsmokers, pushes for laws and public ordinances to segregate smokers, and establishes smoke-free work areas.

GASP is a nonprofit environmental action group concerned with the hazards of tobacco smoke. It has many offices throughout the country, and is conspicuous in educational and legal efforts to protect the public from sidestream smoke.

To help you protect yourself in your work environment or in public places you frequent, you may want to contact ASH, GASP, or another organization that is active for nonsmokers. They may be able to monitor the area in question, initiate legal actions, or help you organize reforms that keep your work environment clear of irritating and dangerous smoke. People with asthma, allergies, emphysema, or bronchitis can be made sicker in a smoke-filled room; they are especially entitled to live and work in spaces free of this hazard. For more information on ASH or GASP, you can find the address and telephone in Appendix 3.

On your own, don't be afraid to speak up and protest when friends, family members, co-workers, or even strangers pollute your environment with smoke. You have a right to insist that you not be a victim of someone else's habit. For those of you who smoke, become a nonsmoker and join the ranks of the public action groups. But first you can stop and congratulate yourself on a difficult job well done.

10

Alcohol and Recreational Drugs

With so much attention focused on smoking and diet, few people are aware that high alcohol consumption drastically increases our risk of several cancers—especially if combined with smoking. Fewer still are aware that certain recreational drugs may increase cancer risk because they diminish the potency of our immune reactions.

I am not equipped—nor do I wish—to deal here with alcoholism, a real disease/addiction that is best addressed by alcoholism counselors and recovering alcoholics, with their nationwide organization Alcoholics Anonymous. AA can offer the best support for those suffering from this disease, with their thousands of support groups, recovery centers, and educational materials available throughout the world. Most admitted alcoholics are aware of the many health threats he or she faces. We now know that the list includes cancer.

What I want to address primarily is the threat of drinking for those who drink fairly heavily but are able to cut back on their consumption—those who can control the number of drinks they take. This group may not be aware of the cancer risks, and can moderate their intake accordingly, perhaps without additional outside help.

ALCOHOL AND CANCER

Alcohol is not, in a strict sense, a direct cause of cancer. In laboratory studies with animals, ethanol alone does not trigger malignant growth. Scientists believe that alcohol acts rather as a co-carcinogen—or promoter—enhancing the effects of other carcinogens, especially tobacco smoke. Alcohol can also suppress the immune system.

The link between alcohol and malignancy is strongest in cancers of the mouth, pharynx, larynx, and esophagus—sometimes referred to as

172

"cancers of the head and neck." Recently, breast cancer was added to the list. The highest risks for contracting these cancers occur when one drinks *and* smokes. By drinking heavily, you may increase your risk two to three times over that of nondrinkers. Drinking *and* smoking do not just add to your risk; they multiply it!

The more you drink, the greater the danger. Two drinks a day probably don't increase cancer risk if your nutrition is good, and alcohol, in moderation, may have some relaxing benefits. Three or four are enough to increase your risk slightly, but the risk rises sharply at more than six drinks per day. For the most part, studies to date show that the amount, not the *type*, of alcoholic beverage makes the difference. One 1981 study did indicate that beer and wine increased risk of oral cancers more than hard liquor. But a 1980 study concluded that whiskey was more likely to raise the risk of laryngeal cancer. And a 1978 population study of black men in Washington, D.C., correlated the very high rate of cancer of the esophagus there (28.6 per 100,000) with a much higher rate of alcohol consumption than the national average for black males. Hard liquor in particular was implicated, as it has been in other population studies that have connected drinking with cancer of the esophagus.

Other cancers that have been linked, though less strongly, to alcohol are liver, pancreas, stomach, thyroid, and colorectal cancers.

Here is a breakdown of cancers associated with drinking and some of the supporting evidence for linkage:

Oral, pharynx, and larynx: An estimated 75 percent of these cancers are due to a combination of smoking and drinking.

Breast: A recent study of the Harvard School of Public Health, published in the *New England Journal of Medicine,* followed nearly 90,000 women between 34 and 59 years old. Women who consumed 0–2 drinks a week had no increased risk of breast cancer; 3–9 drinks a week drove up risk 30 percent; and 9 or more drinks increased risk by 60 percent. Younger women appear to be most affected.

Esophagus: Cancer of the esophagus is twenty-five times more likely to occur in heavy drinkers than in the nondrinking population.

Liver: Primary liver cancer is rare in the U.S. However, cirrhosis of the liver appears to be a risk factor for liver cancer, and cirrhosis is frequently caused by heavy drinking. Other possible dangers include the combined effects of drinking and the poor nutrition that often accompanies heavy drinking.

Pancreas, thyroid, stomach, and large bowel and rectum: Evidence for the relationship between alcohol and these cancers exists, though it is less convincing.

HOW ALCOHOL INCREASES RISK

Alcohol can be a tumor promoter. Without question, it acts synergistically to increase the cancer-causing capacity of tobacco. Alcohol acts as a solvent, aiding in the transport of carcinogens across cell membranes. This may explain the powerful carcinogenic effects drinking and smoking have on the oral cavities, where both alcohol and smoke come in direct contact with bodily tissues. By damaging liver cells, alcohol decreases the liver's detoxifying powers and allows exposure to carcinogens, which can't be eliminated by a damaged liver. Some alcoholic beverages contain contaminants—either accidental or added—that can be carcinogenic, such as PAHs, nitrosamines, urethane, and possibly asbestos fibers from filtration processes. (Contact the Center for Science in the Public Interest if you're concerned about a particular brand of liquor or wine—see Appendix 3.) Some studies have associated alcohol's capacity to suppress immunity with the increased risk of cancers of the head and neck.

Recommendations

Restrict your daily intake of alcohol to no more than one or two drinks—liquor, beer, or wine. If you smoke heavily, cut back as much as possible on your alcohol intake.

Pregnant women should not drink at all because of the higher risks of having babies with fetal alcohol syndrome or other physical and mental disorders.

If you do drink, make sure to maintain a healthy diet. Poor nutrition has been identified as a co-factor in alcohol's role as a cancer promoter.

Be sure to eat more foods and take additional supplements of vitamins A, C, and B-complex. Vitamins A and C can combat free radicals produced in the liver through exposure to alcohol. Both A and C have powers to prevent several of the cancers linked to alcohol—including esophageal, throat, and stomach cancers. Vitamins B_1, B_6, and folic acid may be deficient in heavy drinkers, and the latter two are crucial to immunity. Stick with the CPDG and its suggestions for drinkers (see page 128) and you may moderate the damage caused by alcohol.

RECREATIONAL DRUGS

The evidence of links between recreational drugs (such as marijuana, cocaine, or heroin) and cancer is quite indirect. The main problem found with some of these drugs, particularly if abused, is the suppression of immunity. This, we know, represents a weakening of our cancer defense and possible increased susceptability.

People who use hypodermics to self-administer drugs like morphine and heroin are prone to many virulent infections. Doctors believe that unsterilized needles are the primary cause. Now another factor is coming to light: the drugs themselves suppress immunity and make the drug user more vulnerable to any infectious agent.

A recent Italian study examined the effects of morphine on rabbits and mice. When the morphine-treated animals were infected with a common fungus, they had a higher mortality rate than an untreated control group. It was apparent that the morphine damaged the effectiveness of macrophages in their ability to scavenge invading bacteria, viruses, and fungi. The drug also shrank the liver, kidneys, and spleen (where macrophages are stored).

The damaging effect of morphine (and perhaps heroin) on immunity may be another reason, besides infected needles, that intravenous drug abusers are so vulnerable to AIDS. When the AIDS epidemic first struck, and before HIV was implicated as the primary viral cause, there were many theories about the causes of the disease. One early notion was based on the frequency of drug abuse among AIDS victims who were also homosexuals. Although records indicated a high level of recreational drug use among AIDS victims, including marijuana, barbiturates, amphetamines, cocaine, and LSD, one unusual drug turned up with alarming frequency: nitrite inhalants. Large quantities of amyl and butyl nitrites—commonly known as "poppers"—had been inhaled often by these patients. For a short period, speculation abounded as to the possible contribution of poppers to the cause of AIDS.

We now know that HIV is the necessary cause of AIDS, but that other factors, including viral infections, other sexually transmitted diseases, and drug abuse weaken the immune system and leave it incapacitated. These other factors are the fertile ground that enables HIV to replicate and wreak full damage on our immune cells.

Poppers appear to be immunosuppressive, and their use was found to be especially common among the AIDS patients who also suffered from Kaposi's sarcoma (KS). KS attacks the blood vessels, and poppers are known "vasodilators"; they directly affect the blood vessels. The link between nitrite inhalants and Kaposi's sarcoma, though not fully understood, is still strong enough to militate against ever using these drugs.

Amphetamines are often prescribed as appetite suppressants or antidepressants, though they are often abused as recreational drugs. Some studies have linked amphetamines with a high risk of Hodgkin's disease. "Speed," as amphetamines are commonly called, should therefore be avoided.

Marijuana is a tricky question. Although this drug is not considered very dangerous, there is increasing evidence as to its ability to dampen our immune power. The chemical constitutent of marijuana known as THC—delta-9-tetrahydrocannabinol—seems to be the immunosuppressive culprit. A 1979 study at Columbia University showed that a group of chronic pot smokers had much lower blood levels of IgG-type antibodies, which are part of our first-line defense against bacteria, viruses, and other antigens in the blood. Macrophages may also be impaired in their normal activities in the body.

A study at Tufts University showed that THC suppresses the activity of natural killer (NK) cells in rats. NK cells are able to search out and destroy cancer cells, and any loss in their potency is a potential threat to our cancer defense. Interferon, that natural antiviral cell product, is another vital cog in our cancer defense that could be compromised by marijuana. Researchers at the Medical College of Virginia found that THC-treated animals responded very poorly to an incoming virus: interferon production took about six times longer than normal to get started. These same investigators also found impairments in T-cell immunity and antibody production in animals treated with amounts of THC considered high but not far beyond the equivalent, in human terms, of several joints a day.

All of this does not necessarily translate to human beings. There is no hard-core proof that marijuana suppresses human immune systems in the same manner, though it is likely that some of these effects do occur. How much and how seriously is still unknown. If you use marijuana, you may notice that you are more prone to allergies, colds, or other infections after indulging. You should consider the possibility that your immune system is being compromised and either cut down or quit completely. As for other forms of drug use or abuse, you can now add a damaged immune system to the list of probable dangers to your health.

11

X-Rays and Prescription Drugs

Over the past twenty years, many of us have developed a healthy suspicion of diagnostic x-rays—and not without reason. Former NCI director Dr. Arthur Upton once estimated that diagnostic x-rays cause approximately 3,670 cancer deaths each year in the U.S.

However, there is some good news to report: the amount of radiation released in most common diagnostic x-ray procedures is far less than it used to be. In the recent past, radiologists have employed techniques to minimize the field of x-ray exposure; and lead shields and aprons are used to cover parts of the body, including the reproductive organs, for which no picture is needed. Many new diagnostic techniques are being developed that have no radiation effects at all.

Despite these advances, there still appear to be a surprising number of x-ray procedures conducted without sufficient reason. Some are done for the legal protection of the practitioner, while others are ordered when previous pictures—or pictures from other doctors or institutions—could be made available. In addition, the best-known techniques for limiting the amount of x-ray exposure may not be employed by any given practitioner, and some x-ray units may not be up to current standards required by state laws. For these reasons, *it is still important not to expose yourself to more x-rays than are absolutely necessary.*

In radiation therapy, which is used to treat cancer and other diseases, the exposure is considerably higher, but the higher risks must be balanced against the potential benefits. The same is true of some prescription drugs—estrogen, the immunosuppressive drugs, and certain anticancer agents. When these medical treatments are prescribed, the benefits usually outweigh the risks involved, though sometimes they don't. It is very important to discuss the benefits-versus-risks issue fully with your doctor before undergoing radiation, transplantation, or various forms of chemotherapy.

THE DANGERS OF X-RAYS: RECENT REVELATIONS

X-rays, which are a form of ionizing radiation, were first discovered in 1895 by Wilhelm Conrad Roentgen, professor of physics at the Bavarian University of Würzburg. Although x-rays had probably been produced by a number of physicists since the latter part of the eighteenth century, Roentgen was the first to recognize the power of his materials and how they could be put to use.

Medically, x-rays were employed rather widely in the early part of this century—especially with skin diseases—but the hazardous, long-term effects weren't fully recognized at that time. Between the 1930s and 1950s, numerous studies were made that showed the danger of too many exposures to x-rays. From 1935 to 1954, a group of women underwent fluoroscopy, an x-ray procedure designed to assess the effectiveness of their treatment for tuberculosis. The women received high doses of 150 rads (see page 179) to the chest. Ten years later, the women were found to have a higher incidence of breast cancer than normal. In the 1940s, another study found that physicians suffered about twice the incidence of leukemia of the general population. And radiologists, in particular, had a mortality rate from leukemia ten times greater than other physicians.

An early example of the risks of medical radiation therapy occurred before 1950. Children were often treated for various benign conditions of the head and neck, including enlarged thymus glands, with high levels of radiation. Many years later, it was found that these individuals were contracting thyroid cancer and leukemia at a much higher rate than normal.

HOW X-RAYS WORK

X-rays are electromagnetic waves. They are a step shorter than ultraviolet rays and are equally invisible. In this part of the light spectrum, radiation absorption becomes very great. It is because of this property that x-rays can pass through "softer material" such as flesh and stop at denser material, such as bones, or, in the case of stomach or colon x-rays, the denser barium that has either been swallowed or flooded into the lower bowel and colon.

The radiation, absorbed in the tissues as x-rays pass through them, is powerful enough to knock electrons out of their orbit around atoms, producing the unstable molecules that can lead to the formation of dangerous free radicals. Radiation can also cause the chromosome breaks or genetic mutations that sometimes lead to cancer.

Rads

The units that measure the amount of radiation absorbed by body tissues are called "rads" (radiation absorbed dose). Everyone is exposed to about 0.1 or 0.2 rads every year through "background radiation" from natural sources like cosmic rays or radioactive substances in rocks and water. Whole-body irradiation of many hundreds of rads are enough to cause death within a short period—but if radiation exposure is broken up and the whole body is not exposed, the short-term effects are not lethal. In the case of radiation therapy for cancer, patients may receive 200 rads a day to a section of their bodies many times over a period of weeks and months. In these cases, the cancer-causing effects, if any, may not be known for many years.

Diagnostic and therapeutic x-rays are usually measured in millirads (mrads—thousandths of a rad). The number of millirads transmitted in diagnostic x-rays varies greatly from procedure to procedure, and the number can vary for the same procedure given with different equipment in different settings. The amount of skin exposure—though it does not tell you how much various internal organs or bone marrow gets—gives you a general idea of the amount of radiation involved in different examinations. The following table indicates the range per picture of acceptable skin exposures for several routine x-ray examinations (remember, x-ray exams involve more than one picture).

If you are concerned about your x-ray exposure owing to many examinations, ask your radiologist to give you an idea of the number of

Examination	Skin exposure (mrads per projection)
Chest (PA)	12–26
Skull (lateral)	105–240
Abdomen (AP)	375–698
Retrograde pyelogram	475–829
Cervical spine (AP)	35–165
Thoracic spine (AP)	295–485
Extremity	8–327
Dental (bitewing and periapical)	227–425

Table from *Merrill's Atlas of Radiographic Positions and Radiologic Procedures*, sixth edition, by Phillip W. Ballinger, published by the C. V. Mosby Company.

millirads per picture. You may not get an answer, but it is worth a try. You may be able to determine, based on comparison with the above table, whether you're getting more mrads than are considered acceptable.

MAMMOGRAMS

One of the biggest controversies has been waged over the use of x-ray mammography as a means of early detection of breast cancer. Mammograms used to involve high doses of radiation; newer techniques involve levels that can be considered "low-dose"—less than one rad. The primary concern about safety with regard to mammograms is whether you are being screened with the latest low-dose equipment or not.

For women who have no symptoms, the American Cancer Society recommends one baseline mammogram for women between 35 and 39; one mammogram every 1–2 years between the ages of 40 and 49; and annual exams after 50. These recommendations are particularly important for women considered high risk because of a family history of breast cancer. For women who have symptoms—namely, any kind of suspicious lumps—mammography can help with diagnosis.

Given the important role of mammograms in early detection of breast cancer, levels of radiation exposure are of the utmost concern. I asked Jack Edeikan, M.D., Professor of Radiology at the University of Texas/M. D. Anderson Hospital and Tumor Institute, and Chairman of the Education Commission of the American College of Radiology, how women can find out if they're really getting low-dose mammograms.

"The main question you can ask," said Dr. Edeikan, "is 'Do you have a dedicated mammogram machine?' This is your best hint—if the machine is only being used for breast work. The other thing for women being screened to look for, is whether it [the unit] is approved by the American Cancer Society. The American Cancer Society and the American College of Radiology have a review program which establishes quality and dose for screening. If they get approval, then you know you're safe."

Dr. Edeikan also clarified some of the terms used for the newer mammographic equipment. "A 'film/screen combination' gives you the lowest dose . . . and then there's xerography, which is a little higher dose. But the modern xerography is still a low dose." Although there are varying figures for the number of mrads per picture with low-dose mammography, Edeikan said that the breast itself receives about 70–200 mrads. (This is an approximation because the dose to the inside of the breast is hard to measure; the estimate is based on calculations from skin exposure, which is greater.)

The following table gives you representative skin exposures, and approximate glandular exposures (how much the breast gets) for three types of mammography—the old "direct exposure" (too high); xeromammography (low-dose); and screen/film (the lowest dose).

Examination	Skin exposure per projection (mrad)	Approximate glandular dose per projection (mrad)
Direct exposure	6,000–15,000	2,500
Xeromammography	500–1,500	400
Screen/film	200–1,000	75

Table from *Merrill's Atlas of Radiographic Positions and Radiologic Procedures,* sixth edition, by Phillip W. Ballinger, published by the C. V. Mosby Company.

Depending on how concerned and/or gutsy you are, you can also ask your doctor, radiologist, or technician: "Is this machine calibrated?" If the answer is yes, you can ask, "How many millirads will I get to the center of my breast?" According to Dr. Edeikan, he or she should be able to answer this question.

However you decide to approach the problem, you should ask questions based on the above facts and expect answers. As Dr. Edeikan has remarked, "I wouldn't want a woman screened every year if she were getting two or three rads [2,000–3,000 millirads] per exposure."

Remember—as long as you're getting low-dose mammography, regular screening according to the ACS guidelines is recommended for early detection of breast cancer, which can substantially improve the prospects of cure.

PREGNANCY AND YOUNG CHILDREN

There has been evidence showing that prenatal exposure to radiation, occurring when women receive diagnostic x-rays during pregnancy, causes a somewhat higher risk of leukemia to the child by the age of sixteen. For this reason, avoid x-rays during pregnancy at all costs—and if you are prescribed x-rays, be sure to advise your doctor if you suspect you might be pregnant.

Infants and young children are especially susceptible to the ionizing radiation of x-rays. They should not receive any routine or unnecessary x-rays, and be given special protection when they are necessary.

COMMONSENSE GUIDELINES TO FOLLOW FOR X-RAYS

- Make sure that a medical or dental x-ray is absolutely necessary. Don't be afraid to ask your doctor for an explanation as to why he considers it important.
- Ask for lead shields for parts of the body not being x-rayed—especially the reproductive organs and the thymus gland (irradiation of the thymus can cause potential damage to your immune functions). These precautions may or may not be possible, depending on the procedure, but don't hesitate to ask your doctor, radiologist, or technician for a full explanation.
- Avoid repeat x-rays. If you go to another doctor for a second opinion, find out if previous x-rays will suffice.
- Pregnant women and all children should avoid x-rays whenever possible.
- Make sure you are taking the optimal doses of beta-carotene and vitamins C and E suggested in the Cancer-Prevention Diet Guide. These antioxidant vitamins may help protect you from radiation-induced free-radical damage.

RADIATION THERAPY

When radiation is prescribed as a treatment for cancer, very often it is the most effective treatment available and is well worth the risk of later cancer. The risk may be quite small, and is insignificant compared to the benefits of treating your cancer effectively, which may include saving your life.

There is always some risk where radiation exposure is involved. When it is prescribed, discuss all the options with your physician. If it is clearly the best option for the particular stage of your disease, it will be worth the risk. If your doctor or oncologist offers comparable alternatives, consider them seriously.

Two of the guidelines suggested for diagnostic x-rays also apply to people undergoing radiation therapy: request proper lead shielding of other parts of the body, and take the recommended amounts of beta-carotene, and vitamins C and E.

PRESCRIPTION DRUGS

The three main classes of drugs that include known cancer-causing or promoting agents are:

- Estrogens
- Anticancer drugs
- Immunosuppressive drugs

In the past ten years, the estrogens have been the source of major controversy over their possible long-term carcinogenic effects—particularly in regard to oral contraceptives and estrogen replacement therapy (ERT) for postmenopausal women. As scientists have learned more about estrogens and how to combine them safely with other hormones, most of the controversy has died down, and the safe use of them is fairly well established.

Immunosuppressive drugs and certain anticancer agents present a different problem altogether. Here the dangers are fairly well known, but in many cases, the benefits of using them to save a life or eliminate pain outweigh the risks of causing cancer later in life. Certainly any drug that has carcinogenic or immunosuppressive capacities should be avoided, if possible, and alternatives sought. The main point is to be aware of the potential benefits and risks, and to participate in the decision with your doctor. Here my purpose is simply to identify the questionable drugs and urge you to discuss the options with your physician.

The Estrogens

Estrogens, the female hormones, have been a recurring item in the news for the last decade. The question that has stirred debate is: Do estrogens—whether in birth-control pills or in replacement therapy for postmenopausal women—cause cancer? The answer has finally become, if not crystal clear, a lot sharper than it ever was before. If used properly, oral contraceptives and estrogen replacement therapy (ERT) should not cause cancer. In the case of ERT, a proper regimen can actually *prevent* cancer.

"E.R.T. today is very different from the therapy prescribed even a decade ago," writes Dr. Lila E. Nachtigall, Associate Professor of Obstetrics and Gynecology at New York University School of Medicine. "Our knowledge has vastly increased since then and techniques have been greatly refined. Today, E.R.T., according to virtually all of the recent and most respected studies, has been shown not only to be remarkably effective but also remarkably safe." In her book *Estrogen: The Facts Can Save Your Life*, Dr. Nachtigall makes a compelling case in favor of judicious and carefully monitored ERT for women who need it and who have not had breast or uterine cancer. She also cites a major advance—the use of the "transdermal patch," which sticks to the skin and delivers a low dose at a controlled rate—more the way estrogen is released naturally by the ovaries. This method is probably safer than taking pills.

Estrogens are produced mainly in the ovaries and adrenal cortex. They help regulate menstruation and pregnancy, and are responsible for the development of secondary sexual characteristics. There are three different types of estrogens—estradiol, estriol, and estrone. Cells of the uterus, breast, and ovaries contain "receptors" (molecules on their surfaces that "receive") for estrogen, and are therefore estrogen "sensitive." Estrogens can stimulate the glandular tissue of the breast and uterine endometrium in such a way that cells proliferate. If this proliferation goes out of control, a tumor can develop. Progesterone is one type of estrogen that can offset or moderate the stimulating effects of other estrogens.

Estrogens are used in ERT to treat the symptoms of menopause, when the ovaries decrease production of these hormones in the body. A carefully administered ERT regimen will dramatically relieve common symptoms of menopause, including hot flashes and sweating, vaginal atrophy, and osteoporosis. This therapy can truly restore a vital sexuality and stop bone loss in postmenopausal women who suffer from estrogen deficiency. A number of recent studies strongly suggest that estrogen replacement is more effective at reversing osteoporosis than calcium, and that ERT may help calcium to do its job of maintaining healthy bones. The probable reason is that estrogen deficiency—not low calcium—is the greater culprit in osteoporosis.

The use of replacement estrogen has been linked to cancers of the endometrium, which is the lining of the uterus. One early study concluded that women who take estrogen for more than seven years increase their risk of cancer of the endometrium fourteen times. The researchers also determined that women who stopped taking replacement estrogen will decrease their risk of this cancer to normal levels after two years. When estrogen alone is used, the increased risk has been estimated at from two to twenty times that for the average nonuser.

The big breakthrough with regard to ERT has been the use of lower dosages of estrogen, combined, for part of each month, with progesterone. Several major studies have indicated that replacement regimens combining estrogen with progesterone not only eliminate risk of endometrial cancer, they lower it. For example, Dr. Nachtigall followed a group of 168 patients, half on combination ERT and half taking placebos. After ten years, one case of endometrial cancer and four cases of breast cancer turned up in the placebo group, while *no* cases of either cancer turned up in the group on ERT.

There has been a lot of research devoted to finding out whether replacement estrogen therapy increases women's risk of breast cancer. The answer still isn't completely clear. Some studies have shown an increased risk, especially in long-term users, while others have shown a decrease in the risk of breast cancer. Once again, it appears that low-dose estrogen (such as 0.625 to 1.25 Premarin) combined with progesterone is the safest regimen—far less likely to cause breast cancer and perhaps responsible for preventing some breast cancers.

A 1986 study of the Centers for Disease Control, published in the *Journal of the American Medical Association,* compared the medical records of 1,400 breast-cancer patients and 1,600 women without the disease. There was no increased risk for women on ERT, even if they'd been taking estrogen for twenty years. There was, however, a twofold increase of breast cancer among long-term estrogen users who had had their ovaries removed.

Women with a family history of breast cancer, who have benign breast disease, or who have had their ovaries removed should consult their doctors. ERT may not be advisable for them. Women who have had breast cancer need to find out if it is of the "estrogen-dependent" type, which is more common before menopause. If so, they definitely should not go on ERT. If they have had "non-estrogen-dependent" breast tumors, more common after menopause, then ERT can be considered. You must find out from your doctor your tumor type, and whether replacement therapy is appropriate.

Birth-control pills are mainly composed of synthetic estrogens. Most common are combination pills, which contain both estrogen and progesterone. Up until the late 1970s, another form of birth-control pills was available, known as "sequential" pills. Sequential pills provided the estrogen and progesterone separately and in sequences. It was found clearly that the sequential form increased women's risk of cancer of the endometrium, and so they were taken off the market.

Ironically, combination pills, now the most widely used and effective oral contraceptives, may actually protect women from cancer of the ovary or endometrium. The Center for Disease Control estimated in 1983 that such pills might prevent 1,700 cases of ovarian cancer and 2,000 cases of endometrial cancer each year.

However, the pill as it is commonly used today cannot be completely cleared of worrisome health risks. Although the evidence does not point to increased risk of breast cancer for most women, certain subgroups of women may be more likely to develop breast cancer if they've taken the pill for long periods.* Women with a family history of breast cancer, or those with benign breast disease (fibrocystic disease) may add to their cancer risk by taking oral contraceptives. In one study,

*A 1988 study by the Centers for Disease Control and the National Institute of Child Health and Human Development found no evidence that early use of birth control pills increased breast cancer risk. The researchers did not eliminate the possibility that the pill could increase risk after a very long latency period, though they regarded this as unlikely. It was the largest study of its kind.

long-term users under the age of thirty-six who had taken combination pills with a high dose of progesterone had a fourfold increase in breast cancer. Another report showed an increased risk for current pill users over forty-five years old—and especially for those older than fifty-one. There is also concern that long-term birth-control-pill taking is associated with certain very rare liver tumors.

DES (diethylstilbestrol) is a synthetic estrogen. During the 1940s, 1950s, and early 1960s, DES was given to expectant mothers to avert miscarriages. Although laboratory evidence showed that DES could cause cancer, its use continued and was not questioned until the 1970s, when a rare form of vaginal and cervical cancer was found in some of the daughters of women who took the drug during pregnancy. The DES research of the last decade has shown that a carcinogen could travel across the placental barrier and affect the fetus.

It is estimated that between 4 and 6 million people in the U.S.—mothers, daughters, and sons—were exposed to DES during pregnancy. The women who took it may have a very slightly increased risk of breast cancer and cancers of the ovary and cervix. The daughters of mothers who took DES during pregnancy are more likely to contract "clear-cell" carcinoma of the vagina and cervix than those unexposed. It should be remembered, however, that this is still a very rare cancer, even among DES daughters. These daughters are also more likely to have some precancerous cellular changes in the cervix, which may or may not indicate increased risk of cervical cancer. The sons of mothers who took DES have been found to have a greater likelihood of certain reproductive-tract abnormalities, undescended testicles (a risk factor for testicular cancer), and possibly infertility.

Although the FDA has not approved it for this purpose, DES is still being prescribed as a morning-after contraceptive and as a treatment for menopausal symptoms. These uses are questionable. Ironically, this drug, which has caused many cancers and much suffering, is quite effective in ameliorating the symptoms and controlling the growth of prostate cancer in men.

Here is a set of commonsense guidelines for the medical use of estrogens, with special attention to the issues of cancer prevention:

For ERT

- Consider ERT only when it is really needed for symptoms of estrogen deficiency.
- Before starting therapy, have a *complete* medical checkup, including a determination of whether you are at high risk for breast or endometrial cancer. If so, ERT should be avoided.

- ERT is safest and most effective with small doses of estrogen (commonly, between 0.625 and 1.25 mg. of conjugated estrogen [Premarin]).
- Estrogen must be combined with progesterone for part of the monthly cycle.
- Long-term use may be preferable for women suffering bone loss (osteoporosis) and short-term may be preferable for those suffering disruptive symptoms of menopause.
- ERT is not considered advisable for women who have had estrogen-dependent breast cancer, endometrial cancer, coronary artery disease, strokes, blood clots, migraines, or liver disease, or who have had their ovaries removed.
- ERT may not be advised for women with a family history of breast cancer.
- ERT may not be advised for women with fibroids, though you should check this with your doctor.
- Any vaginal bleeding should be investigated, whether before or during estrogen replacement therapy.
- After going on ERT, it is important that you have periodic checkups by your doctor or gynecologist that include complete breast and pelvic examinations.

For Oral Contraceptives

- Birth-control pills are not advisable for the following groups:
  Premenopausal women over age forty-five; especially those over fifty-one
  Young women prior to first full-term pregnancy
  Women with a family history of breast cancer
  Women who have or have had benign breast disease
  Women with a late age of first childbirth
  Women at risk for cervical cancer because of sexual activity patterns (multiple partners)
- Women under thirty should avoid prolonged use of high-potency birth-control pills.

For DES

- Pregnant women should not take DES for any reason.
- Mothers and daughters exposed to large doses of DES should avoid further use of estrogens.
- Mothers, sons, and daughters exposed to large doses of DES should be examined by a doctor for abnormalities of the reproductive organs.
- DES as a morning-after pill is not recommended.

Anticancer Drugs

Anticancer agents save thousands of lives each year. The most common anticancer drugs are categorized as chemotherapy. Chemotherapy agents usually have serious side effects—some more than others—as normal cells are also affected by toxic chemicals intended to destroy the cancer-cell populations.

One particular class of anticancer drugs can increase the risk of second cancers, but remember: most anticancer chemotherapy drugs do *not* have this effect. Drugs of this class are called *alkylating agents*, or sometimes referred to as the *mustard* group. This group is used to treat various cancers, though Hodgkin's disease most often.

Alkylating agents disrupt the genetic machinery of cancer cells, causing them to stop growing and proliferating. Yet these agents can also cause additional genetic mutations, leading to acute leukemias, usually within four to five years of treatment. One study conducted between 1961 and 1973 showed that Hodgkin's-disease patients were developing AML (acute myelocytic leukemia) at a rate much higher than normal, and a chemotherapy protocol used during those years was the suspected cause. This regimen included two agents from the mustard group—*nitrogen mustard* and *procarbazine.* Radiation therapy in addition to this drug regimen increased the risk of leukemia even further.

The drug *melphalan,* another alkylating agent, has been used to treat the type of cancer called *multiple myeloma,* a malignant disease of the bone marrow. Studies have shown that multiple myeloma patients treated with melphalan are at much higher risk for leukemia later on. Women treated for ovarian cancer with melphalan and another drug called *chlorambucil* are also at increased risk of developing leukemia. This problem also exists when alkylating agents are used to treat lung cancer, non-Hodgkin's lymphoma, and certain blood disorders. Another alkylating agent called *semustine* is used to treat stomach and colorectal cancers. One study indicated that semustine used for these cancers multiplied the patient's risk of leukemia by sixteen.

For the most part, these *alkylating agents* have been used to treat very serious or terminal cancers, when the potential life-saving benefits far outstripped the risk of later leukemia. Recently, some new drugs, developed to treat the above cancers, are less or not at all carcinogenic, so in many cases there are alternatives to alkylating agents. However, each individual case is different. If your oncologist has prescribed such an agent, there may or may not be an alternative. But it is an issue you should discuss freely with your doctor.

Immunosuppressive Drugs

Organ-transplant patients must be given special drugs that suppress their immune systems, so they won't reject the incoming foreign tissue. But the immunosuppressive drugs also increase the risk of certain cancers, in all probability because the immune system is also restricted in its ability to combat the rise of cancer cells. *Imuran* (azathioprine) and a number of adrenal corticosteroid hormones have often been used in kidney tranplants, and recently a drug called *cyclosporin A* has been used for this purpose. A 1973 investigation showed that these transplant patients contract a cancer referred to as non-Hodgkin's lymphoma at a rate thirty-two times higher than the normal population. Skin cancers and lung cancers also have occurred at a higher rate among transplant recipients. Kaposi's sarcoma, the cancer that often strikes AIDS patients whose immune systems have been battered by their disease, can occur—though rarely—in transplant patients whose immune systems have been compromised by immunosuppressive drugs.

OTHER DRUGS TO WATCH FOR

- The pain-killing drug *phenacetin* has been linked to kidney cancer.
- *Radioactive drugs* can be used in various diagnostic tests and to treat thyroid cancer, bone tuberculosis, and the blood disorder called *polycythemia vera*. Some of these drugs can concentrate in the tissues and increase the risk of acute myelocytic leukemia, bone cancer, or rare liver cancers.
- *Methoxypsoralens,* used with ultraviolet-A radiation in the treatment of psoriasis, has been linked to skin cancers.
- *Amphetamine* (Dexedrine) is used as an appetite depressant or anti-depressant drug. Amphetamines have been associated with higher risk of Hodgkin's disease, though this finding is still preliminary.

The message I'd like to emphasize is that for some of the drugs mentioned above the cancer risk is very small, while for others the risk is appreciable. Therefore, don't be alarmed if one of these drugs is prescribed for you. Find out as much as you can, and *ask a lot of questions.* The risks may be worth it—or they may not.

12

Suntanning

Surprisingly, suntanning has become an addictive leisure-time behavior for many Americans, on the order of compulsive shopping or TV watching. While the latter compulsions may pinch your pocketbook or dull your senses, suntanning has a different effect: it can increase your risk of skin cancer.

Newsweek, in a June 1986 issue, quotes a California woman: "I tried to stop, but I just can't. I mean, I'll think: Okay, today I'm going to stay inside and watch T.V. But then I'll see my neighbor lying out next to the pool and I'll say, well, five minutes won't hurt. And then it's three hours later and I'm working on the insides of my ankles. I started out like most people—at the beach. But then I began pretending I was going to town so I could sit at the bus stop for an hour or two. One day my husband caught me in the parking lot, trying to catch the reflections off a Porsche. That's when I realized I had a tanning problem."

Such a compulsion may be bred by affluence. Many of us don't have the leisure time to lie in the sun, nor do we all live in climates that enable us to indulge year round. Nevertheless, few of us have really taken seriously the warnings of dermatologists about the long-term (if not short-term) effects of the sun on our skin, and taken the necessary precautions to protect ourselves from cancer. The skin cancers caused by the ultraviolet light of the sun represent the single largest category of malignancies—over 400,000 per year. Most are curable, though they can entail costly, unpleasant, or sometimes deforming surgery. And a small percentage of skin cancers—the melanomas—are truly life-threatening.

SUNNING AND SKIN CANCER

Whether or not you are a sun addict, like the California woman, you are at risk in the sun, even if you tan only now and then—especially if you burn easily. A lot depends on your skin type (see ahead), a lot depends on your geographical location and the time of day you are exposed, and a lot depends on how often and how long you stay out.

Dermatologists now believe that any substantial exposure to the sun starts a cumulative effect that increases over the years and may eventually lead to cancer. If you start suntanning at four, you may be in trouble by the time you're forty. "It's like filling a bottle," says Dr. Henry Wiley III of the University of South Florida. "Last week's suntan gets added to a lifetime's worth of exposure."

All skin cancers have been on a sharp rise in the last fifty years, and malignant melanoma, a very dangerous cancer that can be deadly, has risen 900 percent since 1930, when one in 1,500 people contracted it. Now, one in 100 do.

The much publicized depletion of the atmospheric ozone layer means that we will all probably be exposed to more ultraviolet light, the cause of skin cancer. This is one more reason to protect ourselves.

Tan, the Elite Color

What has caused the tremendous increase in sunning? No one is exactly sure but there is speculation that tan didn't become the chic skin tone until the 1920s, when clothes grew scantier and delicate white skin was no longer a badge of the gentry. For chic, the colors had to change. A bronze complexion, formerly (for whites) the sign of being a farmer or outdoor laborer, soon became the gold medal of the country club set and subsequently the jet set. Hundreds and thousands of people took to the rooftops of New York or the beaches of Morocco and spread out their aluminum foil to get as dark as possible as quickly as possible. Alabaster white now signaled that you were just a factory worker or office drudge. And somewhere along the way a tan became linked to good health—a cultural myth that does not please dermatologists today.

What seems to be happening is that the people who grew up in the twenties are beginning to reach their later years, so that we are now reaping the first generation of light-skinned people whose bodies have been exposed to a lifetime of ultraviolet rays (give or take our cavemen ancestors, who, in any case, had more body hair to protect them!). Before the twenties, you will recall the athletic ladies on the tennis courts enveloped in flowing dresses with high necks and at the beach in knee-length swim costumes—suitably met at the knees with lisle stockings. Even the men wore bathing suits with vests and pants that fell to the knee.

The dermatologists have been trying very hard to tell us that we must begin, in our clothes-liberated age, to protect our skin from earliest childhood with hats and long-sleeved shirts and with sunscreens and sunblockers—appropriate to our particular skin types. Not tanning lotions. They don't really protect us.

UV-A and UV-B

Scientists separate ultraviolet light (UV) into two categories—UV-A (longer wavelength) and UV-B (shorter wavelength). UV-B is thought to be the better tanner—and the primary culprit in skin cancer. It is the strongest at midday (10 A.M. to 2 P.M.) in all latitudes; and stronger near the equator. Other factors, such as sky cover, altitude, and moisture, also affect the amount of UV-B in the atmosphere: the higher the altitude and the drier the atmosphere, the stronger the UV-B rays. Note the burning effects of the dry season in California or the sunny days in the Rockies.

UV-A, which falls more evenly throughout the day and was formerly thought to be a benign form of radiation, is now more suspect. This throws the commercial tanning parlors, who proudly advertise that they use "only UV-A," into suspicion as well. Although this issue has still to be resolved with further experiments, for the time being it's best to err on the side of caution. Certainly, most dermatologists warn against intensive tanning with UV-A.

Wrinkles and Blue-Eyed Blondes

When ultraviolet rays penetrate the skin, they can cause dryness, nodules, wrinkles, benign or malignant cancers, and premature aging of the skin. Indeed, it may be fear of the latter that will finally persuade many in our youth-oriented culture to give up the worship of tanned skin. According to dermatologist John M. Knox of Baylor College of Medicine, the usual signs of aging skin don't take place if skin is kept out of the light. "If you do biopsies on the buttocks of people age 75 and 35, you won't see any differences under the microscope. Skin (if protected) stays youthful much longer than people realize."

Fair-skinned, blue-eyed blonds and red-headed Caucasians are the most susceptible to ultraviolet rays because they lack melanin, the brown skin pigment that is a natural filter against UV. All skin cancers are more common in this group, and least common among blacks.

Dermatologists have broken skin types down into categories:

Skin Type 1. Very fair complexion. Always burns, never tans.
Skin Type 2. Fair skin. Usually burns, sometimes tans slightly.
Skin Type 3. Sometimes burns, usually tans.
Skin Type 4. Almost never burns, always tans.

Skin types 1 and 2 are most susceptible to skin damage and cancerous growths. Those with skins of these types should not even try to tan and should be especially cautious about sun exposure near water, snow (which reflects solar radiation), in dry atmospheres or high altitudes, or in any occupational or recreational circumstance where they are exposed to the sun for long periods.

Those with types 3 and 4 should also be careful, because they are not immune to skin damage and cancer—only at less risk. They should acquire a tan gradually, and follow the guidelines below for sun exposure.

Here are points to remember for all skin types to reduce exposure to the ultraviolet rays that leave them vulnerable to skin cancer:

• Beware of hot sunny days, particularly in high altitudes, near the equator, or in a dry climate. Don't be fooled by haze or clouds. Ultraviolet rays penetrate them, and can burn just as easily, causing the same skin damage. Radiation can also be just as intense on a 70-degree day in July as on a 90-degree day—or, with snow, on a 20-degree day. Take the same precautions on these days as you would on very hot days.

• Try to avoid direct exposure to the sun during the middle of the day, between 10 A.M. and 2 P.M. UV-B rays are most intense during this time.

• Wear a big hat, use a beach umbrella, and cover your arms and legs with white or light-colored clothes. However, even these do not provide optimal protection. Ultraviolet rays reflect from sand, water, and snow, and penetrate light clothing. (Anyone who has snorkeled in clear South Sea waters with a shirt on can attest to this.) Use sunblockers or sunscreens in addition.

• For those who are skin type 3 or 4 and want to get a tan, use sunblockers/screens, and avoid midday sun. In the beginning, tan for fifteen to twenty minutes a day only; work your way slowly up to forty-five minutes, but no more.

• Use sunscreens! *They should be applied by everyone under any circumstance of prolonged sun exposure or tanning, at work or play, on the beach, in the snow, or elsewhere.*

• Wear dark sunglasses if you are out in the sun for work or leisure for very long periods. Dark glasses block ultraviolet rays, which can contribute to or aggravate cataracts. Check the tag for the "transmission" factor; they should transmit only 10–25 percent of visible light; if there's no tag, go for the darkest glasses you can.

SUNSCREENS AND SUNBLOCKERS

- *Sunscreens:* These are gels, creams, oils, or lotions that selectively absorb ultraviolet rays. Most sunscreens contain PABA (para-amino-benzoic acid), generally recognized as the most effective screening element. Some contain benzophenone, which is also effective. PABA products are rated by the sun protection factor (SPF) from 2 to 15 or higher, according to the amount of protection they provide. The higher the number, the greater the protection. The SPF numbers refer to the amount of time you can stay in the sun without burning: 2 means you can stay in the sun without burning twice as long as it would normally take you to burn; 3 means you can stay out three times as long, etc. Sunscreens *do not block* out all ultraviolet light, and do allow tanning in spite of the screen. Therefore, it is important that you still follow the time recommendations above. You can burn with a sunscreen, if you stay out too long.

The Skin Cancer Foundation recommends using sunscreens with a minimum SPF of 15—especially if you are skin type 1 or 2. Sunscreens should be applied a half hour in advance of sun exposure and should be reapplied every few hours, or immediately after swimming or heavy perspiration.

- *Sunblockers:* These products are usually opaque creams that deflect ultraviolet light. They usually contain titanium dioxide, zinc oxide, or talc. Blockers are not practical for applying to the whole body. They are useful for areas of the face—lips, nose, earlobes—that burn and peel easily. You may have noticed Dennis Connor in the 1987 America's Cup races; you almost never saw a picture of him without nose and lips covered with white goo.

Zinc oxide is an effective sunblocker now marketed in many bright colors to enliven the beach scene. SPF-23 and SPF-25 are new products, which just came on the market in late 1986. They are more liquid than zinc oxide and therefore more appropriate for overall body coverage. SPF-23 and SPF-25 are intended to prevent any UV from reaching the skin.

- *Suntan lotions:* Watch out for these products! They contain oils that may help promote tans, but they offer little, if any, protection against ultraviolet light. Some suntan lotions offer minimal protection, but, if the label does not claim protection, it probably does not offer any.

THE SKIN CANCERS

Common skin cancers, such as the type diagnosed in President and Mrs. Reagan and Vice President Bush, account for more than 400,000 new cancers each year. These cancers are primarily basal or squamous cell carcinomas, and are the most benign and easily cured malignancies known. Basal cell cancers are usually uncomplicated, and their surgical removal represents cure, as was the case with the Reagans and Bush. The cure rate is upward of 95 percent.

Solar radiation—ultraviolet rays—is the major known cause of these skin cancers. It may be responsible for 90 percent of all such cases.

One in eight Americans will develop the common skin cancer during their lifetimes, according to the Skin Cancer Foundation. Although these carcinomas are curable at least 95 percent of the time, surgical removal can be disfiguring and costly, and cause more serious damage to local tissues if they are neglected. It is, therefore, very important to catch them early and have them excised when they are small.

Basal cell carcinomas are most often small, smooth, waxlike, raised nodules. Sometimes they are reddish, flat, scaly-outlined patches. The area may become sore, and bleed or crust and not heal. They commonly appear on the face, arms, legs, or other areas often exposed to sun rays. If you notice any small (often white) pimplelike nodules or flat scabs (not from injuries) that don't seem to go away, check with your doctor or dermatologist.

Malignant Melanoma

Malignant melanoma is another case altogether. It is far less common than basal cell carcinoma, and it is extremely dangerous. It, too, seems to be caused by overexposure to ultraviolet rays. Because of the rapid rise in the incidence of melanoma, the need to control the sun factor has become vital. A recent Canadian study indicates that intermittent, intense sun exposure, as with the vacation tanner, may be more harmful than constant exposure, as in daily occupations. The highest risk seems to be in untanned subjects with a history of sunburn. The Canadian researchers point out, however, that the tendency to burn may be more important than the number of times burned.

At this time, melanoma strikes about 27,300 men and women in the U.S. each year and there are about 5,800 deaths annually. If not detected early, it can spread very quickly and aggressively to other parts of the body. Early treatment, however, has an excellent chance of success; the five-year survival rate is 83 percent. *But it must be caught early.*

Melanomas are usually distinguished by change in the size or color of a mole or other darkly pigmented growth or spot. They may be dark brown or black, or multicolored—a mixture of tan, brown, black, or reddish pink. The spots may ulcerate or bleed easily. If you notice any of these, see your doctor or dermatologist immediately. It's likely to be nonmalignant. But by having fast medical attention you will either be relieved quickly of anxiety or receive treatment for a condition that, left unattended, could become serious. For more on early detection, see Appendix 2.

SUNLIGHT AS FRIEND AND FOE

All this sounds as if ultraviolet light is a bogeyman, to be avoided at all costs. This is not the case. We need sunlight to keep us healthy and happy, and to buttress our immune systems. Environmental engineers are now beginning to suggest that we use full-spectrum glass or plexiglass in our house windows to allow ultraviolet light to pass through. They also suggest installing full-spectrum fluorescent lights in our workplaces. It is now suspected that seasonal affective depression (SAD) and other depressive conditions may be caused by the lack of sunlight in our "civilized" indoor lifestyles. In particular, the elderly, who are least apt to go out in winter weather, are urged to spend twenty minutes a day outside in full-spectrum light to help buttress their immune systems and ward off depressive reactions. But you can get plenty of UV on a cloudy day or under a shady tree on a bright day.

Ultraviolet light can be likened to fire. We can't warm ourselves or cook food without fire. But, uncontrolled or improperly harnessed, it burns and destroys. The same holds for the ultraviolet rays of the sun. Sunlight can meet important health and psychological needs, if we limit exposure and take the necessary simple steps to protect ourselves from potential damage and malignancy.

13

Exercise! Exercise!

If exercise could be packaged into a pill, it would be the single most prescribed and beneficial medicine in the nation.

Robert N. Butler, M.D.
Chairman of the Gerald and May Ellen
Ritter Department of Geriatrics
and Adult Development,
Mount Sinai Medical Center, New York, N.Y.

Exercise is wonderful as a preventive—and sometimes curative—measure for countless ailments. Research shows that exercise strengthens your heart and lungs, can lower your blood pressure, protect against adult diabetes, strengthen your bones, slow down the effects of osteoporosis, tone muscles, keep joints, tendons, and ligaments in shape, and relieve constipation.

It helps burn off fat (always a good idea), helps you lose weight and sleep better.

It makes you feel mentally more alert, promotes self-confidence, and seems to bolster the immune system.

What more could you ask for?

There is more. Early studies show that a certain level of activity often modifies some risk factors for some specific kinds of cancer.

A Harvard University study compared alumnae who had been college athletes with their less-active colleagues. Dr. Rose E. Frisch, Associate Professor of Population Science at the Harvard School of Public Health, analyzed 5,398 women who graduated between 1925 and 1981. The results were striking: over the years, the athletes proved two and a half times less likely to develop cancer of the uterus, ovary, cervix, and vagina than their more sedentary counterparts, and nearly two times less likely to develop breast cancer. This proved true even if the woman smoked or used oral contraceptives or postmenopausal estrogen, or if cancer ran in her family.

Many of these women weren't Olympic or marathon types—just biweekly exercisers participating in dance, volleyball, swimming, field

hockey, basketball, and track. Dr. Frisch believes that moderately intense—*but regular*—exercise is what matters, and that its optimum
benefits occur if you start exercising early in life. Most of the active
women in her study were involved in sports starting in high school or
earlier.

Researchers aren't sure why exercise seems to reduce cancer. One
theory is that active women produce less estrogen than inactive
women, which accounts for the lower rate of estrogen-sensitive cancers.
Other evidence suggests that health-conscious athletic women are apt
to eat diets lower in fats and higher in complex carbohydrates and fiber,
and keep to an exercise regimen as they grow older.

Two other studies, reported recently in the *American Journal of
Epidemiology,* found that colon cancer occurred less frequently in men
with active jobs than in those who mostly sat at their desks. Exercise
seems to stimulate muscular action in the colon, thus reducing the time
that feces with potential carcinogens are exposed to the surfaces of the
colon.

Psychological benefits from exercise may help protect the immune
system from stress. For many people, regular aerobics, jogging, calis-
thenics, swimming, stretching exercises, cycling, yoga, or group sports
help discharge tension, reduce anxiety, and improve self-image. Doctors characterize exercise as a "mild antidepressant." Michael Murphy
of the Esalen Institute says sports are "Western meditation," and likens
their effects to those of Eastern meditations, which relax the body and
mind and improve their functioning. Since depression compromises
immunity, exercise may help some people offset immune damage.

Some researchers speculate that the slight temperature rise occurring during vigorous exercise may be akin to an "acute phase" immune
response. Acute immune responses involve the release of a biological
response modifier, interleukin-1 (also called *endogenous pyrogen*) by
macrophage cells. It is the same response that takes place when fever
results from acute bacterial infection. The fever, mediated by interleu-
kin-1, is part of the body's heightened defense against microbial invaders. You will recall the story of Dr. William B. Coley in Chapter 3, "Our
Amazing Defense Systems": his bacterial vaccines induced high fevers
and regression of tumors. It is now believed that Coley's toxins may set
in motion interleukin-1 to induce fever and reawaken a network of
immune reactions against cancer cells. Fever itself seems to have healing properties, if not direct anticancer activity. If this is so, the "heat"
generated by exercise could help keep the immune response in fine
fettle.

Much of this thinking is still speculative. Although enormous research has been undertaken on the effects of exercise on heart disease,
diabetes, and osteoporosis, researchers are just beginning to investigate

its relationship to cancer prevention. However, early results suggest that exercise may have more anticancer benefits than we now know.

If you are not a regular exerciser, start with about fifteen minutes twice a week (five to ten minutes, if you are over sixty), and build up gradually. Eventually, a good weekly schedule should include at least thirty minutes of brisk—preferably aerobic—exercise at least four days a week. Do some stretching as well as warm-up and cool-down mild exercise for five to fifteen minutes to tune up your body before hard exercise and to wind down afterward. There are many good books on how to begin and maintain regular exercises and I have listed a few of these in the Appendix. For those over sixty, the National Institute for Aging has some excellent free or low-cost publications that describe exercise programs. Write to:

Exercise, National Institute for Aging
Building 31, Room 5C35
Bethesda, MD 20205.

Walking is one of the best exercises for everyone and one of the cheapest. It is fast becoming a national fad, surpassing jogging as the No. 1 form of exercise among people of all ages. According to a Harvard research study, a brisk two-mile walk every day can cut one's risk of a heart attack by 28 percent.

If you have any concerns about your health, see your doctor before starting a fitness program. Most people—even those with illnesses or disabilities—can take part in some sort of moderate exercise program, and it will improve your body-mind strength and your sense of well-being.

14

Viruses and Sexually
Transmitted Diseases

At one time, viruses were thought to be a major cause of cancer. With the advent of more sophisticated research tools, it has become clear that the relationship between viruses and cancer is complex—and much more limited than scientists speculated twenty years ago.

As molecular biologists and virologists begin to zero in on the role of viruses, it is becoming clear that, in a few cases, viruses are "necessary and sufficient" to cause cancer. But, in most instances, they are "necessary" but *not* sufficient." In lay terms: other factors must be present in addition to the virus to account for the development of tumors.

The following table shows the viruses associated with different cancers. Several of the cancer-linked viruses are sexually transmitted, and I will describe them and methods for prevention later in this chapter.

Virus	Cancer Type
HBV (Hepatitis B virus)	Primary liver cancer
EBV (Epstein-Barr virus)	Burkitt's lymphoma
	Nasopharyngeal cancer
	Hodgkin's disease
HSV-2 (Herpes simplex-2)	Cervical cancer
HTLV	Leukemias and lymphomas
HIV (or HTLV-III)	AIDS (Kaposi's sarcoma)
CMV (Cytomegalovirus)	Kaposi's sarcoma
Papilloma viruses	Genital warts (precancerous)
	Cervical cancer
	Vaginal/vulva cancer
	Penile cancer

LIVER CANCER

Primary liver cancer is quite rare in the United States, but is one of the most common cancers in Africa, China, Taiwan, and the Philippines. Infection with hepatitis B virus as the cause of liver cancer is nearly iron-clad. A huge 1981 prospective study followed some 23,000 men, 3,500 of whom had hepatitis B antigen in their blood. Forty-one of the full group of 23,000 developed primary liver cancer, and forty of that forty-one came from the group that tested positive for hepatitis B. The authors of the study stated that this was "the strongest [association] ever established between a virus and a human neoplasm." There are several co-carcinogens suspected as allies with hepatitis B in causing liver cancer, including exposure to aflatoxins in grains, nuts and alcohol.

In developing countries, where hepatitis B infection and liver cancer are quite common, the recently developed hepatitis B vaccine is considered the strongest preventive weapon. New diagnostic tests for HBV are now being distributed more widely, so early detection of the virus is another way for liver cancer to be prevented. Antiviral agents such as interferon are also a means of diminishing HBV infection in carriers, and with increasing availability, they will add to the arsenal against HBV and, therefore, against liver cancer itself.

EPSTEIN-BARR VIRUS

Epstein-Barr virus (EBV) is part of the herpes family of viruses. It is best known as the cause of most cases of infectious mononucleosis. For reasons unknown, some people are either more genetically or immunologically susceptible to EBV than others, and may be more susceptible to developing related cancers. EBV infection has been linked to Burkitt's lymphoma, nasopharyngeal cancer, and possibly to Hodgkin's disease.

The two cancers with the strongest connection to EBV—Burkitt's lymphoma and nasopharyngeal cancer—are uncommon in the U.S. Burkitt's lymphoma primarily strikes African children. Telltale genetic markers of EBV have been found in 95 percent of African cases of this disease. A massive prospective study conducted in Africa found that people with antibodies against EBV (meaning they've been exposed to the virus) had thirty times higher risk of contracting Burkitt's lymphoma.

Nasopharyngeal cancer is a tumor of the nasopharynx, part of the passageway from the mouth to the esophagus located behind the nasal cavity. This cancer is rare for most populations, and is seen most often in China. Antibodies to EBV have been found in almost all cases of this cancer, so exposure to the virus is surely a causal factor.

The EBV-Burkitt's-nasopharyngeal connections are a good example of the "necessary but not sufficient" concept scientists and epidemiologists are so fond of. Since the virus has been implicated in such a large number of cases, it can be said that, for the most part, its presence is necessary for the disease to develop. But EBV is probably not sufficient since most people who have been exposed to EBV do not get these cancers. Why do some get cancer while most do not? The answer is that co-factors must be present—genetic or immunological factors, or exposure to co-carcinogens or tumor promoters.

Among patients with Hodgkin's disease, 30 to 40 percent have been found to carry antibodies to EBV. Other viruses and causal factors have been identified in 60–70 percent of Hodgkin's cases. Therefore, EBV infection should be considered only a co-factor in the development of Hodgkin's disease.

Improved hygiene and the utilization of a recently developed Epstein-Barr vaccine are considered the best hopes for prevention of EBV-induced cancers (Burkitt's lymphoma and nasopharyngeal cancer) in developing countries. Theoretically, better nutrition, which boosts antiviral and anticancer immune responses, could also help prevent EBV infection and the resulting tumors.

HTLV

The letters "HTLV" may have a ring of familiarity to them. They stand for "Human T-cell Lymphotropic Virus," and the strain dubbed "HTLV-III" has been implicated as the cause of AIDS. HTLV-III was recently renamed "HIV"—which stands for "human immunodeficiency virus."

The public is less familiar with the fact that the other known types of HTLV (and there are several) can cause certain leukemias or lymphomas that are rare in the U.S. but common in Japan and the Caribbean. HTLV is a retrovirus—a class of viruses that can cause tumors in animals. The cancers caused by HTLV are T-cell leukemias or lymphomas, and 90 percent of the patients with these illnesses have detectable antibodies to the HTLV virus.

How these viruses are transmitted in the high-incidence areas is still uncertain. As with AIDS, sexual transmission and the tainting of the blood supply with viruses from infected donors, as well as other means, are being investigated. If blood banks are implicated, screening measures will be a first method of prevention. When more is discovered about how HTLV is transmitted, and what co-factors may be involved in bringing about T-cell leukemias and lymphomas, a careful strategy for prevention will undoubtedly be devised. The major forms of leuke-mia and lymphoma in the U.S. and most countries are *not* believed to be caused by viruses or transmitted through infections.

SEX AND CANCER

A link between sex and cancer? A more unhappy notion could not have been devised even by the most nefarious advocates of biological war-fare!

However, the connection between sex and cancer *has nothing to do with the natural functions of sex itself.* The cancer agent involved in sex is always a virus that is transmitted *through* sexual contact. Sex itself is a healthy and health-promoting function, and may actually help prevent certain malignancies. As far back as the early 1700s, physicians noted that women who were sexually active and bore children had less incidence of breast cancer than nuns, who were celibate.

The cancer-causing viruses that can be transmitted through sexual contact are avoidable through preventive measures. Abstinence is not called for. But full awareness of the risks and *proper precautions are called for*—and strongly. Almost all sexually transmitted diseases (STDs)—not just AIDS—are proliferating rapidly, for reasons no one is quite sure of. To prevent all STDs, including AIDS, sexual partners of all sexual preferences need to discuss the risks and preventive measures openly and become adept at using condoms, the most effective form of prevention now available. This is not just true for homosexuals and other groups at high risk but also for heterosexuals, particularly those with more than a single long-term sexual partner. According to Drs. Phillip and Lorna Sarrell, the Masters and Johnson sex-counseling team at Yale University, one of the groups that may be transmitting AIDS and other STDs at a considerable rate is married people who, unknown to their spouses, are having extramarital affairs with homosexuals or heterosexuals. The old myth that the respectable middle class is im-mune from infection with any STD is totally without validity.

Cancer of the Cervix

For a long time, scientists believed that cervical cancer was probably caused by exposure to herpes simplex virus-2, commonly called "genital herpes." Herpes-2 causes genital sores, which periodically recur. Herpes simplex virus-1 is the type that causes oral lesions or cold sores, and may cause some genital sores, though herpes-1 genital sores don't recur without another exposure to the virus.

Although there is some connection between herpes-2 infection and cancer of the cervix, it is no longer considered a causal connection. Antibodies to herpes-2 have been found in a fairly high pecentage of women with cervical cancer, and in one study, one in every four women with active genital herpes also showed either precancerous changes in the cervix, early tumors, or invasive cancer of the cervix.

This kind of evidence was enough to make scientists put herpes-2 at the top of the list of suspects, although it was always clear that co-factors were also involved. Sexual activity at an early age, early pregnancy, and a large number of sexual partners are all associated with an increased risk of cervical cancer.

Recently, however, a discovery shed new light on the possible viral causes of cervical cancer. Advances in molecular research technology now implicate the human papilloma viruses (also known as "HPV"), known mainly as the cause of annoying genital warts and some uncommon genital cancers.

Today, papilloma viruses seem to be the fastest-spreading sexually transmitted diseases. A spokesman for the Centers for Disease Control in Atlanta estimated that the incidence of papilloma infection has increased tenfold since the late 1960s. The early suspicion about papilloma was triggered by the observation that genital warts sometimes progressed to cancer. In the last seven years, investigators in North America and Europe have reported the presence of the papilloma virus in about 90 percent of cervical-cancer cases tested. The virus is also turning up in 90 percent of cervical dysplasias, the cellular changes that can precede cancer.

Papilloma research has turned up many fascinating clues about the origins of genital warts, rare genital cancers, and cervical cancer. It seems that the papilloma is actually a family of viruses that includes some forty different subtypes. Certain of these specific types have been found to cause warts, while a few others have consistently turned up in cervical-cancer cases. A simple diagnostic tool to determine presence of the different papilloma types is not yet available, but should be in the near future.

Along with the Pap smear, an early diagnostic test will be of great value, because many people infected with papilloma virus are asymptomatic for long periods; they have no visible lesions or other symptoms that are easily recognized. Catching the virus early will go a long way to preventing cancerous growth (for more on early detection of cervical cancer, see Appendix 2).

Researchers are again seeing a "necessary but not sufficient" scenario with the papilloma viruses and cervical cancer. Though the link between the two is strong, co-factors, such as concomitant presence of the herpes-2 virus or other sexually transmitted infections—and smoking—are important to the development of full-blown cervical cancer.

Women who smoke have approximately four times greater risk of cervical cancer. These findings point out once again that cancer is a multifactoral disease.

Virologists at the University of Minnesota have studied the papilloma viruses in relation to cancers of the vagina, vulva, and penis. All three are very rare—especially cancer of the penis—yet the researchers have consistently found papilloma viruses in patients with these cancers. The virus also causes warts on both the male and female genitalia, as well as flat lesions in men and women (different from warts) that are benign but may lead to the development of genital cancers.

If you have any of the symptoms mentioned, don't be alarmed; genital warts, lesions, or cervical dysplasia caused by the papilloma virus won't necessarily lead to genital or cervical cancer. However, you should see your doctor and find out if you're infected. You will need to find out how to prevent complications, avoid spreading it to others, and receive treatment for your symptoms.

To date, there is no vaccine or other surefire means of preventing the spread of the papilloma virus. Although an antipapilloma vaccine will be hard to develop, such a possibility offers hope for a powerful weapon against cervical and genital cancers. Antiviral agents that attack the virus or prevent viral replication, such as interferon, are now being tested as possibilities.

The best advice experts can now give about preventing the spread of the papilloma virus—and herpes-2 as well—are caution with regard to sexual partners, and the use of condoms. (See the following section on AIDS for guidelines regarding the use of condoms to prevent STDs.) Don't be afraid to ask sexual partners about their exposure to sexually transmitted diseases. They may not know that they are infected with papilloma or herpes-2, but the presence of lesions of unknown origin should tip you and/or your partner off that the virus could be present. Finding out about the possible viral exposure of a sexual partner is a good idea for preventing all STDs, including AIDS. All women should have Pap smears for cervical cancer detection once every three years after two initial negative tests one year apart. Early detection is all important.

AIDS

AIDS—which has received the most media attention of all the STDs, and rightly so, has now reached epidemic proportions in the Western world and in Africa. It is the cause of an increase in the incidence of a host of opportunistic diseases, including a rare and deadly cancer, Kaposi's sarcoma.

AIDS must be preceded by exposure to the virus HIV (or "human immunodeficiency virus." It was previously referred to as HTLV-III or LAV.) But again, HIV seems to fall into the "necessary but not sufficient" category. In order to contract AIDS, you must have the HIV virus, but many people who check out positive for HIV antibodies (meaning they have been exposed to the virus) do not necessarily acquire AIDS. It's possible that the HIV alone is "sufficient" to cause AIDS when it is transmitted through the blood (as in transfusions), although researchers are not yet certain why this should be so.

One of the factors that makes this issue cloudy is that the incubation period between being exposed and acquiring AIDS could be very long, and we do not know what will happen to those who currently test out as HIV positive and yet are otherwise completely healthy. However, it now appears extremely unlikely that all of the people who test positive for HIV will go on to acquire AIDS. Why do some resist the disease while others do not? No one is quite sure.

In most AIDS cases, a combination of other factors makes the person susceptible to contracting the disease. Perhaps the clearest co-factors include exposure to a variety of other STDs and infections through multiple sexual contacts. These other viral or bacterial infections further weaken the immune system and make it all the more vulnerable to the effects of HIV, which can act as the final straw that breaks the camel's back. HIV attacks a crucial subset of T-helper cells that are needed for healthy immune reactions, leaving the individual finally vulnerable to all manner of infectious diseases and cancer.

Any drug abuse further compromises immunity, and repeated ingestion of semen from multiple sexual partners has also been found to tax the immune system.

Perhaps the least-considered powerful co-factors are *psychosocial*. Psychological states and social factors contribute to our health and immunity through specific neurological pathways. Homosexual men, in particular, have been subject to a great deal of psychosocial stress, in part from built-in cultural prejudices that existed long before the AIDS epidemic, and in part from the AIDS epidemic itself. People in high-risk groups should seek counseling, social support, or psychotherapy in addition to the best possible medical help—whether they have suspicious symptoms or are simply frightened about the specter of AIDS. Psychological health is as important as proper nutrition if we are to maintain an immune system capable of meeting the challenge of infectious agents. (See Chapter 19, "How the Mind Influences Immunity," for my discussion of the link between mind and immunity. Also, see Appendix 3 for a listing of AIDS support organizations.)

The causes, treatments, prevention, and social ramifications of AIDS and its proliferation are well beyond the scope of this book, but many AIDS books and materials are now available on the market. Here, I would like to discuss AIDS in its relation to Kaposi's sarcoma, a rare disease that has now suddenly and tragically begun to flourish. For the most part, you are only susceptible to this cancer if you have contracted AIDS.

Kaposi's sarcoma is a skin cancer characterized by flat or raised red or purplish lesions. Previously, Kaposi's was common only in parts of Africa, though it occasionally occurred in transplant patients whose immunity was compromised by immunosuppressive drugs. Suddenly, a few years ago, it began to appear with frequency in homosexual men in the Western world, and the U.S. in particular. No one could understand this sudden outbreak until AIDS itself was discovered and described.

The AIDS complex is characterized, as its name suggests, by the near total breakdown of a person's immune system. And it is this breakdown of immunity that leaves the person susceptible to other infections and cancer. In AIDS patients, the most common cancer is Kaposi's sarcoma. According to one estimate, about forty-five percent of AIDS patients contract Kaposi's sarcoma, while between 65 and 80 percent acquire PCP (Pneumocystis carinii pneumonia), an often lethal form of pneumonia. A large number of other opportunistic diseases also plague AIDS victims, and many acquire more than one.

Why some AIDS patients contract Kaposi's while others do not is still uncertain. One theory is that other sexually transmitted diseases among homosexual men may be co-factors in the development of Kaposi's sarcoma. One such virus is cytomegalovirus (CMV), found in a high percentage of AIDS patients and a very high percentage of Kaposi's sufferers. Further support for this theory is the fact that other groups of AIDS patients—such as intravenous drug users, transfusion recipients, or hemophiliacs who contract AIDS from tainted blood products—rarely get Kaposi's sarcoma.

Therefore, safe sex is the best form of prevention not only for AIDS and all STDs, but for Kaposi's sarcoma as well. AIDS and STDs are spread through the exchange during sex of bodily fluids—namely, semen and blood. The following safe sex guidelines should therefore be followed by everyone, with special relevance to high-risk groups.

Safe Sex Guidelines

- *Limit your number of sexual partners:* The more sexual partners you have, the higher your risk of exposure to HIV and other sexually transmitted diseases.
- *Avoid an exchange of bodily fluids:* If you are in a high-risk group,

and/or have multiple sex partners, avoid exchanging bodily fluids (especially semen). The AIDS virus and other STDs may be present in semen, blood, and perhaps, in very small amounts, in saliva. These fluids should not enter orifices or contact open wounds. Anal sex is the highest-risk sexual activity because slight tears in the rectal mucosa may enable viruses present in semen to enter the bloodstream. Oral sex and vaginal intercourse also permit viral transmission.

- *Use condoms:* Condoms are a well-established, if not foolproof, way of preventing the transmission of HIV and other STDs. Semen is the most common carrier of HIV, and tests have shown that condoms block the virus in semen from entering the partner's body. Condoms can be used to prevent AIDS in vaginal intercourse, anal intercourse, and oral sex as well. Here are some rules concerning the proper use of condoms.

1. Unroll the condom over the erect penis all the way down to the bottom of the shaft.
2. Leave half an inch or so of slack at the tip, to hold the semen.
3. Proper lubrication is important to prevent breakage; if additional lubrication is needed, use only a water-soluble lubricant. Oil-based lubricants such as petroleum jelly can damage the condom.
4. The condom should be applied before coming into any contact with external genitalia, mouth, or rectum.
5. The penis should be withdrawn while still erect, and the base of the condom held during withdrawal to prevent slippage or leakage.
6. Many spermicides contain a mild detergent called "nonoxynol-9," which happens to be able to kill the AIDS virus. Its use is recommended, especially for vaginal intercourse.
7. To block viral transmission during anal sex, the toughest condoms available are recommended to prevent any chance of breakage.
8. Never use condoms more than once. Throw a used condom away and apply a new one if sexual activity is resumed immediately.

Intravenous drug users are also at "high risk," through sharing their needles without sterilizing them between injections. Hemophiliacs also have contracted HIV through treatment with tainted blood-clotting factors, but the incidence of this is now decreasing with better control of blood products, particularly the careful screening with the currently available HIV antibody test. As with hemophiliacs, transfusion subjects who have contracted AIDS acquired it from blood that had been contaminated. As the blood supply is purified through the HIV screening procedures, these cases will become fewer.

If you need a transfusion or are a hemophiliac, and are worried, make inquiries to assure yourself that the blood products you use have been properly screened; no doubt they have been. No matter what the purpose, hypodermic needles should only be used with the greatest of caution, including proper sterilization procedures.

We are in the midst of a lethal epidemic of tremendous proportions, which includes increased risk of cancer in addition to many other opportunistic diseases. All of us—homosexuals and heterosexuals alike—should take every available precaution.

15

Protecting Yourself at Home

Air pollution is the big issue both at home and at work (see next chapter). It's growing worse as our houses and offices become more energy efficient. There's a catch-22 here: the tighter and better insulated your house (or office) and the lower your fuel bills, the greater the possibility that noxious gases from chemicals will be trapped inside. A leaky house is good for your health. It keeps the air moving. The "sick-building syndrome" is a modern phenomenon and refers most specifically to the newer office buildings, whose windows are permanently sealed shut, and which lack proper ventilation, thus trapping inside all sorts of air pollutants, including some possible carcinogens. Be sure your house doesn't become similarly sealed. Whether or not you have air-conditioning, leave some windows open for an hour a day. In winter, be especially careful that, unless you have good old cracks and leaks to let in air, some windows are left open for a period each day. Under no circumstances, keep your windows shut all year round.

RADON, THE INVISIBLE, ODORLESS SPECTER

Radon is the most dangerous of all the house pollutants, but its threat depends on just what part of the country you live in. Although it sounds like something from a grade-B horror film, radon gas is a hazard to millions of American homeowners. This invisible, odorless gas, produced by the decay of uranium deposits in rock and soil, is the second leading cause of death from lung cancer, after cigarette smoking. Estimates range from 5,000 to 30,000 lung-cancer cases each year from radon in the home. The Environmental Protection Agency (EPA) estimates that radon-caused cancer kills as many as 20,000 people in the United States each year.

Radon seeps into basements through cracks and pipes. According to the EPA, all American homes have some radon. Although 88 percent of these homes fall within safety guidelines, an estimated 8 million houses are situated on earth containing dangerous levels of radon contamination. Certain parts of the country have higher known concentrations of radon than others. Presently the worst known areas are Maryland, eastern Pennsylvania, New York, New Jersey, and specific communities in Montana, North Dakota, Colorado, and Washington. The EPA is continuing to uncover new hot spots all the time.

Considerable controversy exists over the issue of how much radon is dangerous. The gas is measured by picocuries per liter (pCi/l). Some scientists believe that exposure to 4 picocuries will cause one lung cancer case per 100 people. The EPA considers 4 picocuries the threshold of concern. Others contend that there is no danger under 10 picocuries; no one disputes the danger of more than 10. According to the EPA, residents of homes with more than 100 picocuries face an enormous risk. Between one in three and two in three of them may contract lung cancer.

If you are concerned about radon levels in your house, the first step is to find out what level of the gas is present. You can take several routes:

1. Contact your state EPA office for advice.
2. Ask the EPA to recommend either a contractor who has testing equipment, or to provide a list of distributors of home testing equipment.
3. Purchase one of the commercially available testing devices.
4. Send away for a home radon-testing device.

There are two types of commercially available home radon detectors: "alpha-track devices" and "activated-charcoal detectors." The charcoal types, which range from $12 to $50, give faster readings and are recommended for an early warning. The alpha-track detectors (around $25) may require three to six months for an accurate reading, but the reading they provide may be more precise.

For a complete report on commercially available radon-testing devices, see *Consumer Reports,* July 1987, or ask your local or regional EPA office for information.

An activated-charcoal detector can be obtained through the mail from Dr. Bernard Cohen, Department of Physics, University of Pittsburgh, Pittsburgh, PA 15260. Enclose a $12 check payable to the University of Pittsburgh and you will receive a testing container with instructions. Return the container and you will receive a report from the lab. In addition, your test will contribute to their research.

If you discover high levels in your home, what can you do? You can install a ventilating system designed to reduce seepage by creating a suction around the basement to collect and draw gas away from the house. These systems have proved to be partially effective. You can strategically place fans in unfinished basements to draw radon away from the house. Neither basement sealing nor conventional ventilation is foolproof but they might help. More complex—and expensive—systems of ventilation, blockage, or removal can be installed. There are a variety of effective systems that are recommended for serious radon problems, which require professionals for construction and installation. Contact your state or local EPA office for more information on radon detection and reduction methods (see Appendix 3 for EPA information address and phone).

Although there is reason for widespread concern about the radon problem, the government has only recently begun to commit itself to the issue. Grassroots movements are attempting to grapple with the problem. We need a national information, detection, and control program. Until we have such a program, you should ask questions about your house, test for radon, and take steps to secure your safety.

KEEP THE AIR CLEAN

Organic compounds, cigarette smoke, airborne bacteria, and combustion by-products are the major types of indoor pollutants. Some of these pollutants are carcinogenic; some cause other health problems; all of them irritate mucous membranes and respiratory systems. You should consider the possibility of air pollution at home or at work if you suffer from unexplained eye, nose, throat, or skin irritation, breathing difficulty, headaches, or nausea.

A recent EPA study reports connections between the presence of certain building materials, cleaning agents, paints and solvents, and chemicals in indoor air. Some of these chemicals, including *benzene* and *carbon tetrachloride,* are known carcinogens. Products created to bring "industrial-strength" cleaning power to our homes are *not* necessarily safe. Some of the agents in these products present a minimal cancer risk, but why chance long-term effects when it's easy to eliminate potentially unhealthful substances?

Government agencies, including the Food and Drug Administration (FDA), the Environmental Protection Agency (EPA), and the Consumer Product Safety Commission (CPSC), set standards and regulate harmful and potentially hazardous chemicals and products that contain them. They are prompted and aided by consumer action groups like the Environmental Defense Fund, the Consumer Federation of America, and the Health Research Group of Public Citizens. Unfortunately, the current administration has made it difficult for regulatory agencies to

be vigilant and to enact new statutes based on the latest research findings.* Thousands of new chemicals are introduced into the marketplace
each year. A latency period of many years can exist between exposure
to these chemicals and the manifestation of cancer. Therefore, many
suspect products may never be banned and others not until they are
proven to be dangerous. We must press for more efficient chemical and
product testing from the EPA, FDA, and the CPSC. We should push for
federal protection against carcinogens. But until that is effected we
must learn to protect ourselves.

The first step in protecting ourselves is to eliminate suspected carcinogens from the house. *Read labels* to be sure that suspect chemicals
are not included in the cleaning, cosmetic, or house-repair products you
buy. Look for alternatives. If you must use suspect chemicals, be sure
to do so in a ventilated space. Open windows to create good cross drafts.

The second step is to make certain your house is properly ventilated. Use exhaust fans and air-to-air heat exchangers that function by
heating the air coming in with warm outgoing air. You can purchase
ventilation systems that ventilate the entire house. Indoor air filters also
help. Commercially available air filters include electrostatic, fiber, and
charcoal filter devices, which can be very efficient in removing fine
particles from the air. Each device has its own advantage. See the
January 1985 issue of *Consumer Reports* for an evaluation of air filters
then available on the market.

CLEANING PRODUCTS

Check labels on all cleaning products for:

- Benzene
- Carbon tetrachloride
- Perchloroethylene

Benzene is a chemical solvent often found in household cleaning
products, spot removers, solvents, and glues. Gasoline contains 8 percent benzene. The raw material is used in the synthesis of chemical
compounds; transformed benzene is used in a wide variety of products
ranging from adhesives used in shoemaking to pesticides, inks, and
paints.

Benzene has been linked to an increased risk of leukemia, particu-

---

*The EPA announced its intention, in early 1988, to review its estimates of the cancer
risks of many chemicals in products and in the environment. The agency contends that
prior standards have overestimated the risk of some chemicals, while environmental and
health groups are arguing that this is but another stage of government relaxing its regulatory policies.

larly in industries where the chemical is used in extremely high concentrations and where workers have been exposed to it for long periods of time. Examples of such industries are oil refineries and all situations where there are coke-oven emissions.

Avoid using cleaning products containing the known carcinogens *carbon tetrachloride* and *perchloroethylene.* Do not buy these products; if you have them in the house, get rid of them. If you must use any of them, make sure that the room is extremely well ventilated.

INSULATION, PLASTICS, AND FABRICS

Chemical carcinogens in home construction and home use products are often difficult to identify. Synthetic fibers, plastics, and rubber products are made with chemical compounds that might contain some level of carcinogenic material. Heightened awareness of the potential risks to workers and to consumers has led to some regulation and reduction of the use of these compounds.

AN, or *acrylonitrile,* is used to make acrylic fibers and is found in consumer goods, such as plastic kitchen and dinner ware, food and beverage packaging, toys, luggage, automotive parts, small appliances, and telephones. Studies in the early 1980s confirmed AN as a carcinogen.

In 1977 the FDA did not approve the use of AN in soft-drink and other beverage containers. In 1979, the FDA began consideration of various manufacturing plans designed to reduce residual levels of the chemical. In 1980, the CPSC said that consumer exposure to AN through migration to food from packaging is low, but still a "cause for concern." Finally, in 1984 and 1987 the FDA established tighter regulations on the amount of AN that could be used in beverage bottles. People who live near manufacturing sites run the risk of vapor inhalation or absorption through the skin.

Asbestos is the generic name for a group of naturally occurring chemicals composed of silicate fibers. Long-term inhalation of asbestos fibers that have escaped into the air can cause asbestosis, a diffuse, chronic inflammation and scarring in the lung. In the late 1970s, Dr. Irving J. Selikoff of New York's Mount Sinai Medical Center published studies directly linking a high incidence of lung cancer with asbestos exposure among industrial workers. The latency period for asbestos can be between twenty and forty years.

A staple of the construction industry since World War II, asbestos is found in flooring materials, thermal and electric insulation, wallboard, floor and ceiling tile, caulking, gaskets, automobile clutch and brake linings, plastics, textiles, and fireproof theater curtains. Asbestos has been used to fireproof thousands of schools and other public buildings.

The greatest asbestos hazard in our homes probably stems from insulation, floor and ceiling tiles, or other construction materials set in place before governmental limitations were enacted. Renovation and repairs, or simply the breakdown and crumbling of old plaster and insulation, can cause the release of asbestos fibers, which then can be inhaled.

Even though the risk seems remote, exposure to small concentrations of asbestos in spackling, patching, and jointing materials commonly used in home repair could increase cancer risk. Try to find and use home-repair products that do not contain asbestos.

Over the years, asbestos has been regulated in industrial settings and banned from clothing, fireproofing materials, wallboard patching compounds, and gas heaters. It has been removed from electric hair driers. The National Institute for Occupational Safety and Health (the research arm of OSHA) recommends that all nonessential uses of asbestos be eliminated. As late as 1979, 600,000 tons were consumed in the United States, and it is still used in a variety of products.

On the positive side, asbestos production has decreased significantly. Local school systems are required to report asbestos dangers to parent-teacher groups, although there still is no federal injunction to do so, and many have begun removal procedures. Nevertheless, asbestos production has yet to be fully regulated and asbestos still exists in many of our homes.

What should you do about asbestos in construction materials or insulation in your house? *Do not disturb old asbestos or material suspected of being asbestos.* Send for the Consumer Product Safety Commission guide for handling asbestos (see Appendix 3 for address). If your situation requires action, contact a licensed, experienced asbestos crew. In some cases it may be better to wrap or seal crumbling material instead of removing it.

It is preferable that the job be done by professionals, but if you work with asbestos yourself, follow these guidelines:

1. Seal off the entire repair or removal area.
2. Wear protective clothing and a respirator.
3. Ensure proper ventilation.
4. In order to prevent fibers from entering the air, wet the material before moving it.

PCBs (polychlorinated biphenyls) are a family of synthetic compounds that have been used for over fifty years in a variety of products. We do not know the extent to which we are exposed to PCBs in our air, water, and food, places where they pose the greatest danger. We *do* know that PCBs are extremely toxic and have wide-ranging health effects. Animal studies show their potential as carcinogens. Scientists report that the manufacture of PCBs, which are nonbiodegradable, has left traces in water, soil, air, and human tissue, but it will be years before the effects of sustained exposure in humans will be known.

In 1973, the FDA set limits on PCBs in foods. These limits were strengthened in 1979. At the same time, after years of regulatory debate, the EPA finally banned the manufacture, processing, and distribution of PCBs.

Before 1972, PCBs were commonly used in the manufacture of hydraulic fluids, transformer coolants, lubricants, and plasticizers. Today they may be present in the home in plastics, coatings, adhesives, sealants, and printing inks, which were manufactured over a decade ago.

There is not much we can do about PCBs in these substances, both because determining their presence is difficult and because the only way to destroy them is to burn them in a special incinerator, which generates temperatures of 2,000–3,000 degrees Fahrenheit. However, the threat of PCBs in the home appears to be minimal. Its greatest threat was to those living in close proximity to PCB incinerator sites.

A 1975 report by Karl E. Bremer of the EPA, listed these products, some of which were manufactured with PCBs at that time or earlier:

laminate, the layered covering of ceramics and metals;
washable wall coverings;
coatings for ironing-board covers;
flameproofer for synthetic yarns;
waterproofing for canvas;
additives for paints and varnishes;
protective lacquers;
insulating tapes;
additives in toner for Xerox machines;
"carbonless" carbon paper.

Formaldehyde, that favorite of high school biology, is valued by industry for its properties as a bonding agent and preservative. It is used in over three thousand products, from permanent-press fabrics to room deodorizers. Formaldehyde poses a health risk because it can irritate the skin, eyes, nose, and throat and can cause severe allergic reactions. Formaldehyde can cause cancer in laboratory animals exposed to its fumes. The Consumer Product Safety Commission has asserted that some cancer risk to humans is probable.

Formaldehyde is most commonly found in pressed-wood products—particle board, fiberboard, waferboard, flakeboard, and plywood—and in a wide variety of paper products, including paper towels and milk cartons, room deodorizers, furniture, and permanent-press clothing. The amount in permanent-press clothes is probably not enough to be carcinogenic, but may cause other allergic reactions among people who are sensitive. If you suspect this problem, the only way to find out if the article of clothing contains formaldehyde is to contact the manufacturer. Other products that *might* also contain formaldehyde include:

new car interiors,
shampoos and toothpastes,
indoor paneling and insulation,
carpets,
kitchen cabinets and counter tops,
emissions from gas stoves, incinerators, auto exhaust.

Apparently, the highest levels of formaldehyde emissions are in homes newly renovated with pressed-wood products, or in homes built with these materials. Pressed-wood products are used in constructing mobile homes, which are often poorly ventilated. Any pressed-wood products that are used in construction should be the kind that are specified as "low-emitting." Problematic pressed-wood surfaces can be "sealed" with varnishes, insulating paints, or polyurethane. There still may be a threat posed by overall emissions from a variety of sources in your home. It certainly isn't necessary to rip out your kitchen counter tops and cabinets, or to try to find out if your carpet contains formaldehyde. However, it is important to be aware of the level of formaldehyde emissions in your indoor air. You can have an air-quality consulting firm monitor levels in your home. Inexpensive formaldehyde monitors are available on the market. Of course, ventilation is important, especially on hot and humid days, and air filtration is an alternative when formaldehyde problems have no other solution.

In 1982, urea-formaldehyde foam insulation (UFFI) was banned by the Consumer Product Safety Commission and labeled a serious health threat owing to its high emissions. Until that time UFFI had been used as insulation in thousands of new homes. The CPSC ban has been overturned, but this product is rarely used. Do find out if UFFI insulation exists in your house and, if you aren't sure, have your home tested. Even if this form of insulation was used, you may not have to worry since emissions decrease with time. Contact the CPSC for further information (see Appendix 3).

Vinyl chloride is a gaseous raw material used in the manufacture of plastics. Polyvinyl chloride (PVC) is the primary plastic produced from vinyl chloride. Both the gas and the plastic are established carcinogens. PVC appears in food packaging such as plastic bottles, "blister" packs used for luncheon meats, and other pliable but preformed plastic wraps. Improved manufacturing processes have limited the migration of polyvinyl chlorides from packages to foods, but some consumer groups claim that PVCs still present a considerable danger and should be banned entirely.

PAINTS, THINNERS, AND STRIPPERS

"Do it yourself" renovations and repairs often require the use of a number of products that will interact with the environment. When using solvents, chemical cleaning products, acrylic paints, and protective sealants, *always* keep the windows open, take frequent breaks and wash carefully afterward.

Methylene chloride is considered the best liquid paint remover (stripper) available and is also used as a compound in the aerosol propellant for pesticides, paints, and lubricants (see gardening chemicals, page 221). Paint strippers are usually 50 to 90 percent methylene chloride; some, which may be labeled "nonflammable," are 100 percent. Spray paints may contain up to 33 percent of the chemical.

Recent testing has prompted the Consumer Product Safety Commission to move to designate methylene chloride as a "hazardous chemical," thereby subjecting its manufacture and use to federal regulation and, possibly, to federal banning. The commission has concluded that cancer risks from exposure to methylene chloride are "among the highest ever calculated for chemicals from consumer products." Unlike some other carcinogenic chemicals that appear in small quantities in household products, methylene chloride presents a greater risk since it is often highly concentrated. Lung cancers have developed in laboratory mice exposed to high levels of methylene chloride. Testing for the cancer risks of this chemical disclosed that it can cause other serious health problems as well. People who inhale the fumes of chemical paint strippers suffer effects that may indicate damage to the central nervous system. Symptoms include dizziness, nausea, headaches, and a "drunken" feeling, with light-headedness and confusion.

Consumers can protect themselves from the chemical's possible effects by eliminating the use of those products that list it in their contents. *As always, be a label reader.* If no other products can effectively substitute for one containing methylene chloride, be sure to wear a protective face mask and gloves when working with it. Make absolutely certain that you have *adequate ventilation,* and that the vapors are blown away from your face. If the stripper is poured into a tray or jar, make sure that the larger can is closed or covered during the time it takes to finish the job. Store methylene chloride paint and stripper products outside and be careful to dispose of all used brushes or rags.

Again, try to clear your shelves of all aerosols that may contain methylene chloride and use pump sprays and other liquid dispensers instead.

Another note about methylene chloride: it is also used to remove caffeine from coffee. Since it is employed in the decaffeinating processes for some of the most widely known brands of decaf coffee, many restaurants and grocery stores have now introduced coffee that has been decaffeinated through a nonchemical water process. *Avoid chemically decaffeinated coffees.*

MICROWAVES

Microwave ovens have become increasingly safe and popular in recent years. Their design and safety features have improved and they now boast some economic and health advantages as well. Microwaves save energy and, if used properly, can minimize the nutritional damage done to foods cooked by more conventional means.

Microwave ovens heat food quickly and from within; their short cooking process preserves vitamins and protein. Manufacturer instructions should be followed closely when cooking meat and poultry to destroy microorganisms normally exposed to external heat.

Microwave ovens use a form of non-ionizing radiation that is far less potentially damaging than the ionizing form found in x-rays. Nevertheless, animal studies suggest that non-ionizing radiation can cause severe damage to various tissues. Excessive radiation leaks were the biggest danger in early oven models. In 1971, the FDA established safety standards: today the ovens cannot emit substantial microwaves unless the door is not firmly locked. Ovens must have two interlocks and a circuit that checks them, shutting off the oven if a lock fails. Still, there may be a tiny emission of microwaves within a foot of the oven. The best safety advice is simply to remain more than two feet away, thus reducing exposure.

For safe cooking:

- Use only uncracked cookware, dinnerware, paper and plastic containers intended for microwave cooking.
- Leave metal out of the oven.
- Don't place foods packaged in plastic coverings in the oven.
- Don't heat baby foods or formula in the oven, since they can become very hot.
- Never remove food from the oven while holding a baby.
- Plug the oven into a polarized and grounded outlet.
- Avoid overcooking food.

WATER

Industrial waste—chemicals, gases, plastics, etc.—that was never intended for human or animal consumption is a big source of water contamination. Domestic sewage, agricultural runoffs, and pesticide residues add to it. Cancer-causing chemicals such as asbestos, bromoform, benzene, vinyl chloride, carbon tetrachloride, bis (chloromethyl) ether, cyanide, dieldrin, and PCBs contaminate waters across the country. Cancer-causing metals such as arsenic, cadmium, chromium, lead, nickel, and mercury are prevalent in drinking waters where industrial processes, seepage from soil, or mineralization from rocks occur. Nitrates that can be transformed into carcinogenic nitrosamines in the body also exist in some waters. In areas with hazardous drinking water, the incidence of stomach, intestinal, and urinary-system cancers greatly increases.

When industrial plants dispose of wastes either in water or in the ground, water can become chemically contaminated. Disposal sites can leak, causing groundwater to become contaminated with toxic chemicals. Radioactive substances, such as strontium and radium, sometimes leach into local waters when local hospitals, certain industries, and nuclear power plants practice improper disposal methods. The chemical industry has been prompted to help communities reduce health risks, but often companies do not want to spend large sums to alter their production processes. EPA regulations and public action groups have helped, but governmental commitment to safe drinking water has wavered, and so the threat of contaminated water will remain with us for years to come.*

If you live near industrial sites, or have some concern about the purity of your water sources, contact your local EPA office to get an assessment of local drinking water. If it cannot provide one, you can ask where you can get your water tested locally. Ask for a water-quality testing laboratory.

The EPA has guidelines for levels of toxic contaminants, including carcinogens, in our water supply. The agency has begun to enforce statutes requiring safer disposal of hazardous wastes. It monitors water and regulates levels of certain chemicals; unfortunately, widespread contamination still exists in some industrial areas. It is difficult to assess the cancer risk from these contaminants, but when carcinogens in water are known to exist, precautions should be taken.

*Good news comes in the form of final ratification of the EPA's Safe Drinking Water Act of 1986. The agency is required to regulate at least 83 drinking water contaminants (including carcinogens) by 1989. Though one EPA official doubted their capacity to meet this deadline, there is no doubt that the safety of drinking water in some regions will be much improved by the early 1990s.

City or town filtration and purification systems may not provide adequate protection. Filtration systems do filter and treat water to minimize the risks from bacteria, other dangerous microorganisms, and active chemicals, but they also can go awry. The central problem with water-purification systems for large populations is the very chlorination process used to kill the bacteria that cause diseases such as typhoid, cholera, and dysentery. When chlorine reacts with organic compounds in water, carcinogenic chemicals called trihalomethanes, or THMs, may form. If this seems like a catch-22, it is: the product (in this case a process) eliminates one threat but poses another. Water made available through complex and sophisticated purification and distribution methods may be unhealthful.

If you have determined that your water is bad, or if you merely suspect that it is, you may choose to buy bottled water. Some of these are naturally carbonated and others—if we are to believe the advertisers—are bottled by loving mountaineers somewhere in the great green hinterland of the United States Northwest or in the French Alps. There's little question that, if tap water is questionable, these products provide us with a fine, if expensive, alternative. But a water filter may work just as well. Tap filters use activated carbon filters to remove contaminants. Some are installed under the sink while others attach right to the faucet. Certain models can be relied upon to do a reasonably good job, though some people consider them inefficient. See the February 1983 issue of *Consumer Reports* for their assessment of the best water filters. (This should be available at your local library.)

GARDENING CHEMICALS AND PESTICIDES

All aerosol products probably contain some carcinogenic chemicals, since compounds of lethal chemicals are used in their production. *Methylene chloride* and *vinyl chloride,* defined carcinogens, exist in some aerosols. Improper ventilation increases the risks involved in using these products. Most commercial pesticide products that are packaged in aerosol cans contain freon propellants. Freon has been linked to liver tumors in tests using laboratory animals. When tending your favorite spider plant or coaxing the flowers from your African violet, use *nonaerosol products* that spray with a pump from a plastic container, rather than aerosol cans.

We also know that the fluorocarbons contained in all aerosol products are ruining the ecosphere, so we should not use them for that reason as well.

Arsenic is the deadly poison that has finished off characters in more than one murder mystery. But this chemical is used as more than a dramatic device. Arsenic occurs naturally in some foods but it also appears in chemical compounds in pesticides, glass, ceramics, paints, dyes, and wood preservatives.

Arsenic is especially dangerous in industrial settings where these products are manufactured, or in metal smelting plants with high levels of arsenic exposure. Studies have shown that high levels of exposure increase the risk of lung, lymphatic, and other cancers. A recent *New York Times* report indicated that some arsenic-based pesticides have been withdrawn from the market but may reappear when others are withdrawn.* Avoid pesticides or other products that contain arsenic compounds like *arsenic trioxide.*

Dioxin is a contaminant that results from the manufacture of some herbicides and defoliants that are used commercially to kill weeds on pasture and range land. Dioxin is found in Agent Orange, used in Vietnam, and in 2,4,5-T, used as a commercial weed killer in the United States. Although dioxin is a suspected carcinogen, its use remains unregulated while the danger to humans is investigated. Federal regulations do limit its waste disposal, and 2,4,5-T has been regulated. Consumer exposure through food and water contamination has not been estimated. *Common sense indicates that herbicides and defoliants suspected of containing dioxin should be avoided.*

EDB, or *ethylene dibromide,* has been used as a pesticide and preplanting soil fumigant in agriculture, especially with citrus crops. In September of 1983, the EPA banned the use of EDB as a soil fumigant when it became clear that it could possibly persist and contaminate fumigated and stored fruit and grain. Before EPA regulation, hundreds of thousands of people came in contact with EDB in the form of pesticides on fruit and, also, in leaded gasoline.

DDT, a pesticide that is a chlorinated hydrocarbon, was the subject of tests conducted from 1947 to 1969 and was banned in 1974 because of its carcinogenic nature. Before 1974 the entire population was exposed to DDT, and today traces of the water-insoluble pesticide remain in the environment.

The EPA has banned other chlorinated-hydrocarbon pesticides, namely *aldrin, dieldrin, heptachlor, and chlordane.* The two former pesticides have been banned except for termite control by certified technicians. Heptachlor and chlordane are also used for termite control, but they show up in commercial pesticides as well. Any products you have containing these pesticides should be disposed of. They should only be used for termite control by certified personnel.† Even when

---

*In addition, amid much controversy, the EPA has just substantially lowered its assessment of the risks of arsenic.

†Recent update: As of April 15, 1988, the EPA has totally restricted use of all four above-mentioned pesticides—including in termite control. Remain alert, however, for their presence in older commercial products.

production and use of a product has been banned, it is important that residents and homeowners remain vigilant about identifying the pesticides that may have affected their communities and homes. There still may be some carcinogenic commercial pesticides on the market. Watch out for the pesticide *alachlor,* also called *alanex, lasso,* or *lariet.*

Disposal of commercial pesticides—or any other potentially dangerous chemical products in the home—should be carried out this way: leave the product in its container, with the label, and wrap carefully in a plastic bag. Then dispose of the product(s) at your local landfill (not in your own trash can!). Leaving the label on will enable environmental workers to identify the agent in the event that the container is crushed and contents released. You may also want to contact your local health department to find out if they have a "pick-up day" for questionable materials (if they don't, you should encourage them to start one). This method is advisable only for home products; the recommendations for *industrial* waste disposal are entirely different.

COSMETICS

Formaldehyde occurs in extremely small amounts in a variety of cosmetics, including lipstick. The FDA considers these amounts too small to regulate. Nevertheless, some studies point to increased cancer rates among beauticians. Although currently available cosmetics are, for the most part, considered safe, some products, like fingernail hardeners, can contain formaldehyde and should be avoided.

Permanent hair dyes, used by millions of women in their homes, contain a suspected carcinogen known as *4-MMPD (4-methoxy-m-phenylenediamine),* which may be linked to breast and bladder cancer. The FDA has proposed a warning label indicating whether a hair dye contains this chemical. As of this writing, a challenge to the label requirement has held it up, though some manufacturers have voluntarily removed the compound from their products. Be cautious and check labels; if the manufacturer is stupid enough to market the product and list 4-MMPD, you should find another dye.

16

Protecting Yourself at Work

Air pollution is the major problem at work, just as it is within the home. The danger of pollutants in industrial plants has been heavily publicized over the last twenty-five years, but much less has been said of the increasing threat of office pollutants. I will therefore begin this chapter with the office and take up industrial hazards afterward—though not in great detail. Many excellent books have been written on industrial hazards, and occupational health groups are the best resources for workers with questions about safety on the job.

CANCER RISKS IN THE OFFICE

The "sick-building syndrome" goes into full effect in skyscrapers or small office buildings whose windows are sealed, and whose ventilation systems aren't up to snuff (and many of them aren't). Some of the same hazards that exist in the home may exist in the office building—asbestos, radon, formaldehyde, benzene, PCBs, and, perhaps worst of all, cigarette smoke. As in houses or apartments, sealed work places pose real health problems. Cancer risk may not be the most common of these problems, but it must be considered. *Offices must be properly ventilated.*

Be sure to take this matter seriously. If you or your co-workers suffer from minor symptoms such as coughing, allergies, asthma, eye, throat, and skin irritation, you may be the victims of sick-building syndrome. If you believe that you are, let others know, and put pressure on your employer to make the necessary changes. You do not need to stalk the halls and back rooms of your office looking for sources of pollution. Simply exert pressure for proper ventilation and, if necessary, air filtration.

As you do so, be aware of other sources of office pollution:

Photocopiers, a staple in every office, pose a small potential carcinogen problem. There are two possible sources: the oxygen energized by high voltages in the photocopier causes the formation of ozone, a sweet-smelling gas. Ozone is probably a mutagen and possibly a carcinogen. You can usually smell ozone at levels below that considered hazardous; this is one way to tell if you have a problem. Any doubts should lead office workers and managers to insist on proper ventilation. Keep workers at a reasonable distance from the machine where emissions come from exhaust. Make inquiries about the availability of filters that can be installed in your copier to block ozone from entering the air.

Another problem with copiers could stem from the toner, the fine chemical powder used in all these machines. Toner is made of a substance called carbon black, which contains contaminants shown to be mutagenic and possibly carcinogenic, though the risks from exposure are small. Copier maintenance personnel run the highest risk, and they should avoid changing toner without wearing a mask. Recently, Xerox has made an effort to remove the dangerous contaminant from toners supplied for its machines, though it is difficult to know whether any given product has had the culprit removed. Read safety information supplied with your toner.

"Carbonless" copy paper usually contains PCBs or formaldehyde, an irritant and potential carcinogen. This paper should not be used.

Fluorescent lights, so common in offices today, can create health problems such as skin rashes and headaches. In addition, a recent study in the British medical journal *Lancet* indicated an association between fluorescent light and melanoma. If you can arrange for alternative lighting, by all means do so.

Video display terminals (VDTs), found in almost every modern office, cause eye strain and stress in those who use them constantly. There is evidence of small emissions of both ionizing and non-ionizing radiation from VDTs. An FDA report has stated that the danger of ionizing radiation—the potentially cancer-causing kind—from VDTs is slim, and that they "emit little or no harmful radiation under normal operating conditions." However, criticism of that report points out that the FDA did not test a wide enough range of models. Many fully tested models have been proven to emit a level of radiation equal to the background count—considered to be a safe level. You will be safest working on a machine whose manufacturer has provided emission-level data showing that the level is at or below the standard set (.5 millirems per hour). VDTs may also emit low-frequency levels of *non-ionizing* radiation that should not be cause for much concern in terms of cancer risk.

Here are a few basic guidelines for safe VDT use:

- Machines should meet the minumum standards for radiation emission.
- Machines should be shielded with a metal casing or special paint to minimize radiation emissions.
- Do not use any machine that is not operating properly—it is more likely to emit radiation.
- Stay at a normal distance from the terminal.
- Take reasonable time breaks.

INDUSTRIAL CANCER

In the latter half of this century, with the growing sophistication of the sciences of epidemiology and toxicology, we have begun to grasp the extent of the threat of occupational cancer. Industrial workers exposed to high levels of carcinogenic agents over many years have developed cancers at staggering rates. The industries with high potential cancer risk are those in which carcinogenic chemicals are either produced or used in the manufacturing process, where dusts and fibers, metals or wood products are made or used.

The government's regulatory agency, the Occupational Safety and Health Administration (OSHA), has helped limit and ban many industrial carcinogens. Unfortunately, the government often has handcuffed OSHA or limited its power, bending to industry lobbying. Thus workers must be knowledgeable and organized around issues of their own health and safety, both to keep pressure on for proper regulation and to safeguard their own health in immediate, practical ways.

Which Industrial Agents Cause Cancer?

Since 1971, an organization called the International Agency for Research on Cancer (IARC), under the aegis of the World Health Organization, has published reviews of major cancer-causing agents. Based on an amazing amount of data gathered from sources that include human and animal tests and population studies, the IARC put these agents into the following categories:

Group 1 for chemicals, chemical groups, or industrial processes clearly causing cancer.
Group 2 for those considered *probable*.
Group 2 is split into
  2A for probable carcinogens with high potential risk
  2B for those with less potential risk.

For easy identification of major chemicals or chemical agents that are known or likely carcinogens, here is a summary table of the IARC's findings. These are the substances you should look out for:

CANCER-CAUSING INDUSTRIAL/CHEMICAL AGENTS

Table I	*Known Carcinogens*

Group 1: Industrial processes and occupational exposures causally associated with cancer in humans:

Auramine manufacture
Boot and shoe manufacture and repair (certain occupations)
Furniture manufacture
Isopropyl alcohol manufacture (strong-acid process)
Nickel refining
Rubber industry (certain occupations)
Underground hematite mining (with exposure to radon)

Chemicals and groups of chemicals causally associated with cancer in humans:

4-Aminobiphenyl
Arsenic and arsenic compounds
Asbestos
Benzene
Benzidine
N,N-Bis(2-chloroethyl)-2-naphthylamine (Chlornaphazine)
Bis(chloromethyl)ether and technical-grade chloromethyl methyl ether
Chromium and certain chromium compounds
2-Naphthylamine
Soots, tars and oils
Vinyl chloride

Table II	*Probable Carcinogens*

Group 2A: Chemicals, groups of chemicals or industrial processes *probably* carcinogenic to humans with at least limited evidence of carcinogenicity to humans:

Acrylonitrile
Benzo(a)pyrene
Beryllium and beryllium compounds
Diethyl sulphate
Dimethyl sulphate
Manufacture of magenta
Nickel and certain nickel compounds
ortho-Toluidine

Table II	*Probable Carcinogens*

Group 2B: Chemicals, groups of chemicals or industrial processes *probably* carcinogenic to humans with sufficient evidence in animals and inadequate data in humans:

Amitrole
Auramine (technical grade)
Benzotrichloride
Cadmium and cadmium compounds
Carbon tetrachloride
Chlorophenols
DDT
3.3'-Dichlorobenzidine
3.3'-Dimethoxybenzidine (*ortho*-Dianisidine)
Dimethylcarbamoyl chloride
1,4-Dioxane
Direct Black 38 (technical grade)
Direct Blue 6 (technical grade)
Direct Brown 95 (technical grade)
Epichlorohydrin
Ethylene dibromide
Ethylene oxide
Ethylene thiourea
Formaldehyde (gas)
Hydrazine
Phenoxyacetic acid herbicides
Polychlorinated biphenyls
Tetrachlorodibenzo-*para*-dioxin (TCDD)
2,4,6-Trichlorophenol

Tables I and II from U.S. Dept. of Health and Human Services, NIH Publication No. 85-691, *Cancer Rates and Risks,* 3rd ed., 1985.

The above table does not split agents into classes or categories, such as metals, fibers and dusts, solvents and chemical compounds. Here are examples from each category.

Dusts and Fibers

Asbestos, a group of substances composed of silicate fibers, is the number one fiber presenting serious cancer risk in the workplace. In the construction industry, asbestos is used for insulation, cement sheets and piping, ceiling and floor tiles. In the shipbuilding industry it has been used for fireproofing and insulation. It is also used in the manufacture of automobile clutch and brake linings.

Workers exposed to asbestos for long periods with little protection have a cancer rate three times greater than those never exposed. Lung cancer is the biggest threat, though other cancers, including mesothelioma, a rare cancer of the lining of the chest and abdominal cavity, have been linked to asbestos.

OSHA has leveled a number of regulatory actions at asbestos in the workplace. Some manufacturing processes, including fireproofing of high-rise buildings, and use of asbestos as a component in wallboard patching, have been discontinued. In general, industry limits its use to 2 asbestos fibers per cubic centimeter of air. As of this writing, a proposal to lower it to .5 fibers is still pending owing to industry lobbying. The EPA recently called for a near total ten-year phase-out of all manufacturing uses of asbestos.

Chemicals

Some chemical carcinogens have been banned outright or severely limited in their industrial use: *TRIS*, which was used in textiles, fabrics, toys, and wigs, is one of them. *Acrylonitrile (AN)*, a substance used in the manufacture of synthetic fibers, plastics, and rubber, has been partially regulated, and OSHA requires workers who handle AN to wear protective clothing and respirators.

Benzene, a clear, transparent liquid, is widely employed as a solvent in the chemical and drug industries. It is an additive in some gasoline, and is found in oil-refinery and coke-oven emissions, pesticides, inks, paints, and shoe manufacturing. Eight million tons are produced annually in the United States.

In 1977, OSHA imposed a 90 percent reduction in the levels of benzene permitted in factory air, but the courts did not uphold the reduction. The previous ceiling—ten times higher than OSHA's 90 percent recommendation—stayed in effect in spite of the fact that a recent study indicated a two to eightfold increase in leukemia deaths among workers exposed for a decade to currently allowed levels. Water contamination with benzene disposal has been regulated since 1980. Industrial workers exposed even to low levels of benzene should take protective precautions (see guidelines, page 230).

Metals

Metals are used in many types of manufacturing, especially in the smelting and metallurgic industries. Workers commonly exposed include boilermakers, machinists, sheet-metal workers, steelworkers, aluminum-mill workers, plumbers, welders, and metal molders.

These are examples of carcinogenic metals in industry:

- *Arsenic.* It is estimated that 545,000 U.S. workers are exposed. Regulations have limited smelter air emissions and industrial water effluents. Since 1978, health monitoring and protective equipment have been required for exposed workers.
- *Cadmium.* Used in the rubber industry, in plastics, soldering alloys, pigments, and batteries. One study showed that cadmium workers and miners have a twofold increase in lung-cancer rates, plus a significantly higher incidence of prostate cancer.
- *Chromium.* Chromium compounds are used to make stainless-steel and other alloys, and in the manufacture of glass, bricks, and ceramics. High lung-cancer rates have been seen among workers in these industries.
- *Nickel.* Approximately one million workers are exposed in industries such as shipbuilding, aerospace, electroplating, ceramic and paint manufacturing. Cancers of the lung and nasal passages are found among those heavily exposed. OSHA has placed some regulatory limits on nickel.

Wood Products

No one knows exactly what causes higher cancer rates among woodworkers. The problem was first noted in the furniture-making business. Around the world carpenters, furniture makers and refinishers as well as paper-mill workers have turned up with higher incidence of cancers of the nasal passage, larynx, lung, stomach, and lymphatic system. The breakdown of wood—especially hardwood—seems to be responsible, as airborne dusts are inhaled. The predominance of certain cancers in woodworking industries may also be related to various chemical processes involved.

Airborne dusts in these industries can be controlled through adequate ventilation of the workplace; masks or respirators should be used when exposure is intense.

SEVEN SIMPLE GUIDELINES FOR INDUSTRIAL EXPOSURE

If your work exposes you to any of the chemicals, metals, dust or fibers, to any of the agents in the IARC table, or to any other suspected carcinogen, take the following steps:

1. Wear protective clothing.
2. Wear a mask or respirator during prolonged exposure.
3. Keep work clothes separate from street clothes.

4. Vacuum or clean work clothes before putting them on or taking them off.
5. Dispose of work materials that can't be cleaned. Check with your occupational safety personnel to determine the safest means of disposal.
6. Contact your union, and/or OSHA, for more information about the nature of the problem where you work, and what you can do on an organizational level to limit or eliminate exposure of you and your fellow workers.
7. Be informed.

V

THE PSYCHOLOGICAL FACTOR

17

Cancer and the Mind

Facts . . . in respect to the agency of the mind in the production of the disease (cancer) are frequently observed. I have myself met with cases in which the connection appeared so clear that . . . questioning its reality would have seemed a struggle against reasoning.

Walter Hyde Walsh, M.D.
The Nature and Treatment of Cancer, 1846

There's been a huge transformation in the way we view the relationship between our mind and good health, our mind and disease. In many ways, it's nothing short of a revolution.

Robert Ader, M.D., 1979

The link between mind and body may be as old as history itself—certainly as old as the days of Hippocrates, when the imagination was considered the primary cause of disease.

Throughout the centuries, the mind-body link has been debated—and generally supported—until the advent of scientific bio-medicine in the late nineteenth century, when it disappeared entirely from Western mainline thinking (Eastern philosophy and medicine *never* separated body and mind; nor did it, like the West, invent antisepsis or institute public-health practices). Now, it has reemerged—this time with some backing from the bio-scientists themselves. But, in the years between the remarks of Walter Hyde Walsh and those of Robert Ader (above) mind-body connections were pooh-poohed or bypassed entirely by much of the medical establishment. So much so that Ader can now say the transformation is "nothing short of a revolution."

And to many of us who've been schooled in the Western scientific principles, the idea does seem strange, if not deeply suspect. We've become used to the notion that if someone is tense and driven he may contract an ulcer or set himself up for a heart attack. But the idea that *all* the mind's processes—thinking, feeling, remembering, imagining,

235

experiencing—can deeply influence all the body's processes seems far-fetched. And surely the mind can't affect cellular diseases like cancer!

Yet the concept that emotional factors play a part in the onset of cancer dates at least as far back as the second century A.D. Galen, ancient Greece's most highly regarded medical specialist, whose book was regarded as a classic for fifteen hundred years, was perhaps the first to recognize the connection. He observed that breast cancer occurred more often in women with a "melancholic" rather than "sanguine" temperament. In 1759, the surgeon Richard Guy wrote that women susceptible to cancer were "of a sedentary, melancholic disposition of mind, (who) meet with such disasters in Life as occasion much trouble and grief." In 1870, the famous British physician and surgeon to Queen Victoria, Sir James Paget, made a similar observation: ". . . the cases are so frequent in which deep anxiety, deferred hope and disappointment are quickly followed by the growth and increase of cancer that we can hardly doubt that mental depression is a weighty addition to the other influences favouring the development of a cancerous constitution."

Descriptions of this sort have been recorded throughout medical history. In the nineteenth century alone, the medical literature is stuffed with clinical observations and statistical investigations. One brilliant study by Herbert Snow in 1893 reported that out of 250 women with uterine or breast cancer 156 had experienced some significant problem—often the loss of a loved one within a short period before their diagnosis of cancer. Snow said, ". . . the number of instances in which malignant disease of the breast and uterus follows immediately [upon] antecedent emotion of a depressing character is too large to be set down to chance."

Physicians and scientists in the many years before the twentieth century foresaw what our present-day mind-body researchers are now developing more scientifically: emotions and character traits don't directly *cause* cancer, but can contribute to the risk and to the prognosis. In view of these early reports, it is rather amazing that today's researchers investigating the mind-body link must fight an uphill battle simply to have the notion taken seriously.

But history is full of pendulum swings. And, during the last century, mind-body links were completely ploughed under by the extraordinary advances of bio-medicine: The microscope was invented; germs were discovered and the germ theory was born; the cell became the locus of biological research; dramatic vaccines were developed and, shortly after, the curative miracle drugs like penicillin. Hygiene was instituted, antiseptics introduced, and drinking water was cleaned up. Descartes's philosophy was in vogue: the body was a machine; the separate "soul" or "mind" was "immaterial substance." Says psychologist-historian Lawrence LeShan, "The physician's job (at that time) was that of a mechanic—to fix up any broken down parts of the body. Medical research's principal aim was the identification of the specific cause of each disease: a specific disease in a specific organ must be caused by one specific (exterior) organism." For any ailment, there was "one cause and one cure." Everything was duplicated and "proved" in the laboratory; any disease that couldn't be duplicated was dismissed as "unreal." If a doctor had evidence that a patient was "only nervous" and his symptoms—no matter how acute—had no evident physiological basis, his disease was considered "imaginary" and the patient himself was considered to be "malingering" or accused of "deceiving the doctor."

Only a few lonely voices called for a deeper look at mind-body links—most of them from the developing field of psychiatry. There was Freud, of course, but he was largely dismissed by the mainline physicians as someone who treated female hysteria and other conditions that weren't *"real* diseases—*only mental* ones."

A few other researchers held their ground and did so specifically on the mind-cancer link. In a book published in 1926, the Jungian psychoanalyst Dr. Elida Evans reported that cancer patients were often individuals who had invested all hope and found their full identity in one role or relationship. Before the onset of cancer, that role or relationship was somehow lost, and the person reverted inward, became unmoored, and gave up hope. Dr. Wilhelm Reich, a controversial psychoanalyst in Freud's inner circle, who later broke away to pursue biological energy research, published a book in 1948 entitled *The Cancer Biopathy.* In this original study (which was much maligned—and often by people who never read it), Reich asserted that resignation and an inability to "reach out" emotionally and sexually can lead to a withdrawal of "life energy" from areas of the body. The result, claimed Reich, is fertile ground for cellular disorganization and a greater vulnerability to cancerous growth. But Reich was generally dismissed and his cancer work had little impact.

More in the mainstream, psychiatrists like Franz Alexander (known today as the father of psychosomatic medicine) and his colleagues Nolan D. C. Lewis, Gotthard Booth, and Flanders Dunbar pressed the issue further by suggesting that many diseases had both physical and emotional aspects. They listed fourteen disease entities* as psychosomatic and recommended that patients suffering these diseases be treated with psychotherapy as well as medicine or surgery.

Although some doctors listened, Alexander remarked that most "regular doctors" were still more comfortable "in leaving the mind out of it all," and in restricting psychology to a "healing art." Psychological

---

*Among them: ulcers, hypertension, colitis, rheumatoid arthritis, hyperthyroidism, asthma, and neurodermatitis.

treatment was to be kept distinct from "scientific" therapy based on chemistry, anatomy, and physiology. Even today some physicians believe that psychosomatic phenomena are "logically impossible."

THE GERM AND THE TERRAIN

"We've lived too long with the idea of 'one cause, one cure' and it's not easy to break away from it," says LeShan. "We like magic bullets. They're simple. But there is no 'one cause' for disease—for any disease, really—but especially not for the degenerative diseases like cancer. There's always the combination of a specific agent or germ *and* the person's condition."

The French physician Claude Bernard used to say, "Diseases float in the air; their seeds are blown by the wind but they only take root when the terrain is right." And Pasteur's last words were reported to be "Bernard was right—the germ is little, the terrain all." It's the germ *and* the terrain. But, in the last 100 years, we learned to ignore the terrain—the person—and think only of the specific cause. Only just now are we beginning to pay attention again to the person and to use not only the mainstream medicine's understanding of "the germ" but also bring to bear all the other resources to strengthen the defenses of the terrain: nutrition, exercise, psychotherapy, and developing a person's spiritual abilities. We are learning that cells don't get cancer. That's only where it shows. *People* get cancer and *people* must be treated—and that's what good medicine is all about.

R. D. Smithers, former president of the British Cancer Council, remarked in 1979, "Cancer is no more a disease of cells than a traffic jam is a disease of automobiles. Both traffic jams and cancer are problems of the ecology—of an entire organism, in the case of the city, of the whole person, in the case of cancer."

Once germs have taken hold in the terrain, they must be destroyed, but it's less damaging if you can buttress a human being's innate ability to weed out the intruders before they take hold.

Immunology research tells us that the "terrain"—the body-mind—is manned by an interacting network of defenders against outside invaders. Biological cancer research tells us that a host of carcinogens, like the germs in LeShan's metaphor, can enter the terrain and either be eliminated or start the malignant process. How well the terrain is defended is as important as the "germs" (carcinogens) that penetrate our body's barriers. The strength of the terrain depends on many factors, including genetics, diet, emotions, personality traits, and the power of the attacking carcinogens.

MODERN-DAY RESEARCH IN CANCER AND THE MIND

Reintroducing the concept of mind-body relationships has been difficult. Today the relationship between cancer and the mind stirs up strong waves of controversy.

During the past thirty years, psychological researchers have been busy investigating the connections between emotional states and susceptibility to cancer. They have developed a body of highly suggestive data, illuminating a pattern of shared characteristics among those who develop cancer (see next chapter). Responsible researchers in this field do not assert—or even imply—that tumors are direct reflections of mind states. They have demonstrated the possibility, however, that how we think and feel affects our cancer defenses, and thus contributes positively or negatively to cancer risk. But many of the biological scientists found psychological issues too vague and the instruments to measure mind states too imprecise. They wanted proof on a cellular level of just how emotions affect the body's processes.

The debate went back and forth, and for years the psychologists appeared to be making little headway with the somatically oriented medical researchers. Now, however, investigators in entirely new fields—such as psychoneuroimmunology (PNI)—are beginning to discover the *biological mechanism* by which the mind influences the body. Research on many fronts is unearthing a complex web of interactions between states of mind, the functioning of our nervous and endocrine systems, and the response of our immune systems. Nevertheless, many doctors remain skeptical and won't be content until the mind-body link is "proved absolutely."

Faced with this conflict, a patient—particularly a cancer patient—finds himself in the awkward position of being torn between his belief in the traditional medical approaches of surgery, chemotherapy, and radiation, and the possibility of additional therapies that often deal with mental states and emotions. There should be no either/or. Traditional medicine treats the tumor and adjunct therapies treat the whole person; neither should be bypassed. It's tragic that rigidity on both sides of this debate so often excludes the other. If the new "revolution" is on target, biomedicine and mind-body approaches are both needed for full recovery—and for prevention, as well. Says Richard Grossman of Montefiore Hospital in New York, "What we need is ecumenical medicine."

NORMAN COUSINS

More than anyone else, it was Norman Cousins who introduced the public to the healing possibilities of activating the mind-body link. His first article on this subject appeared in the *New England Journal of Medicine* and was later expanded into a 1979 best-selling book, *Anatomy of an Illness.* In it, he told of his struggle to overcome ankylosing spondylitis, a degenerative disease of the connective tissue of the spine. His prognosis was dismal; he was given minimal chance for full recovery.

With full belief in the body's regenerative powers when properly allied with the mind, Cousins decided to design his own course of therapy. He was backed by an unusually responsive and supportive physician. Cousins's plan was to summon up his "positive emotions," which, he believed, would have the effect of strengthening his immune defenses. He asked for a projector in his hospital room, watched his favorite Marx Brothers movies—which made him laugh—and sought out the best collections of humorous stories he could lay his hands on. (Later he "moved his act" out of the hospital and into a hotel room.) Based on his own research, Cousins believed that massive doses of Vitamin C might ameliorate his condition, and with the help of his doctor he arranged to receive the vitamin intravenously. Within days his symptoms improved; within months he was fully recovered.

Cousins supported his own ideas about the mind's healing powers with reports of ongoing scientific research into the placebo effect; of the relationship between creativity, the will to live, and healing; and he attempted to bridge the gap between holistic and traditional Western medical practices. *Anatomy of an Illness* broke through many barriers and stimulated new dialogues between doctors and their patients. Unfortunately, many have simplified Cousins's ideas and missed his point. Laughter and vitamin C are not necessarily the answers for everyone. Taking charge of your own health is. Trusting your own sense of what is good for you, making conscious decisions together with your doctor rather than passively accepting a prognosis, and creating an environment that you enjoy are all ways to strengthen mind-body interactions. The principal issue is to do everything possible to gain a sense of being in charge of your body—in command of your fate.

Cousins's ideas have been applied to the question of cancer more than to any other disease. And, without question, his approach is as applicable to the prevention of disease as it is to the cure.

AND WHAT ABOUT GUILT?

In another book, *Illness as Metaphor,* author Susan Sontag seeks to explode myths about cancer, which, in her view, include ideas about cancer and the mind. Her theme is the folly and danger of metaphors about illness that have flourished in life and literature. She focuses on nineteenth-century myths about TB and twentieth-century myths about cancer, which she compares and contrasts. She hammers home the point that these myths are often moralistic, punitive, and unrelated to "objective" medical truths.

Sontag performs a valuable service in undermining those myths about cancer that "put the onus of the disease on the patient," or otherwise blame the victim. She rightfully scolds those who might see cancer as stigma. Her most trenchant prose is reserved for literary and political metaphors that use cancer as a symbol of all that is negative: "The people who have the real disease are . . . hardly helped by hearing their disease's name constantly dropped as the epitome of evil."

In the process of exploding myths, however, she creates a few of her own—notably, that the people who see a connection between cancer and the mind are blaming the victim. According to her, such folk— physicians or laymen—embrace the idea that cancer represents a fatal inadequacy of the human spirit. While there may be a few individual doctors, patients, or others who hold such harmful views, responsible psychological theories of cancer are *not* based on the idea that people must be held responsible for psychological conditions that may increase their risk of cancer.

Most psychologists and cancer specialists who are seriously exploring this problem do not make judgments—implicit or explicit—about people who have cancer. Lawrence LeShan, who has spent over eight thousand hours in psychotherapy with cancer patients, comments,

> We are long past the stage where we should believe that because there are emotional factors pressing on us, that it's our fault. When a patient asks if it's true that I'm causing cancer in myself, or my attitudes are causing cancer, the answer I give is "absolutely no." I am only saying that we all fall into emotional traps when we are young—when we have very little experience to guide us, when our brains are still technically unfinished—and we are wounded by life in certain ways and don't know how to handle it. Our bodies react to the stress. Our abilities to maintain health are weakened. But we can't *cause* cancer. Nobody's that good.

Contrary to the belief of many physicians, cancer patients rarely blame themselves, even if they believe that their lifestyles or emotional states have contributed to their illness. Many view the issue as an opportunity to do something themselves to improve their prognosis. In writing of her experience with nodular lymphoma, Lycia Hayden, a young Californian, wrote:

> I had always sensed that my cancer was not caused simply by an invader that had chosen me at random. Nor was it just a set of cells gone spontaneously cuckoo. I felt I was plagued with some interior aggravation that influenced my energy, my thinking, my emotions. But, until I began to read the Simontons and LeShan, it didn't occur to me that there was anything I could do to help myself. It was a relief to learn that there might be therapies—other than my passive acceptance of radiation—that I could undertake actively to help myself. If, as suspected, my outlook on life had contributed to weakening my defenses against the disease, then by making changes, I might help diminish its effects. I went into action.

The notion that a patient might feel—or should feel—blamed because he has suffered psychological wounds that lowered his resistance is an idea as antediluvian as the belief that someone should feel responsible for a genetic predisposition to disease. It is also not too different from the stigma once associated with seeking psychotherapy.

The issue of psychological factors in disease can be thorny, and it must be handled delicately by doctors, therapists, and patients alike. The problem of some patients suffering guilt needlessly may, in fact, have arisen because most doctors are not trained to deal with psychological issues in cancer. Trying to cope with them only complicates their job; they prefer to concentrate on cell pathology, about which they know much more. As a result, most sidestep psychological factors or dismiss them with a simplistic piece of advice to their patients: "You've got to have the right attitude." And then, if the patient can't suddenly produce the "right attitude," he or she might indeed feel guilty!

THAT WORD "RESPONSIBILITY"

There's another area where we sometimes run into semantic and moralistic trouble—and this can be laid more at the feet of the eager New Age types than at those of traditional doctors. That overused statement "You are responsible for your own health" can so easily be turned into an implied "If you become ill, there's a flaw in your character"—which is really not much different from the Bible thumper's "God is punishing you because you are a sinner." The distinction between moralism and support may lie in the difference between "being held responsible" and *"taking* responsibility." To "be held responsible" implies that some outside authority—relatives, doctors, society, or God—is passing judgment and deciding that, single-handedly, you must lift yourself up by your own bootstraps out of the muck of illness and back into that rarefied realm of "health." Not a very inspiring prospect.

"Taking responsibility" on the other hand implies—or should imply—going into action in your own behalf in ways that are appropriate to you and you alone, and, if desired, seeking help in doing so. It has nothing to do with blame. Nor does it mean that if you "fail" you have not taken "enough responsibility" or not done so in good faith. It means that you are "doing the best you can" (a phrase that will never top the charts) to alter damaging processes that have occurred beyond your control, and to engage the powers of the mind so that they are again in sync with the needs and sensations of the body.

This process spans the spectrum from changing habits, like nutrition, exercise, and stress, to reevaluating one's life and liberating desires and emotions that may have been held in check for years. It's no easy process, nor does it ensure success. But, above all, it's *no test of character* whether or not cancer—or any other illness—is prevented or overcome through such efforts.

Perhaps the word "responsibility" should be trashed altogether in this context. The key words are "action in your own behalf" or "taking enlightened command of your own health and body," which, after all, belongs to you and no one else. Many of us are simply—and innocently—unaware of the healing or regenerative powers we have.

THE TIME LAG OF OFFICIALDOM

In regard to prevention, the medical establishment is loath to make recommendations about cancer risk factors until "all the evidence is in." Part of the reason, of course, is political pressure from such groups as the cigarette or meat lobbies, but part is the training of scientists not to make suggestions until something is "proved absolutely."

This makes good—if not vital—sense, of course, in regard to synthetic drugs, which may have complicated side effects, and in protecting the public against charlatans and fads. But it shouldn't hold true for benign suggestions if they have already been shown to have other health benefits, such as good nutrition.

Only many years after much nutritional research pointed to the possible anticarcinogenic effects of foods high in vitamins A, C, and E and the importance of a high-fiber, low-fat diet did the National Cancer Institute and the American Cancer Society dare to suggest that nutrition might be a major factor, and then call for further research. In the meantime, the nutritionists were simply recommending a healthier diet, which could only reap physical benefits, whether or not it reduced (as the nutritionists believed it did) the risk of cancer. Now the scientific evidence for the cancer-preventive role of these dietary prescriptions is overwhelming. We could all have benefited from less of a time lag.

Psychological research on health and disease is in a similar position today. Not much is yet air-tight but the evidence is highly suggestive and it's time to pay attention. Many therapists, researchers, and patients have devised therapies and self-help antistress methods that may well bolster our immune systems. Unquestionably, there are some kooky ideas out there, but responsible adherents are not calling for arcane measures or treatments with dubious values and possible side effects. The few suggestions I will make in Chapters 20 and 21 for antistress techniques and for better psychological health do not guarantee cancer prevention, but they have their own intrinsic rewards. Better coping mechanisms, improved outlets for emotional expression, and a commitment to living one's life fully and joyfully are important goals in and of themselves.

But, in the next two chapters, let's look at what results the psychological and psychoneuroimmunological researchers have unearthed to date.

18

Is There a "Type C" Personality?

In a small southern Connecticut hospital, Jim Baily, a fifty-two-year-old patient recovering from colon surgery, was talking casually with his nurse, Lelia, about cancer. "You know," said the nurse at one point, "there are people who believe it's the nice guy's disease." Jim was struck by the comment. He asked the nurse how she came by this information. He wanted to find out whether it was simply one of those clever little remarks tossed off by people who like to make easy psychological equations or whether the idea had any scientific backing.

Lelia seemed to know quite a bit about the subject. She told Jim about a number of scientific studies that had shown a clear association between certain personality types and susceptibility to cancer. She said that none of the researchers implied that personality or emotional factors actually *caused* cancer, but rather that they contributed to a person's vulnerability to contracting it. A "nice guy" personality, she said, often seemed to be associated with increased cancer risk: the kind of person who wants to please others to the detriment of his own desires; the type that holds in his needs, frustrations, and anger, and goes out of his way to avoid troubling friends, family, or strangers.

Jim was amazed. This sounded uncomfortably like a description of an aspect of his own personality that had always troubled him. He knew that he was polite to a fault and that, in situations that angered him, he reverted to even nicer behavior in fear that he might alienate the person who had, in fact, disappointed *him*. He was even aware that he added insult to injury by blaming himself for being so nice all the time.

During their talk, Lelia mentioned Dr. Bernie Siegel, the Yale surgeon who runs special groups for cancer patients to help them explore the psychological factors contributing to their illness—all as part of a comprehensive program to help them rally their anticancer defenses. After he left the hospital, Jim decided to join Siegel's group in

New Haven. His experience there confirmed his own insights into the origins of his illness. Four years after his surgery, he is convinced that this group, and the subsequent changes he made in his life and his behavior, have helped keep him cancer-free.

Jim's story is a true one. Only the names have been changed. However, the "nice guy" theory is just one facet—though often a central one—of an evolving picture. It seems that there are a complex of personality characteristics associated with increased cancer risk. Some researchers have begun to use the term "Type C" to describe this complex, much the way behaviorists and heart specialists coined "Type A" for personality factors associated with heart disease. There is still no clear consensus as to what exactly comprises a "Type C" personality, or indeed whether such a term is meaningful at all in discussing the psychological factors in cancer. For the moment, it is a controversial yet potentially useful way to refer to the characteristics that many researchers have seen time and again when studying cancer patients.

The two major questions for study and speculation regarding psychological factors and cancer are: (1) to what extent do personality and emotions contribute to the *initiation* of cancer? and (2) to what extent do emotions and attitudes alter the *progression* of cancer after it has already begun? Researchers are vitally interested in the latter in order to determine the particular states of mind that can help or hinder the cancer patient's efforts to become well again. Tremendous controversy has surrounded this research. One side of the debate points to results that would validate the need for psychological intervention in addition to conventional medical/surgical treatment. The other side, which debunks the role of the mind in fighting cancer and disputes the effectiveness of psychological treatments for cancer patients, was given a prominent voice in an article and editorial in the *New England Journal of Medicine* for June, 1985. At that point, the two factions locked horns. I will describe this controversy more fully later in the chapter.

Because the central concern of this book is to present ways to prevent cancer from developing, let's look first at the relationship between the mind and the onset of cancer.

LIFE HISTORIES, EMOTIONS, AND CANCER RISK

In-depth scientific research on cancer and the mind began during the 1950s, accelerated in the 1960s and 1970s, and has found new life and a new scientific foundation in the 1980s. There have been several parallel tracks of this research, which can and should be looked at as the important parts of an intriguing whole. They can be loosely categorized in terms of the relationship between cancer risk and:

- emotional states and early life experiences;
- stressful events or recent losses of significant relationships; and
- personality traits.

Much has been written and many studies made about the connection between the loss of a "significant other" and the onset of cancer. Without question, this is one of life's most stressful events. However, Hans Selye and others have indicated that it's not so much the loss itself but how it is experienced and handled by the bereaved person. And this brings us directly into a consideration of the personality traits and early-life experiences of the person involved, which appear to be more significant than the fact of loss in and of itself. From the studies, it appears that certain experiences and characteristics leave a person more cancer-prone than those with other life experiences and traits—whether or not they have experienced loss. However, loss may often tip the scale toward cancer vulerability if the personality factors are present as well. To generalize, researchers often note:

- People who go on to contract cancer often recall a difficult childhood, characterized by a lack of closeness to one or both parents. As a result, they feel alienated and alone, and often experience later difficulties in establishing close and fulfilling relationships.
- Many cancer patients suffer a profound feeling of hopelessness and despair about achieving any meaning in life—whether from relationships, creativity, or work achievements. This feeling seems to have existed long before any cancer was diagnosed. Often, it was present as far back as the patient can remember.
- The expressions of emotions—especially anger—are characteristically suppressed or repressed. Such people, like Jim, seem to deny their own needs and hold in their anger from an early age for fear of rejection by others.

KISSEN: SMOKING AND PERSONALITY

Some of the earliest and most systematic, controlled studies in this field were carried out in the 1950s and '60s by the late Dr. David Kissen, a chest physician from the University of Glasgow, who was also the specialist for the Scottish mining industry.

Kissen began by studying miners who were also heavy smokers. He administered psychological tests to study subgroups who contracted lung cancer, those who contracted other lung ailments, and those who remained healthy. Kissen wanted to see if there were psychological answers to the age-old question of why some smokers contract lung cancer while others, who smoke just as much, do not. What he found was that the people who had contracted cancer had "poor outlets for emotional discharge." They were, in general, much more prone to deny or repress their feelings. This factor was an even stronger determinant of cancer risk than smoking.

BAHNSON: UNINVOLVED PARENTS

Psychologist Claus Bahnson, while at the Eastern Pennsylvania Psychiatric Institute and Jefferson Medical College, was a pioneering investigator of the early life and emotional makeup of cancer patients. Using a battery of accepted psychological tests, he noted differences between the backgrounds and emotional states of cancer patients, patients with other illnesses, and a control group of healthy individuals. He determined that "cancer patients, unlike persons in three control groups, remembered their parents as noninvolved, cold and not participatory in their early emotional lives." As a result, Bahnson believed, those who go on to contract cancer are often out of touch with their own needs, and "present a realistic and *pleasant* (italics mine) interpersonal attitude, even though they seem to live a constricted and bleak life."

SCHMALE AND IKER: LOSS AND CANCER

Dr. Arthur H. Schmale and Dr. Howard Iker of the University of Rochester began their investigations after noticing a pattern among cancer patients: almost all had experienced a loss or other stressful circumstance to which they responded with a sense of hopeless frustration. To test the validity of this notion, they selected a group of women whose Pap smears revealed some abnormal cells. They then administered psychological tests to determine if there had been such a loss or event that evoked an already existing feeling of utter hopelessness or helplessness. On the basis of their findings, Schmale and Iker attempted to predict which women would be found to have cancer after further medical tests were conducted. *On the basis of the psychological information alone, they were able to predict accurately 73 percent of the time.*

Schmale and Iker's research was especially important for one key reason: they made clear the distinction that stress itself and the loss of a key relationship or role are not in themselves risk factors for cancer. People feel stress and suffer losses all the time and don't become seriously ill. It is the individual response to stress, conflict, or loss that determines how our health and cancer risk are affected.

RETROSPECTIVE STUDIES AND PROSPECTIVE STUDIES

To date, most studies have been *retrospective*—they've looked back at the cancer patient's emotional life histories before they became ill, in search of a pattern. These studies have not been taken as seriously as perhaps they should be by scientists, who point out that the results and conclusions may be skewed by a variety of factors. Cancer patients' responses to psychological tests and the remembered view of their lives before diagnosis may be biased because of their current level of distress. Moreover, they say, slow-growing cancers (which may have existed many years before being found) theoretically could affect emotions by subtle shifts in hormones or nervous-system changes caused by the presence of a tumor. These arguments have yet to be settled.

So, many critics say the retrospective studies prove nothing. What's needed are *prospective* studies that follow for many years a large healthy population whose psychological characteristics have been defined at the outset. Investigators can then determine if those who go on to contract cancer had common traits not seen in the groups that stay cancer-free. A few such studies have been made, which I will detail, and unquestionably, there will be more. Nevertheless, it is important that the retrospective studies not be ignored. What they represent are the collective attempts of investigators to find out what the inner experience of the cancer patient is all about, and it is somewhat closed-minded for certain scientists to claim that studies of the emotional lives of cancer patients are entirely invalid because "how can they [the patients] be objective? how can they know how they felt *before* diagnosis?"

Self-reports are not completely objective, and the stresses of having cancer may, indeed, affect self-perception. But, for the most part, I believe that cancer patients—no matter how depressed or frightened— can to a considerable degree report honestly about their lives and how they felt long before they found out they had the disease. Their own experience and self-assessment are real, human data, and should not be ignored or pooh-poohed. Investigators such as Kissen, Schmale and Iker, Bahnson, and Lawrence LeShan all used established procedures and based their conclusions on both careful clinical observation and the results of proven psychological testing measures.

Psychiatrist Steven Greer—perhaps the leading British researcher of cancer and the mind—has pointed out that retrospective studies are especially useful because they provide important clues to look for in prospective studies. The specific traits that have been discovered from studies of cancer patients will be the factors to look for in healthy populations followed for decades. If people with these traits do end up with a much higher risk of cancer, then the earlier studies will have been validated. Such would be the additional evidence needed to satisfy the strictest criterion of scientific inquiry.

DR. CAROLINE THOMAS—"STRIKING AND UNEXPECTED FINDINGS"

One well-known prospective study has already led straight down this path, although such was not its original intent. Starting in 1946, Dr. Caroline Bedell Thomas of Johns Hopkins University began following a group of thirteen hundred medical students. She wanted to see if there were psychological or behavioral clues or precursors for coronary heart disease. She decided to take complete medical histories, gave the students a battery of psychological tests to determine a range of traits and emotions, and interviewed each to obtain a complete family history. In following them, she watched not only for heart disease but also for hypertension, mental disorders, suicide, and cancer. Ironically, she had no expectation whatsoever that there would be any important link between cancer and psychological factors.

In 1978, Dr. Thomas collected all her data and was able to draw some "striking and unexpected" findings. Two hundred of the students had serious diseases; forty-eight of them had cancer. Among those who had cancer, a look back at their answers to the psychological questionnaires and personal interviews turned up a consistent pattern. Those who had fallen prey to cancer were not, by and large, close to their parents when young; were themselves emotionally detached or "low-gear"; and had generally negative feelings about early family life.* The cancer patients' psychological profiles were most similar to those of the students who had committed suicide.

Dr. Thomas's surprising findings echoed many of the conclusions of the retrospective researchers, especially those of Bahnson and LeShan.

LAWRENCE LESHAN: "THE SENSE OF HOPELESSNESS AND HELPLESSNESS"

Lawrence LeShan, author of *You Can Fight for Your Life,* is a pioneering researcher of the emotional factors involved in cancer. LeShan's work developed through several stages. In the 1950s, he began intensive psychotherapy with seventy cancer patients, many of whom he followed for over twenty-two years. At the same time, he was treating eighty-eight patients without any known malignancy, and they served

---

*A recent review of the same data by Graves and colleagues (*Psychosomatic Medicine,* Nov./Dec. 1986) reanalyzed the subjects' initial Rorschach tests and found that the cancer patients, in contrast to all others, gave responses indicating far less satisfactory interpersonal relationships in general.

as an informal control group, enabling him to determine differences between the life histories and personalities of those with cancer and those without.

LeShan's first step, however, was to do a formal study: he administered baseline psychological tests to a group of 250 people diagnosed with cancer, none of whom were yet in therapy with him. He took personal histories, and held structured interviews with this group of cancer patients.

He took special care to conduct the interviews in a manner that did not call special attention to psychological factors, so that there would be the least distortion from patients seeking to "give the interviewer what he wants." As mentioned earlier, LeShan also established a control group of disease-free individuals with whom to compare results.

The emotional pattern that emerged from LeShan's studies pointed to a number of factors:

- "Terminal" cancer patients exhibited an underlying loss of hope or a "reason for being" that existed long before they were diagnosed with cancer. Part of this loss of hope included a loss of faith in the possibility that things could change.
- Many patients had experienced the loss of a central relationship with a person or group that had provided a "reason for being." In LeShan's initial phase of research with 152 patients, 72 percent reported such a loss, compared with 12 percent in the control group.
- Many patients showed an inability to recover from loss, along with a chronic feeling of isolation and helplessness, despite the fact that they maintained relationships and were functioning "reasonably normally" in the world.
- Many patients possessed an inability to express anger or resentment on behalf of themselves. LeShan found this trait in 47 percent of his patient group, compared with 25 percent of his control group. A "façade of benign goodness" was common.

In his book, *You Can Fight for Your Life*, LeShan discusses what he found in explorations with his patients. It is a poignant account of the nature of a specific form of suffering that seems to contribute to our susceptibility to cancer. No quick and easy testing procedures could have evoked the human data that LeShan's psychotherapy was able to bring to the surface. We have not reached—nor will we ever reach—a time when blood fractions or Rorschach statistics will tell the full story of a person's character and life history. If, as LeShan and others contend, there is a true link between character, life events, and cancer risk, then his method may prove to be as effective as any other in bringing out these relationships—if not more so.

In summing up his insights from over thirty years of work with cancer patients, LeShan said recently: "The single most significant fac-

tor in the weakening of the cancer defense mechanism is the loss of
hope in ever achieving any meaning, zest, or validity in life. It's the
feeling that we can't ever really be ourselves—fully and richly as human
beings—in being, relating, or creating."

LeShan believes that specific personal losses are secondary to this
key feeling. "For example," he said, "you can demonstrate statistically
that the loss of a major relationship is beyond any question a major
factor. However, it seems to me that this is only a contributory factor
to the loss of hope." Apparently there is a kind of predisposition toward
hopelessness in cancer-prone individuals. When the loss of a major
relationship comes, it serves as the straw that breaks the camel's back,
plunging the individual into what he or she sees as a final trap from
which he cannot escape.

LeShan calls this deep-set feeling "despair" and contrasts it to
depression, which he believes is a condition that marks a temporary
period of withdrawal from functioning while the wounded self recovers
from a profound hurt. In *You Can Fight for Your Life*, LeShan describes
despair as a "much more barren and hopeless outlook than that expressed by the usual depressed patient. The alienation felt by the 'normal' depressed, suicidal or otherwise self-destructive patient often allows a continued contact with others, even if it is composed primarily
and consciously of hostile rather than loving elements. The despair of
the cancer patient, on the other hand, brings about a sense of aloneness
that makes it impossible not only for love to bridge the gap, but also
excludes the possibility of fully and satisfyingly relating to others even
in terms of anger, resentment or jealousy." LeShan also notes paradoxi-
cally that those who are subject to this kind of despair often go on
functioning perfectly normally, but with little feeling or connection,
while those who are depressed usually slow down or withdraw from
their normal routines, at least for a period.

Over and over again, LeShan points out that these feelings and
characteristics *predate the development of cancer by years or decades.*
A crisis or loss may have occurred six months or a year before the onset
of disease, but the cancer patients' "world view" existed long before,
sometimes for their entire lives.

LeShan found that this world view usually began in early childhood, often in the first seven years of life. Such children began to feel
that emotional relationships only brought pain and rejection, and as
children are prone to do, they blamed themselves for this state of affairs.
They began to feel lonely and isolated, a feeling that persisted into
adulthood. This, he says, is often the first stage of the cancer "pattern."

The second stage, according to LeShan, "is centered upon the
period during which a meaningful relationship is discovered, allowing
the individual to enjoy a sense of acceptance by others . . . and to find
meaning to his life."

"The third aspect of the pattern comes to the fore when the loss of that central relationship occurs. Now there is a sense of utter despair, connected to but going beyond the childhood sense of isolation."

For most such individuals, psychotherapy may be the only arena in which these feelings can be explored and exorcised. Otherwise, the current loss confirms the initial experience that relationships bring nothing but pain and desolation, and then the third phase becomes one of almost complete resignation. According to LeShan, it is often shortly thereafter that early cancer symptoms appear.

Because these people are so often self-deprecating, nice to a fault, and unable to express hostility in their own defense, the anger and frustration they have toward those who have hurt them has no place to go. LeShan—like Gotthard Booth, David Kissen and others, and later, Steven Greer—noted how emotionally "bottled-up" these patients seemed to be. He described their "benign goodness" as a sign of their lack of hope and of a real belief in themselves.

When I recently asked LeShan about what happened to the life force of this type of cancer patients—where did it go?—he replied, "This type of person still has a strong life force but it's generally blocked. It's buried beneath all this hopeless bleakness."

The cancer-prone personality seems to have more emotions and energy than he is able to express, while other people often have more outlets and demands than they have energy to meet. Part of the reason for the "bottling-up" is the perception of being trapped, the belief that no means of self-expression can bring happiness.

LeShan described the psychological and existential trap in *You Can Fight for Your Life:* "They feel that they can be themselves, and therefore unloved and alone—or, they can get rid of themselves to be someone else and thus be loved. To them it appears that these are the only paths open." Of course, to "get rid" of one's real self in the hopes of being loved is always a disaster. The personalities LeShan describes always end up in despair because efforts to conform to others' expectations to win love and approval can never bring real gratification. It is not the "real self" that is being loved. If one believes that being one's "true self" can only bring isolation and pain, then both roads are dead ends. They see no "third road," no action that can bring about any change, no alternative to despair.

This type of life history—and many of the accompanying personality characteristics—LeShan found in 76 percent of the cancer patients he studied, but in only 10 percent of the control group. He found an even higher percentage among the seventy cancer patients who came to him for intensive psychotherapy.

LeShan's psychotherapy for cancer patients involves searching for the patient's own "song to sing" in life, his special and unique ways of relating and creating. He looks for what is "right" in an individual, not what is "wrong." This leads, he says, to finding and then living the "third road," on which the individual experiences "zest and meaning in life." I will talk about his approach further in Chapter 20, "Psychological Health and Cancer Prevention."

Taken together, the work of Bahnson, Kissen, Thomas, Schmale and Iker, and LeShan presents an overlapping and consistent picture of the life histories, emotional states, and character traits of those who contract cancer.

STEVEN GREER AND THE "TYPE C" PERSONALITY

The concept of a "Type C" personality arose independently from the researchers above. During the 1970s in London, psychiatrist Steven Greer, at the Faith Courtauld Unit for Human Studies in Cancer at King's College Hospital, led a team of investigators that developed a "Type C" profile. Greer's idea of a cancer-prone personality came about through detailed and carefully planned studies of women with breast cancer or benign breast disease.

Greer's first major study, which began in 1971, involved a group of women who came to the hospital with breast lumps. A biopsy examination then determined whether the lumps were benign or malignant tumors. After the biopsy was taken but before the results were known, a series of tests—including a personality profile and an interview—were given to each of the women. In this manner, neither the patient nor the investigators knew whether an individual had a malignancy.

The tests and interview questions included information about eighty different psychological and "psychosocial" variables. Greer suspected from prior studies that the expression of anger might be an important variable, so he took care to develop a rating scale to measure this and other emotional states.

After the results of the biopsies were returned, the researchers were able to compare the group that had breast cancer with the group that had benign lumps. Many of the psychological test categories, including those having to do with stress, recent losses, or other adverse events, came out relatively the same for both groups. The central difference between the two groups was the frequency of "suppression of anger" among those women who were found to have malignancies.

"We often found extreme suppression of anger," remarked Greer, "which we defined clinically as women who had never or had not more than twice in their lives lost their temper in anger. This extreme suppression of anger was confirmed by their husbands, and was significantly more common among the cancer patients than among the controls. About one in two of the breast cancer patients had this history, in comparison with only about one in seven of the women with benign breast lumps."

Greer found that other emotional reactions, including anxiety, were also more often held in check by the cancer patients. The women with breast cancer also ranked lower on a scale that measured general emotional expressiveness. However, the statistical significance of suppression of anger was much greater than that of any other factor.

A cancer-personality picture was beginning to emerge: people who are loathe to express disruptive or hostile emotions; people who tended to be "awfully nice," compliant, and afraid to assert themselves.

It appeared to Greer—as it has appeared to others in the field—that this personality represented a complete opposite from the Type A personality profile. Type A was the term coined by cardiologists Meyer Friedman and Raymond H. Rosenman in their famous 1974 book, *Type A Behavior and Your Heart,* to define a set of behaviors and traits associated with increased risk of heart disease. Type A characters are prone to outbursts of hostility, impatient, aggressive, and often highly competitive. Type B personalities, by contrast, are patient and noncompetitive.

Although the emerging picture of a Type C personality may be diametrically opposed to Type A, Type Bs and Type Cs might appear similar by virtue of their placid exteriors. Nevertheless, with further investigation it became clear that the Type B person and the emerging Type C were just as opposed. Beneath the calm surface of the Type C personality lay huge reserves of unexpressed frustration and hostility, in addition to possible depression and despair. In contrast, whatever adjustment the Type B personality makes in order to function in the world, it involves a much lesser toll on emotional expression and happiness.

A question then arose as to whether Type C people actually have less emotion, whether they are aware of their strong emotions but choose to keep them suppressed, or are, on the other hand, completely unaware of the strong feelings that are unconsciously held in check. Dr. Greer set up some ingenious laboratory situations to investigate.

> We looked at this question by asking a series of patients with breast cancer, and a control group, to look at some videotape films which were designed to provoke anger, and others which are designed to produce anxiety, and still others which are sort of neutral—rather boring travel films. We asked the patients their reactions (self-reports), and at the same time rated their facial expressions, to see how quickly they moved, whether or not they appeared anxious or angry and so on. The findings suggest that they *really do feel* but do not express their feelings. It's not

that they have no feelings—if you look at the data, they say 'yes, we feel angry, or anxious,' but, outwardly, there is no evidence of this.

Because these patients reported an inner response but showed no outer one, Greer sought some form of objective proof that emotion was being experienced on some level of consciousness.

We looked at physiological measurements . . . for instance, the fluctuations of skin resistance. Cancer patients are more likely to show a rise in skin resistance [sympathetic nervous system activity] when shown an anger-provoking film, so we feel that something is going on in terms of emotional arousal.

How does Dr. Greer sum up his appraisal of the cancer-prone personality? He is still cautious about making claims for absolute correlations between personality factors and cancer. He maintains that suppression of anger and the "nice, compliant" characteristics of the Type C profile are still only "possible risk factors." They are not causes, and whether they are true risk factors has yet to be proved in a way that will be fully recognized by the medical community. Greer and his team have distinguished themselves by providing a foundation for the prospective studies that could confirm the strength of the Type C hypothesis.

LYDIA TEMOSHOK AND THE TYPE C PROFILE

Other researchers have produced findings similar to Greer's. Lydia Temoshok, a psychologist at the University of California at San Francisco, may have been the first to elaborate the Type C concept. Her initial work in the early 1980s involved psychological assessments of 150 melanoma patients.

A large number of them did not express negative emotions; even in the face of cancer, they maintained an even temperament, almost never giving vent to anger, sadness, or fear. They tended to worry more about the problems they might be causing to family, friends, or doctors, than about what was happening to them.

Temoshok describes a Type C personality as "cooperative, unassertive, patient; [one] who suppresses negative emotions (particularly anger) and who accepts/complies with external authorities." This description, she says, "is the polar opposite of the Type A behavior pattern which has been demonstrated to be predictive of coronary heart disease."

Temoshok used very sophisticated research tools, including videotaped interviews, to determine emotional states—and their expression or repression—in her melanoma patients. Those patients who clearly exhibited the Type C pattern tended to fare less well and relapse more often and more severely than others. She measured "repressive coping reactions" (suppressing emotion in the face of grave illness), and found that tumor growth was more aggressive and the lesions were thicker in those who rated high in this category. Those who expressed emotion more openly were often found to have less-aggressive tumor growth, along with a stronger immunologic response to their cancer.

Temoshok's findings that expressing negative emotion is related to a stronger immune response against tumor cells and less thick lesions suggests that how a person handles feelings may have a direct effect on anticancer defenses. In another study, melanoma patients who fared well were compared to those who did not, based only on written self-reports. The group with the unfavorable outcome *reported* greater stress, depression, or anxiety. Temoshok explained this result by making a point similar to the one Greer made in his videotape studies: the Type C person experiences negative feelings but doesn't express them. She has speculated that internal anxiety and depression have a negative effect on the defense against melanoma growth; and expressing these feelings openly may buffer this effect and improve the prognosis.

Temoshok has not tried to prove that the Type C characteristics are direct risk factors in the *onset* of melanoma, though her studies tentatively suggest that they may be. Temoshok points out that the characteristic ways that these patients cope with their illness, including the suppression of emotion, usually reflect styles that existed long before a cancer's development. It is possible that these very same factors, holding back emotions, passivity, etc.—are related to the breakdown of the immune system that may have led to cancer in the first place.

In both Greer's and Temoshok's studies, the Type C profile plays a role *predominantly for younger or middle-aged patients. In older patients, age-related factors—*including the breakdown of immunity that comes with age—*seem more significant and psychological variables less so.*

EMOTIONS AND THE PROGRESS OF CANCER: "WE ARE GOING TO GO ON"

Cancer patients with a "fighting spirit"—and those who "misbehave" (complain, gripe, and agonize) in the hospital—have long been known to recover more often and more swiftly than the "good" or "no trouble" patients. Every experienced oncologist and cancer nurse well understands the meaning of the phrases "too good to live" and "too mean to die." Lydia Temoshok's work with melanoma patients confirms this thesis but does so more specifically: expressed emotions—especially anger, loneliness and fear—result in a better recovery. The sense that one has some control over one's body and can fight for one's own recovery is not only a basic tenet of Temoshok and LeShan, but of many other researchers as further studies are completed. The bitching and agonizing, they say, are often healthy signs of the patient's struggling for control.

You might ask how the fighting spirit of cancer patients is relevant to prevention of the disease in the first place. The answer isn't certain, but the question itself is very much worth asking. It may be that healthy people who have the equivalent "piss and vinegar" or "fighting spirit" in meeting the day-to-day challenges of life are less likely to acquire cancer to begin with. This is only an inference. Nevertheless, we stand to learn a lot about what prevents cancer by understanding the mind states that help bolster the fight against cancer in people who already have it.

In a study begun in 1971, Steven Greer reported on a group of sixty-nine women with breast cancer. All of them were interviewed after their diagnosis, and he placed their reactions to having the disease into four categories:

1. Helpless and hopeless: those who felt nothing they did mattered much; they would succumb to the disease.
2. Stoic acceptance: those who were stoic and resigned; they accepted their "fate."
3. Denial: those who would go on with their lives as if they had no malignancies.
4. Fighting spirit: those who believed they could affect the outcome of their illnesses and, with determination, decided they would fight to live.

Five and then ten years later, Greer and his team looked at these patients' survival rates. The results were clear: the "fighters" did best, with the "deniers" a close second. The "stoic" and "hopeless" groups didn't fare well. And, as you might suspect, the "hopeless" had the shortest survival rate.

Some of the results were surprising, in that we tend to think of denial as a form of repression, and that we also tend to view a stoic reaction as one of some strength. Greer described deniers and why he thought they survived longer than the stoics and the hopeless individuals:

> They often show the kind of denial where they say "look, there might have been a few cancer cells there, I don't know, but as far as I'm concerned, I don't want to know about it. I just want to get on with my life."
> I would almost prefer to call this "positive avoidance." They "positively

avoid" in order to lead a normal life. So they are different than those with "fighting spirit" who try to get all the information they can to fight the disease. But they are similar, in that both seem to be saying "we are going to go on."

The stoics seem to be putting up a "nice guy" front to cover resignation. The fighters and deniers are the most energetic, while the stoics and hopeless have withdrawn energy from the life process. "If I were to make a guess," said Greer about the reason for his results, "it's the active response which seems to be related to a better outcome." Lawrence LeShan makes an additional point: Denial may be a psychological defense mechanism in life, but in response to a diagnosis of cancer, it may well be adaptive. It may be healthy to go through a period of denial when faced with a life-threatening illness.

As discussed earlier, suppression of anger and a sense of hopelessness are two factors possibly associated with a higher risk of contracting cancer. It follows that, if people with cancer can summon up an aggressive response "in defense of themselves," with "faith in the possibility of change," they might awaken their own disease-fighting mechanism. This is yet another inference, but it's a reasonable conclusion to draw from the studies mentioned. (See also the next chapter, "How the Mind Influences Immunity," for the biological basis of this concept.)

Many other studies have been made on how personality, behavior, and emotions might affect the progression of cancer. Among the most notable are:

- In the 1950s, Dr. Eugene Blumberg studied cancer patients in a veterans' hospital, and showed distinct differences between those with fast-growing tumors and those with slow-growing tumors, who had a better prognosis. Those with aggressive malignancies again tended to be serious, overnice—bending backward to please—apologetic, and defensive. Those whose cancers developed slowly had more effective methods for handling stress and were more expressive.

- Dr. Bruno Klopfer, another pioneer in the 1950s, was one of the leading experts on Rorschach testing. Using Rorschach tests, he was able to correlate a specific personality pattern with slow-growing versus fast-growing tumors. Klopfer found that patients who were deeply invested in their "ego defenses" were more likely to have aggressive cancers, while those who were less defensive had slower-growing tumors and less recurrence. He believed that the latter expended less energy on defending themselves and therefore had more left over to fight their disease.

- Dr. Sandra Levy, Associate Professor of Psychiatry at the University of Pittsburgh, followed a small group of breast-cancer patients with recurring bouts of the disease, in the late 1970s. A short-term follow-up indicated that those who survived complained of "significantly more distress and unhappiness" in response to their illness than the ones who died. However, Dr. Levy didn't publish these findings, preferring to wait until a prospective study could be conducted over many years. Her second study has just been completed and her findings presented at several meetings. After she had followed thirty-six women for seven years, twenty-four died. Those who survived differed from those who did not in several respects. The two most significant factors were the length of the interval in which patients were in remission, and high scores in a category called "joy" on a scale used to measure moods. Although it is difficult to explain these results, and too early to extrapolate, one can speculate that expression of emotions—whether negative or positive—bodes well for recovery.

FOLKLORE OR SCIENCE? THE MIND-BODY CONTROVERSY

The mind-body researchers and some bioscientists locked horns when, in 1985, the *New England Journal of Medicine* published a study and an editorial that questioned the role of the mind in fighting cancer. The study, headed by Dr. Barrie Cassileth at the University of Pennsylvania Cancer Center, followed 204 patients with advanced cancers, and another 155 who had been treated for breast cancer or melanoma—conditions that often recur. The patients were all given psychosocial questionnaires about their lives and attitudes, and were rated on various categories of psychological responses. After following the patients for three and a half years, Cassileth and her team concluded that there was no connection between positive outlook and survival or recurrence.

The *Journal* also printed an editorial by deputy editor Dr. Marcia Angell, asserting that the entire mind-body approach to healing had been oversold: "It is time to acknowledge that our belief in disease as a direct reflection of mental state is largely folklore."

That statement by Angell, along with her comment that "medical literature contains very few scientific studies of the relation, if there is one, between mental state and disease," struck an odd chord. The mind-body researchers experienced her comments as a rather shocking example of how far some in the modern medical establishment will go to belittle to scientific inquiry into the mind-body relationship. The phrase "disease as a direct reflection of mental state" is a complete misrepresentation of the complexity of the mind-body link, a complexity that is fully acknowledged by researchers in the field. Moreover, the assertion that there have been "very few scientific studies" of the relationship between mental state and disease is a gross misstatement, discarding decades of published work in psychosomatic medicine and the recent breakthroughs in psychoneuroimmunology.

The problems with Cassileth's study are several. One is conceded by the researchers themselves: the study "did not address the possibility that psychosocial factors or events might influence the cause of the disease or the outcome for patients with more favorable diagnoses." This comment referred to the fact that all the 204 patients were in the far-advanced stages of cancer, where *any* intervention is less likely to bring about improvement. No advocate of psychological cancer therapy that I know of claims that his approach is likely to reverse cancer in the later stages, when widespread metastases are already present.

A second point: the best retrospective studies gather comprehensive life histories, and develop sensitive measurements of psychological states, including suppression of emotions such as anger or anxiety. In this study only seven factors were measured: social ties and marital history, job satisfaction, use of psychotropic drugs, general life evaluation/satisfaction, subjective view of adult health, hopelessness/helplessness, and adjustment to diagnosis. These were measured with single "self-report" scales, considered by many a superficial approach.

A slew of letters to the *New England Journal,* many from renowned psychosocial researchers, criticized the methods used in the Cassileth study. Dr. Sandra Levy and several of her colleagues, whose claims about the role of the mind in cancer progression are modest but precise, said in a joint letter that the Cassileth study "was methodologically limited on two counts: the patient sample and the measures that were used."

POSITIVE ATTITUDE: WHAT DOES IT MEAN?

Dr. Angell began her editorial in the *New England Journal* by saying: "Is cancer more likely in unhappy people? Can people who have cancer improve their chances of survival by learning to enjoy life and to think optimistically?" She then embarked on a critique of mind-body concepts and research. Her implication was that most investigations of cancer and the mind can be boiled down to these two simple questions. In doing so, she has fallen into the trap of the popularizations that misinterpret and simplify mind-body approaches to: "All you've got to do is have a positive outlook." The *New England Journal of Medicine*'s editorial hung the whole field of mind-body healing onto this erroneous interpretation.

There is little question that following the simplistic prescription "Just have a positive outlook" can be dangerous—a point that Dr. Angell makes in her editorial and correctly so. If given as a prescription, it calls for a stiff upper lip, and a denial of the individual's real emotions—both attitudes that most cancer-mind researchers claim only lead to greater decline. But Angell misses the greater point: feelings, however tumultuous they are, must be recognized, if not expressed, and new roads must be sought that will bring genuine, individualized enjoyment and pleasure. There's no faking it. The "positive outlook" must be real—not play-acted consciously or unconsciously. And no one should feel guilty if he doesn't have the "right attitude."

Recently, I discussed this issue with Dr. Stephanie Simonton-Atchley who is currently on the staff in the Department of Otolaryngology at the University of Arkansas for Medical Sciences. She treats cancer patients and conducts clinical research on cancer and the mind-body link. Formerly, Dr. Simonton-Atchley worked with the radiation oncologist O. Carl Simonton, who gave up his radiology practice because he believed so strongly in offering cancer patients the "adjunctive" techniques of psychotherapy, meditation, and visualization, with conventional medical treatment. In the early 1970s, Stephanie and Carl started the Cancer Counseling and Research Center in Dallas, to offer these therapies, and later wrote the exceptional book *Getting Well Again*. They now work separately but in the same field. Stephanie Simonton-Atchley gave me perhaps the best explanation I've heard about how the notion of "positive mental attitude" has become so misinterpreted: "I think that it [positive mental attitude] has been promoted by a lot of non-psychologically trained physicians and nurses who have latched onto this theory, and simplified it from a medical perspective and then say, 'Oh, just have the right attitude.' They're sympathetic to the general concept, but often don't understand anything about how to develop a positive attitude."

"A lot of people are confused in this area," she continued. "They say if a person is hurting and depressed, aware of it and talking about it, that they have a 'bad attitude.' Really, I can get on a soap-box about what people do with that nonsense called 'white-knuckled optimism'! I don't encourage people to deny their feelings in an effort to be optimistic. I've always made the distinction between depression and denying depression. Sometimes the most appropriate way patients can be is hopeless, overwhelmed and grieving. If they can go into these feelings and experiences and find support, they will generally come out the other side to a *realistic optimism.*"

LONG-RANGE PROSPECTIVE STUDIES:
THE WAVE OF THE FUTURE

Retrospective studies can be said to be strongly suggestive, but long-range studies that follow healthy populations are needed to investigate the Type C cancer connection and pinpoint possible characteristics that can be truly predictive of increased cancer risk.

Caroline B. Thomas's prospective study with medical students (see page 250) was important but the number of people who developed cancer (forty-eight) is considered too small for definitive conclusions.

Here are the other major prospective studies that are noteworthy:

- Dr. Otto Hagnell conducted a survey of 2,550 people in Sweden. A personality test was given to them twenty years before the group was assessed for incidence of cancer. The findings indicated that women who eventually contracted cancer were more often those of the "substable" personality type, and more prone to "depressive" moods or attitudes. These assessments were made long before the onset of cancer.

- University of Chicago researchers Linas Bieliauskas and Richard Shekelle were able to take advantage of the information provided by a long-term study of 2,010 middle-aged employees of a Chicago Western Electric plant. Starting in 1957–58, these men were given the Minnesota Multiphasic Personality Inventory (MMPI), the well-established psychological test that measures a variety of personality attributes, including depression. They analyzed the health of this group at intervals over twenty-five years. By then, sixty men had died of cancer. Those who died were twice as likely to have scored high in the "depression" category than those who didn't contract cancer. This association remained strong, even when drinking, smoking, age, and a family history of cancer were taken into account.

- Dr. Ronald Grossarth-Maticek investigated the relationship of psychosocial factors to cancer mortality in a prospective study of 1,353 healthy inhabitants of a city in Yugoslavia. The subjects were given a comprehensive interview and questionnaire covering over one hundred items and measuring a variety of emotional responses, defense mechanisms, coping styles, etc. A decade after the study began, 166 people had died of cancer. The key finding was this: 158 of the 166 cancer deaths scored very high in a category called "rationality and anti-emotionality" (R/A, for short). This refers to the built-in tendency to suppress emotions, especially anger, and maintain control over so-called "irrational" or "hysterical" impulses.

Of the 32 men who had died of lung cancer, 31 of them were, as you might expect, heavy smokers. Of all the heavy smokers in the study, 139 had been rated very high in R/A, while 179 were rated in the low-mid range of R/A. All 32 men who died of lung cancer were from the high R/A group. *Perhaps the most striking finding was that not a single one of the 179 heavy smokers who rated in the low-mid range of R/A acquired lung cancer!* Naturally, Grossarth-Maticek concluded that suppressing emotions and rigid self-control are contributing risk factors for cancer. Combined with smoking, he claimed, it increases the risk some forty times. He also found that "long-lasting hopelessness" is associated with cancer risk, though not as strongly as "rationality/anti-emotionality."

- Grossarth-Maticek reviewed the same data to see if the cancer-prone personality had a particular style of interpersonal relating. What he found was that those who went on to contract cancer were more likely to be the passive receiver of "interpersonal repression." According to Grossarth-Maticek, this means they "can be described as submissive, nonaggressive, suppressing their perceived needs . . . [a] set of characteristics that predisposes them to be a 'receiver of repression,' and thus to be exposed to feelings of helplessness, of giving up and depression." On the other side of the coin, the more aggressive Type A individual, with increased risk of heart disease, was more likely to be an "emittor of repression"—someone who actively tries to "dominate other persons at least in more intimate social relationships by attitudinal, verbal, and behavioral means."

A superficial reading of Grossarth-Maticek's findings, and other Type C studies, might give the impression that if you suppress your anger you're more likely to acquire cancer; and if you release your anger you're more likely to have a heart attack. But that's not quite it; the truth lies in between. A lifelong suppression of anger is unhealthy (Type C); compulsive "acting-out" of anger is also not very healthy (Type A). Awareness of anger and expressing it appropriately in daily life brings greater balance, contentment, and health. No great surprise.

In spite of the interesting findings from these prospective studies, there is still a long way to go. It will be necessary for a very large group—perhaps ten thousand healthy people—to be followed for some twenty years, to yield the numbers and wealth of data that scientists look for in this type of epidemiological research. When and if such studies emerge, the Type C profile may become as much an accepted part of the medical parlance as Type A is today.

19

How the Mind Influences Immunity

Thinking means connecting things, and stops if they cannot be connected.

G. K. Chesterton

From a scientific standpoint, all the relationships demonstrated between personality factors and cancer risk would amount to nothing more than a hill of beans if a lot more connections weren't made.

What connects psychological factors with tumor growth on the biological level? How might things like despair or suppression of anger affect our bodies in such a way as to cause normal cells to develop into cancer cells and then grow into tumors? This has been the crux of the matter for years, and without answers Western biomedical scientists would continue to think of the link between cancer and the mind as nothing more than fanciful speculation. "Demonstrate a biological connection and we'll listen" is the unstated chorus of the skeptical scientific researchers who require more than just "psychological" studies.

That chorus is finally beginning to be answered. The notion of a link between cancer and the mind—and all the psychosocial studies which have been carried out to wit—are being buttressed by research on the biological bridges that exist between psyche and soma.

In fact, entire new fields of research on the mind-body connection have formed in the last decade. Almost all of them have tongue-twisting names, like psychophysiology, neuroendocrinology, and neuroimmunomodulation.

But one field has become predominant, and to a certain extent its name now serves as an umbrella term for all the others: psychoneuroimmunology, known as PNI. If you break it into its three components—psycho, neuro, and immunology—it is clear that the field concerns itself with the bridges between one's psychological state, central nervous system, and immune system.

Although the term psychoneuroimmunology does not directly refer to the endocrine system (endocrine glands and the production of hormones), research in PNI often involves hormones because of the many roles hormones play in linking the mind, the nervous system, and the immune system. I once heard a mind-body researcher say that, if you were going to use an accurate term for the new research, it would be "psychoneuroendocrinimmunology." He doubted that such a term would ever make it into everyday parlance—or even that of doctors.

MEDICINE'S NEW REVOLUTION: PSYCHONEUROIMMUNOLOGY

The major discovery that has opened up new vistas to mind-body researchers—and is revolutionizing our whole approach to medicine—can be summed up in one sentence: the immune system does not act alone. This system—sometimes referred to as a "liquid army" because it consists of roving cells circulating in fluid—was formerly thought to be completely independent of any other biological system. It is now clear that it acts in concert with other systems, particularly the endocrine and central nervous systems. The immune system receives cues from the brain, and is partially regulated by it and by products of the nervous system, as well as by hormones, products of the endocrine system.

The links between the mind and the central nervous system and the endocrine system have been known about and studied for decades. The big news is that these systems are also connected to the immune system. The major connections look something like this:

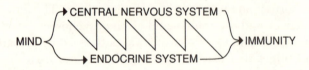

Several pathways also intertwine the central nervous system and endocrine system. What this means is that we all have an interlocking network of biological systems that make up the whole person, where attitudes, emotions, sensations, growth regulation, internal homeostasis (balance), and internal defense and surveillance, are subtly interrelated functions. We all respond to stimuli and experience on many levels at once—and all levels affect one another. It is a holistic vision of human biology, and one that is now being affirmed on the molecular level.

This breakthrough came as a great surprise to many biologists. What all this means for us (I have said this before but wish to reiterate it here in the context of PNI) is that mind and health and mind and disease are so intimately connected that many diseases we formerly thought were "purely mental" or "purely physical" are, in fact, an interwoven admixture of the two. And any therapy, to be effective, should address the needs of both body and mind. Or therapies must be combined to meet the needs of both.

Indeed, the mind seems to have powers over the body which few Westerners deemed possible. It seems that all the mind's processes—thinking, feeling, imagining, experiencing—profoundly affect all the body's processes and systems, including the immune system.

The founding principle of PNI is the idea that the brain can regulate the immune functions and that the immune system is altered by mental and physiological stress.

Dr. George Solomon, a professor of psychiatry at UCLA, and one of the first great PNI pioneers, recently listed "22 hypotheses" on the links between the immune and central nervous systems. In my somewhat simplified language, here are ten of Solomon's key points:

- Personality characteristics influence the susceptibility of an individual's immune system to be influenced by environmental factors.
- Emotional upset or distress will affect the incidence, severity, or course of those illnesses that either (a) result from defects of the immune system, such as autoimmune diseases, or (b) have the possibility of being stopped by the immune system, such as infections or cancer.
- Stress, conditioning, and early experience can alter a person's immune system.
- Manipulating parts of the central nervous system (such as the hypothalamus) will affect the immune system.
- Hormones regulated or produced by the central nervous system can influence immune mechanisms.
- Immune cells, including lymphocytes (the critical cells of the immune system) should have receptor sites for neurotransmitters, neurohormones, and neuropeptides. This implies that products of the nervous system play a role in regulating the activity of key immune cells.
- Feedback mechanisms regulating the immune system should run (in part) through the central nervous system.
- Substances produced by the immune system can affect the central nervous system.
- Biochemical similarities exist between substances that are produced by (and govern) the central nervous system and those produced by the immune system.
- Behavioral interventions—such as biofeedback, imagery, hypnosis, relaxation techniques, and psychotherapy—should be able to enhance immune functioning.

All this sounds somewhat complex—and indeed it is—but if you hang in with me, you will begin to have an idea of the new discoveries in the biological, not just psychological, connections between body and mind.

THE PNI PIONEERS

George Solomon was perhaps the first researcher to validate PNI hypotheses: the immune system can be altered by psychological states and the brain helps regulate immunity. Working at Stanford University in the late 1960s, Solomon was treating patients with rheumatoid arthritis, an "autoimmune" disorder, in which the immune system attacks the person's own joints. He knew that rheumatoid arthritis was also a condition responsive to stress; the symptoms usually became worse when someone was anxious or under pressure. This connection—stress and immune malfunction—prompted Solomon to begin experimental animal research on the link between stress, the brain, and immunity.

Together with immunologist Alfred Amkraut, Solomon created stress in rats by shocking them and housing them in crowded cages. He then implanted tumors in the animals and compared the results with a control group of nonstressed rats. The tumors in the stressed animals grew more rapidly—a sign that the immune system was less active against cancer cells than in the nonstressed rats. It was becoming clearer that stress was directly influencing immunity. But just how? Could the brain be involved?

To find out the answer, Solomon and Amkraut followed a hunch, based on prior Soviet research with rabbits, that the part of the brain called the *hypothalamus* might be a control center for immune functions in the body. They used an electric probe to burn out portions of the hypothalamus in rats to see if their immune systems changed. As they suspected, some of the rats' immune functions became significantly suppressed.

Robert Ader and the Influence of Behavior on Immunity

This "psychoimmunology" research, as it was called by Solomon at that time, took a further leap in the early 1970s with the inspired work of psychologist Robert Ader at the University of Rochester. What Ader discovered was that immune functions could be conditioned, in just the way Pavlov's dogs were conditioned to salivate at the sound of a bell even after a reward was no longer offered.

Ader stumbled onto this finding while conducting a Pavlovian type of experiment. He was trying to develop an aversion to saccharin in rats by injecting a drug that induced nausea after the saccharin was ingested. When many of the rats died during the experiment, Ader found that the nausea-inducing drug he had been using also suppressed the immune system. With this realization, Ader went a step further: he wanted to see if he could "condition" this immunosuppression in rats. Indeed, he was able to associate the drug with the taste of saccharin so that a taste of saccharin alone—without the drug—would be enough to bring about a suppression of the rat's immune system. He had "taught" the rats to alter their immunity, and he later found that rats conditioned this way were more susceptible to infectious diseases. In further experiments, Ader used the same technique to enable rats to overcome autoimmune disease: he trained them behaviorally to inhibit their immune response in order to alleviate the symptoms of a form of lupus erythematosus.

The fact that the immune system could be conditioned behaviorally proved to Ader that the mind and central nervous system were connected to immunity. He coined the term "psychoneuroimmunology," based on his early research and the conviction that this work was the beginning of an entirely new realm of mind-body science.

With regard to cancer, the bridges being uncovered by PNI and other related fields of research are clues to how our anticancer defenses can be influenced by thoughts, feelings, and behavior. I will describe these bridges and how they relate specifically to cancer and the mind. But let me start first with the earlier research on stress and the immune system that eventually led to PNI.

STRESS AND IMMUNITY

Stress is one of those words that confuses. What is stress? Is it a circumstance that causes people to feel taxed, pressured, anxious? Is it the feeling of discomfort that accompanies difficult experiences in daily life? Or is stress only an individual's personal experience of a situation that may—or may not—be objectively difficult or painful?

Stress is not a very precise term, but it is a useful one. Certain situations in life are invariably stressful. The death of a spouse or close family member, divorce, separation, illness, loss of a job, or just physical crowding, noise, or temperature change. Extremely happy events—marriage, pregnancy, a promotion at work—can also be stressors, because they involve change, which in and of itself causes some emotional upheaval.

More and more, it is being accepted that a certain amount and a certain kind of stress are healthy. "Healthy" stressors can be joyous events, transforming events, or are just the friction of daily life that presents healthy challenges. Finally, though, it is an individual's *perception* of an event that determines how negatively stressful any situation will be. The meaning of a typically stressful event differs from person to person, and each person has different mechanisms for coping with stress, which are more or less effective. How our psyches and somas respond to events we consider stressful depends on a host of unique personality factors—some would say, "prior conditioning."

When a person experiences stress, specific physiological responses *always* occur. Dr. Hans Selye, the celebrated biochemist, is considered the foremost biologist and philosopher of stress and its effects on the human animal. Selye followed the work of Walter B. Cannon, who first illustrated the body's neurological response to stress, commonly called the "flight or fight" response.

Flight or Fight: Cannon and Selye

The autonomic nervous system, which involves all involuntary activities, is divided into two main branches—the sympathetic and the parasympathetic systems. The sympathetic nervous system is the one that prepares the body for the flight-or-fight response by increasing heart rate and blood pressure, and regulating certain hormonal secretions. The parasympathetic branch directs involuntary behaviors, including digestion and excretion, and slows the body down when necessary. Cannon first defined the flight-or-fight reaction as our sympathetic nervous systems' built-in tendencies to respond to threatening or potentially painful circumstances by signaling us either to defend ourselves aggressively or make a quick getaway. But it was Selye who took the study of the body's stress response further by uncovering the complex hormonal system that is simultaneously triggered.

Selye found that stress leads to a "cascade" reaction of hormones in the body. To use a corporate analogy: as soon as the brain registers danger or difficulty, a stress message is "written" and then passed by various messengers from one neural or hormonal office to another, each time stimulating a different functional responsibility. The process begins deep within the brain, in the hypothalamus, which sends a specific neurohormone (one of many hormones produced by or stimulating the nervous system) signal to the pituitary gland, the small oval gland at the base of the brain. This master gland of the endocrine system is then activated to secrete more hormones, including the powerful ACTH (adrenocorticotropin).

ACTH is the prime messenger acting on the adrenal glands, the two triangular glands that sit atop the kidneys. The adrenals have an inner portion, called the "medulla," and an outer layer, called the "cortex." Each section produces a different set of vital hormones. When

ACTH reaches the adrenals with its "stress message," the outer cortex is stimulated to secrete a group of hormones referred to as the "corticosteroids." These compounds (which include cortisone) reduce inflammation in the body but, under prolonged stress, they also suppress immunity.

Selye observed the effects of stress on experimental animals, and found that when their adrenal cortexes became enlarged, they often developed stomach ulcers, and their thymuses, spleens, and lymph nodes shrank. The latter three glands are the primary "organs" of immunity; their atrophy under stress was an early clue to the intimate relationship between the nervous, endocrine, and immune systems. It was Selye who first established the idea that our immune systems are imperiled by the effects of long-term stress.

The hypothalamus is also hooked up to the inner portion of the adrenals, the medulla, where the other key group of stress hormones are made—the catecholamines. The most important catecholamines are epinephrine and norepinephrine, which are also referred to as adrenaline and noradrenaline. These hormones act in concert with the sympathetic nervous system. Epinephrine makes the heart beat faster, quickens and deepens breathing, triggers the release of stored sugar from the liver, and helps cause the blood to flow away from the skin and in toward the brain and skeletal muscles. Norepinephrine is manufactured not only in the adrenal medulla, but is also secreted by sympathetic nerve endings. Like epinephrine, it also increases the rate of breathing and, by constricting the small blood vessels, leads to a rise in blood pressure. Norepinephrine increases blood flow through the coronary arteries, slows heart rate, and relaxes the smooth muscle in the intestine.

The catecholamines have been implicated as the stress hormones leading to the damage of coronary arteries that presages heart disease. When stress is considered one of the contributing causes of coronary problems, it is the catecholamines that are the hormonal link between psyche and soma. Type A coronary-prone personalities have been found to have higher blood levels of these hormones.

Now, PNI research is also implicating catecholamines as part of the big picture of how chronic stress leads to cancer susceptibility. Epinephrine, in particular, may impair the proliferation of lymphocytes in the body and may also specifically increase the number of T-suppressor cells—both leading to a loss of T-cell immune defenses. Such a loss can leave the individual more vulnerable to malignant cell growth.

We now know that Cannon's description of the flight-or-fight response initiated by our sympathetic nervous system and Selye's cascade of stress hormones are both interacting parts of the whole that is the mind-body reaction to acute (short-term) stress. We know, too, that when we're exposed to continuous and intense stressors, the condition known as chronic stress begins, which often has a depressing and dangerous impact on our immunity.

Experiments have also been made demonstrating the immune system's ability to recover after long-term stress. I will return to this point later.

Vernon Riley and Mice on the Turntable

The late Vernon Riley of the Pacific Northwest Research Foundation was a pioneer experimental researcher of stress, immunity, and cancer. Riley conducted tests with a strain of mice bred to develop breast cancer. He carefully protected them from any stressful environmental effects whatsoever. Then he subjected them to varying degrees of stress through an ingenious method: he put them in cages on turntables. He assumed that the faster the speed of the turntable the greater the stress would be. He divided the mice into several groups. One group was left quiet. The other groups were placed in cages and spun on the turntable at varying speeds. The results were astonishingly consistent with the idea that the greater the stress the weaker the immune system became. The groups of mice on the fastest turntables developed the largest tumors, and their tumors grew the fastest.

In another experiment, Riley found that a group of the mice genetically predisposed to cancer could still be protected from tumor growth by being kept in a stress-free environment. Ninety-two percent of those exposed to stress grew tumors, while only 7 percent of the protected mice developed cancer. He also showed that conditions of stress resulted directly in an increase in the release of corticosteroids, which in turn injured the mice's immune systems markedly. To drive the point home, Riley was able to help restore their immune functions by injecting the mice with a corticosteroid antagonist.

Because of the effects of stress on the nervous system, the endocrine system, the immune system—and in a secondary way on other biological systems, such as the circulatory, respiratory, and digestive systems—our bodies under stress are more vulnerable to a host of diseases.

The remarkable connections made through PNI research have forced a complete reassessment of the relationship between stress, personality, moods, and disease. As I mentioned earlier, leaders of the new mind-body research now believe that most if not all diseases are *multifactoral*. Stress and psychosocial factors may play a role in all physical disorders. Even infectious diseases, "caused" by a single bacterium or virus, must be viewed in the new light of PNI research. It is possible for healthy immune systems to resist infectious agents under the right circumstances, and we know that suppressed immune systems succumb more readily to such agents. How far this finding can be taken is left to future research. At this point there is no telling how much we can do to protect ourselves from the entire spectrum of human illnesses just by taking care of our psychological and social needs.

IS THE BRAIN LINKED DIRECTLY TO IMMUNITY?

The claim that our immune systems are modified by our nervous systems brings up one question: are there control centers within the brain linked directly to immunity?

The answer is, unquestionably, yes. I've already mentioned that the hypothalamus sends out hormones that eventually influence immunity. But PNI research has uncovered much additional evidence about the intricate hookups between the brain and immune system.

With the exception of the nervous system, the immune system is the body's most complicated network. Now it's clear that these two systems—which earlier biologists believed never touched each other—are intimately linked through the brain and other neural pathways. Because both systems are so complex, discovering and mapping the fine connections is a labyrinthine process, which will occupy researchers for many years to come.

The Hypothalamus, a Busy Messenger Center

The hypothalamus appears to be crucially involved in immunity. This small piece of brain tissue is located deep in the forebrain and can be thought of as a busy headquarters and central interchange for incoming information and outgoing orders. Besides sending out hormones that influence the endocrine system (the pituitary and adrenal glands are activated by hypothalamic messengers), this tiny portion of brain matter also controls body temperature, thirst, hunger, and sexual function. It is the center that integrates the signals from the autonomic nervous system with hormonal activity and plays an important role in emotional activity. The fact that the hypothalamus is the part of the brain most closely linked to emotion is an anatomical clue to the relationship between emotions, immunity, and cancer susceptibility.

Soviet researchers were the first to show that both T-cell and antibody immune responses could be suppressed by damaging portions of the hypothalamus. One of the Soviet studies showed that electrical stimulation of a portion of the hypothalamus increased antibody responses. George Solomon duplicated many of the Soviet findings, and also demonstrated that the thymus, the master gland of immunity, became impaired when parts of the hypothalamus were destroyed.

By studying guinea pigs sensitized to a specific antigen, Dr. Marvin Stein and his research associates at Mount Sinai School of Medicine in New York have found that the anterior or forward portion of the hypothalamus is directly related to immunity. The guinea pigs were sensitized so that, if they had normal immune systems, a second exposure to the antigen would cause "anaphylactic shock," a lethal form of severe allergic reaction. This is just what happened to almost all those in a control group. Another group of guinea pigs, which had also been sensitized but whose anterior hypothalamus had been burned out, were protected from a fatal reaction because their immune systems were no longer operating as expected. Although the researchers are not sure exactly which immune function is inhibited by damage to the anterior hypothalamus, they believe it may be normal antibody production and/ or the action of chemicals in the lung that facilitate the "anaphylactic" immune reaction.

As far back as 1970, Stein also demonstrated a link between the brain and cell-mediated (T-cell) immunity. He reported that lesions in the forward portion of the hypothalamus suppressed skin-test responses to the tuberculin antigen, a measure of T-cell reactions. Then in 1980, Stein, Steven J. Schleifer, Steven E. Keller, and their colleagues took a close look at the immune cells from guinea pigs that had lesions in the same area of the hypothalamus created by delivery of electric current. When their lymphocytes were cultured in whole blood and challenged with a variety of antigens, the guinea pigs were discovered to be markedly less active in their immune responses than normally would be expected.

Swiss researcher Hugo Besedovsky has shown, rather dramatically, the connection between the hypothalamus and the humoral (antibody) immune response. Besedovsky decided to measure the electrical activity of the brain in rats, during the course of an immune response. He hooked up his equipment, then injected the rats with powerful antigens that stimulate an antibody response. He found there was a dramatic increase in the firing rate of neurons in the hypothalamus during the immune reaction, and a more than 100 percent increase in electrical activity. Besedovsky's finding indicated that the brain sends out signals to the immune system and probably also receives signals back in a total feedback loop. In essence, the brain sends out neurohormones to regulate immunity and, in return, receives messages from the immune system that "inform" the brain about what the immune system "knows" and is doing. The brain processes this information based on what is happening in the body. For example, an immune response may need to be heightened quickly or gradually, or it may need to be dampened to prevent a dangerous overreaction. That's why such reciprocal communication between brain and immune system is necessary.

A great deal of worldwide PNI research has been devoted to the neural and biochemical "language" that enables the brain and the immune system to communicate. The complex findings are just now beginning to pour in.

Further Brain Connections

The brain-immune connection does not stop at the hypothalamus. French brain researchers have found that, in mice, the left cerebral cortex is necessary for the production of factors that motivate T-cells to take action. Removal of part of the left hemisphere resulted in fewer T-cells in the spleen and weaker cellular immune reactions.

Researcher Karen Bulloch at the University of California at San Diego studied the thymus, the "master gland" of the immune system, for clues to central-nervous-system linkages. She discovered that the rat thymus is covered with nerve endings from the vagus nerve, which is connected directly to the brain. Human thymus glands are also laced with nerve endings as well. Investigators at Indiana University have gone a step further: following the microscopic pathways of nerve fibers, they have been led not only to the thymus but to the spleen, bone marrow, and lymph nodes as well. Clearly, the body's immune "hot spots" are replete with nerve endings, where central-nervous-system messages are probably processed through chemical messengers called "neurotransmitters."

PNI investigator Nicholas Hall has found that a hormone secreted by the thymus, called "thymosin," known to influence the growth and activity of T-cells, acts also as a neural "messenger" sending signals back to the brain. Hall believes that thymosin may help the brain regulate immune responses in the body—another example of nervous, endocrine, and immune system linkage.

Endorphins are the powerful natural painkillers secreted by the pituitary gland. When we are threatened or stressed, endorphins are released, and they act as a kind of biological version of morphine, helping us endure and function. In laboratory tests, experimental animals were stressed, causing them to release endorphins. These tests showed that the animals had a lower level of activity among their "natural killer cells" because of the endorphins in their system. Endorphin-blocking drugs were then given to help restore the strength of their natural killer cells. This is a potent example of how the brain reacts to distress by releasing a natural drug with a very serious side effect: it reduces immunity.

From the research to date, it does not seem as if our brains control the immune system purely and simply. The brain and the immune system function independently, but they receive cues and signals from each other, and "modify" each other's activities, all in the name of protecting us from any harmful agent from within or without. The immune system has been referred to as another "sensory organ" for picking up stimuli on the molecular level; like any other sensory organ, it "talks" to the brain and receives replies that guide its actions and reactions.

LINKING THE NERVOUS, ENDOCRINE, AND IMMUNE SYSTEMS

Scientists searching for molecular evidence that the immune system is regulated by other systems may have struck gold. They have discovered that lymphocytes—the critical cells of the immune system—have receptor molecules on their cell surfaces designed exclusively to receive chemical "messages" from the nervous system.

A variety of products of the nervous system—called *neurotransmitters, neurohormones,* and *neuropeptides*—fit directly into certain lymphocyte receptors, in a lock-and-key fashion. These receptors—each of which receives only one particular neurotransmitter chemical—tell us that the immune cell can be changed or influenced by products of the nervous system. Substances from the nervous system that can be "received" by immune-cell receptors include corticosteroids, beta-adrenergic agents, growth hormones, acetylcholine, and methionine-enkephalin, to name only a few.

Some of these neurotransmitters or neurohormones have been shown to play a role in the activity and proliferation of lymphocytes. In other words, these chemicals can latch onto immune-cell receptors and cause a change in the cell's growth or actions. This is a vital discovery. It provides clues to the biological process through which stress or emotions can filter down to affect the immune functions on the microscopic level.

Molecular biologists and immunologists are not yet sure how all this works. Which neurotransmitters are the most important? Do they primarily boost or dampen immune responses? Exactly how do they function? Much more work needs to be done. Such molecular research will ultimately provide the underpinning for the human and animal clinical studies showing the effect of stress on immune defenses.

PNI RESEARCH AND CANCER

Specific studies in PNI research confirmed what the clinical psychological studies had suggested about emotions and cancer. As you read in

Chapter 18, "Is There a 'Type C' Personality?," the psychologists associated a sense of "hopelessness and helplessness" with susceptibility to cancer. But how can such seemingly intangible feelings alter our cancer defenses on the cellular level?

Looking for answers to this question, psychologists Lawrence Sklar and Hymie Anisman studied two groups of mice. One group received electric shocks that the mice could stop by their own efforts. The other received shocks but were given no way to stop them. The researchers then implanted cancer cells in both groups. They found that the group that had no control grew tumors more quickly and died sooner than the group that had some control over their "stressor." Psychologist Martin Seligman of the University of Pennsylvania ran a similar experiment with rats, and he too found that the "helpless" group grew tumors more readily than the group that had some power to change their environment.

University of Colorado researcher Steven Maier looked at the direct effect of helplessness on the immune system in rats. Two groups were compared. The rats were tested in pairs—one rat from each group would receive an electric shock at the same time. The only difference between the two groups was that one rat could turn off the shock by turning a wheel, while the other was helpless to change anything. In order to be saved from shock the "helpless" rat had to wait for the other rat to turn the wheel. Maier found that the group that was powerless to turn off the shocks—even though they received no more shocks than the first group—ended up with far fewer active lymphocytes than the group that could control their destiny. Helplessness had caused a direct depletion of immune-cell activity.

Psychologists have also associated depression with vulnerability to cancer. Dr. Steven J. Schliefer and his colleagues at Mount Sinai Hospital conducted studies to find out if clinically depressed patients who were hospitalized (though not on drugs) had any differences in their immune functioning, compared to controls matched for age and sex. They found out that the depressed individuals had fewer lymphocytes, fewer T- and B-cells, and their lymphocytes were less responsive to a variety of challenges than the controls.

The work on depression exemplifies PNI research. It has been well established that depression can diminish the number of white cells and their strength. The question is: how does this occur? Remember the relationship between stress and the release of corticosteroid hormones from the adrenal glands? It seems that people who are clinically depressed often have malfunctions of the hypothalamic-pituitary-adrenal axis that I described earlier. The result is that they produce abnormally large amounts of corticosteroids. Corticosteroids are known to suppress the immune system, so these adrenal hormones may be the link between psychological depression and immunological depression.

Because some psychological studies have shown a strong link between cancer and the loss of a loved one, many PNI studies have been devoted to the biological effects of bereavement.

A group of Australian researchers, headed by Dr. R. W. Bartrop, studied a group of bereaved spouses. They took blood samples from this group and from a similar group who had not suffered a loss. The immune cells from the bereaved group showed no marked differences from the control group when tested two weeks after death of the spouse. However, six weeks later, tests showed that the lymphocytes of the bereaved were much less responsive than those of the control group.

Dr. Steven Schliefer and the Mount Sinai research team studied the immune power of widowers. They ran a series of immunological tests on a large group of men whose wives had breast cancer and then continued with follow-up tests for a year on those men whose wives eventually died. Schliefer found that the widowers' immune responsiveness dropped after the loss, and remained low for about two months thereafter. Over many months, most of the widowers slowly regained their immune power, although some men had still not returned to their earlier level a year after the loss.

If one combines a predisposition toward hopelessness or helplessness with the severe blow of loss, it's not hard to imagine the strain on the immune system.

In the last chapter I spoke about how early life experience can create a pattern of despair or resignation. This may be the origin of a weakened immune system that later in life can't cope with major stresses and is more prone to collapse. Steven E. Keller and his colleagues at Mount Sinai studied rats that had been separated prematurely from their mothers and found that, as adults, they ended up with fewer and less vigorous T-cells.

Natural killer cells and interferon are critical to our anticancer defenses. Stress can cause our pituitary glands to secrete pain-killing endorphins, which, in turn, reduce the potency of our natural killer cells. PNI investigator Steven Locke of Harvard University examined a group of students and found that those who could be classified as "poor copers" (they were more anxious or depressed in the face of problems) had fewer active natural killer cells than those who were good copers. Studies of mice under stress show that they make less interferon. It is possible that the catecholamine stress hormones (epinephrine, norepinephrine) are responsible for the decrease, because animals given these hormones directly show a sudden drop in interferon levels.

PNI research is in its infancy. It is just beginning to fill in many of the missing biological pieces in the vast and fascinating puzzle of cancer and the mind. What it has shown is that critical parts of our anticancer defense—the strength and number of T-cells and natural killer cells, the production of interferon—are weakened by stress and emotional states. Helplessness impairs our immune systems and, in animals, enables tumors to develop and grow more readily. Depression and bereavement stultify our immune reactions. Early separation or loss can lay the initial groundwork for a weakened defense system.

PETTINGALE AND THE ROLE OF HORMONES

Keith W. Pettingale, a research scientist at King's College Hospital in London and a collaborator of Steven Greer's, is a dissenting voice—at least partially so. He is convinced that the immune system plays less of a role in modulating cancer growth than the endocrine system and its barrage of hormones. He bases his argument on the uncertainty that still exists about whether most types of cancer actually can be held in check by the immune system.

Pettingale believes that psychological factors have more impact on hormonal activity and other anticancer defenses than on the immune system itself. In a recent paper, he outlined the following factors as possible keys to the cancer-mind connection:

- Vitamin A, stored and released from the liver, has the ability to inhibit the enzymes that the carcinogenic "promoters" need in order to turn a cell cancerous. Psychological factors may have an impact on the hormones that control vitamin A metabolism, and thereby influence—positively or negatively—our vitamin A defense against cancer.
- Although little is known about our DNA repair mechanisms (see Chapter 3, "Our Amazing Defense Systems"), they consist of certain enzymes and may be able to repair genetic damage to cells before the cells turn malignant. It is possible that psychological disturbance could alter the hormone balance and block efficient DNA repair.
- A host of hormonal growth factors are required for cells to proliferate. Cells turning malignant may exploit these growth factors to their own end: continued and unstoppable reproduction ("immortality"). Pettingale believes that it is possible for "stress hormones acting on growth factor formation in many tissues" to cause an early expansion of a malignant clone of cells. In other words, stress may encourage the growth and multiplication of cancer cells.
- Natural cell death has been given a name—"apoptosis." Pettingale and others believe that apoptosis occurs "during the normal turnover of cells within a tissue" and is a form of deletion that keeps growth

under control. Apoptosis could also involve the deletion of cells with altered or damaged DNA, including cancer cells. Since hormones probably play a part in initiating apoptosis, this may be another psyche-to-hormone-to-cancer defense connection. Pettingale argues that apoptosis is a significant cancer defense mechanism, because it can operate at a very early stage of malignant transformation—long before even the immune system can pick up any change on a cell's surface.

- Pettingale also posits a theory about how psychological and hormonal mechanisms might influence the growth of a tumor once it has been established. Pettingale and his group at King's College Hospital are currently conducting hormonal profiles of people with Type C personality profiles—especially those who are inclined to suppress emotion. He tests them under both normal and stress conditions. The group is exploring the impact of hormones—especially stress hormones—on various tissues, immune cells, and "biologicals" to see how these hormones participate in cancer progress or the cancer defense.

Certain cancers—primarily breast, endometrial, and prostate cancer—depend on hormones for continuing growth. Both breast and endometrial cancers are either caused or exacerbated by estrogens, and prostate cancer depends, at least in part, on androgens, the male sex hormones. Hormonal imbalance either initiates or feeds malignant changes that lead to cancer in these "hormone-sensitive" organs. Psychological distress is one of several factors that affect the sex-hormone balance.

Although most mind-body researchers disagree with Pettingale's deemphasis on the immune system's power to fight cancer cells (the evidence in favor of this ability has become overwhelming), his work on hormonal factors adds greatly to our knowledge of the complex interaction between psyche and soma. Hormonal effects on tissues sensitive to them are unquestionably one way our state of mind could influence the very *genesis* of tumor growth.

The immune system goes into operation after cancer cells have appeared. Mechanisms by which mind alters immunity relate to how well we can fight off cancer cells once they have arisen. Theoretically, we should be able to resist any aberrant cell growth that occurs. If our immune systems can't or don't do this job, we need to find out why. Stress and emotions are now a major part of the answer.

PNI AND CANCER PREVENTION

In terms of cancer prevention, the PNI research—as well as the psychological studies—implies that we must take stress and our psychological health seriously. We must find therapies that help us reduce stress and improve the balance and effectiveness of our hormonal and immune systems. Like other systems of the body, these systems are extremely capable of bouncing back from arduous challenges.

If, from early life experiences, we can "learn" such feelings as hopelessness and helplessness, we can "unlearn" them as well. We can learn control over our lives and revitalize our biological defenses. Robert Ader's research suggests that eventually we may be able to control directly our own immune functions, in much the same way that biofeedback now can help us take control over our heart rate or our stomach's secretion of acid.

Unquestionably, many new therapeutic approaches will be developed to help us master mind-body interactions. Research in PNI, though still young, will guide us toward methods that are verifiably powerful. It shouldn't lead us into blindly accepting any loosely justified "alternative" mind-body approach; rather, this young field should lead us knowledgeably into new territory. The physical power of our highest emotions and instincts are gradually being validated on the molecular level. We have only to gain by finding out as much as possible about the healing powers residing within, how they function, and how we can harness them.

In the following chapters, I will describe an approach, and a number of integrated mind-body therapies that have helped arrest the progress of cancer and may contribute to prevention as well.

20

Psychological Health
and Cancer Prevention

*[L]et me speak to you regarding the things of which
you must most beware. To get angry and shout at
times pleases me, for this will keep up your natural
heat; but what displeases me is your being grieved
and taking all matters to heart, for it is this, as the
whole of physic teaches, which destroys our body
more than any other cause.*

From a letter by Maestro Lorenzo Sassoli, written to a
patient in 1402*

In a scene from *Manhattan,* Woody Allen is told by his girlfriend (Diane
Keaton) that she's jilting him for his best friend. Then, adding insult to
injury, she begs Allen to "get angry so that we can have it out, so that
we can get it out in the open."

Allen replies defensively, "I don't get angry, okay? I mean I have
a tendency to internalize—that's one of the problems I have. I—I grow
a tumor instead."

Is this dialogue funny because the idea is so absurd? Or because,
although oversimplified and exaggerated, it strikes so near the truth?

And what about the advice given by Maestro Sassoli in 1402?

There is still no absolute proof, as I've said earlier, that psychological states—such as repressed anger and "taking all matters to heart"—
makes us more susceptible to physical ailments, including cancer. But
early clinical records such as Sassoli's letter and a body of recent psychological and psychoneuroimmunological research certainly point in that
direction.

From this research and their own clinical experiences, a pioneering
handful of psychologists in the U.S., Great Britain, and Europe are
creating special therapeutic approaches for cancer patients. These ther-

*Cited by Laurence LeShan in his paper, "Psychological States in the Development
of Malignant Disease: A Critical Review," *Journal of The National Cancer Institute,* vol.
22, no. 1, January, 1959.

apies are relatively new—none more than thirty years old—but they are developing rapidly. Because these therapists best understand the personality patterns and life histories of cancer patients, they and their therapies can offer us many clues to prevention.

Among the more prominent developers of therapeutic approaches for cancer patients are the U.S. psychologist Lawrence LeShan; the radiologist O. Carl Simonton and psychologist Stephanie Simonton-Atchley; and the British psychiatrist Steven Greer. The surgeon Bernie Siegel of Yale University, author of the best-selling book *Love, Medicine and Miracles* has devised a special group program for "exceptional" cancer patients, but it is not considered within mainstream psychological research because he is not a trained psychologist or psychotherapist and undertakes no formal clinical studies. He works with effective, enthusiastic energy and intuition, but many researchers feel his results may depend more on his own personality than on an approach that subsequently can be taught and passed on to other therapists.

If the current medical controversy is hot and heavy about whether or not cancer is a "purely physical" disease or whether psychological factors may play a part, you can well imagine that the controversy over psychotherapeutic treatment is even hotter! You will remember (from Chapter 18, "Is There a 'Type C' Personality?") that the 1985 editorial in the *New England Journal of Medicine* states absolutely, "It is time to acknowledge that our belief in disease as a direct reflection of mental state is largely folklore."

Lycia Hayden, the young woman with lymphoma mentioned earlier, fell into the center of this controversy when her renowned lymphoma specialist at Stanford discovered that she had attended a Carl Simonton workshop in Santa Barbara. She describes this in her book, *Beating the Big C.* "My doctor blasted out, 'Simonton's a quack,' and turned on me as if he'd caught me in a felony. Fixing me with his eyes, he warned, 'These groups lure patients away from conventional methods with no basis of proof that they can make the cancer go away. Besides, they're expensive and I don't like to see cancer patients taken advantage of.' He did allow, however, that if I didn't take these groups too seriously, and went to the Simonton Workshop simply to improve my morale, then that was another matter altogether."

Three rather interesting—and not infrequent—misconceptions appear in the Stanford oncologist's statements. The truth is: (1) Reputable cancer psychotherapists—and certainly Carl Simonton—never steer patients away from conventional treatment. They see their role as adjunctive to traditional therapy, not opposed to it. They see their therapies as a way to encourage the patient to fight for himself. (2) No reputable cancer psychotherapist suggests he or she can make cancer go away—or prevent it—only that he or she can help the patient fight on his or her own behalf. Of course, there are those who make wild claims, but they are not found among the serious cancer psychotherapists any more than they are found among the serious oncologists. (3) "Don't take it seriously" translates into: "You can't really do anything for yourself; your mindset is unimportant to the outcome of your disease. But it's nice for us if you keep your morale high and follow our instructions."

Even the most conservative hospitals have cancer support groups, usually run by social workers. These can be most helpful in allowing patients to share their fears of cancer, radiation, surgery, and in helping build morale. But such support—as helpful as it may be—is *not* what the serious psychotherapists are talking about. They're talking about a structured and systematic therapy that will bring about *fundamental changes* in patients' lifestyles and outlooks, which will help reduce current stress and stresses that were present before the disease began— changes that may actively buttress a patient's immune responses, instead of dragging them down.

So how can all this be translated into preventive measures? Obviously, few people are going to enter psychotherapy simply because it may help stave off cancer. But, say the researchers, a severely stressed or depressed existence should be addressed for its own sake. Why be stressed? Why be miserable? And, if change or therapy improves your immune status as well, so much the better.

In preparing this book, I sought out a number of psychotherapists with many years of experience in treating cancer patients successfully. I chose to interview at length two of them, LeShan and Simonton-Atchley, because both have given considerable thought to prevention and have, in print and in public appearances, proved highly articulate about the emotional conflicts that can help initiate or exacerbate cancer.

LESHAN AND THE LUST FOR LIFE

LeShan describes the type of "crisis psychotherapy" he uses with cancer patients in a dozen professional papers in such journals as *The American Journal of Psychotherapy* and in his book for the public, *You Can Fight for Your Life*. His method is basically geared toward uncovering the origins of the loss of the real self, and an almost relentless pursuit of that self, with all its idiosyncrasies, emotions, and desires.

As I described in Chapter 18 ("Is There a 'Type C' Personality?"), many people who contract cancer seem to be out of touch with emotions, and have lost any hope of the possibility of change. LeShan believes that this loss of hope stems from an "untenable" situation the person has been subjected to, often since early childhood. Being true to oneself was often met with hostility, rejection, or indifference. Not being oneself—complying with the wishes of others—led to acceptance, but with it came a deep despair born of the loss of the real self. This leaves such a person with a history of early shattered attempts to be himself that gradually gave way to the freezing of his real desires and yielding to the roles and expectations placed upon him by others.

Underneath the despair that accompanies this kind of "existential trap," there lies a self that has been dormant since childhood. It *can* be reawakened, if only the person can find his way to a third road—an alternative to the two paths of either thwarted desires or unfulfilling accomplishments. In his psychotherapy with cancer patients, LeShan tries to reawaken what is unique in each individual—his "special song to sing"—which has long been lost. In an effort to get at the real self that has long been stifled, he doggedly asks patients, "What do you want out of your life?" Frequently, his patients discover life plans, dreams, creative desires, and career goals that are completely at odds with their present lives.

LeShan helps his patients go back in time to uncover the circumstances that brought about their own rejection of vital parts of themselves. LeShan's purpose is to help them recognize and empathize with the inner child who gave up parts of the self to hold on to the acceptance of others. Then patients can recover the lost shards—so important to the whole of who they are.

After patients learn to recognize these lost parts, the therapist can help clear an opening to a "third road" and encourage the first tentative steps to take their knowledge of the lost self out into the world for testing—not for approval, but for experience.

Linda, a patient of LeShan's, had wanted to go to college. Instead, she followed the wishes of her parents by marrying a man who met all their criteria. She was a "good wife and mother" of four children, but felt caught in a trap she had not wished for. In her frustration, she fell in love with another man, who encouraged her individuality. Her husband and parents reacted with outrage and harassed her into returning to the family fold. Out of great guilt, she did so, and four months later was diagnosed with breast cancer. After surgery, she was told that her cancer had spread and was beyond treatment. It was then that she sought out LeShan and began psychotherapy. He helped her buck her family's expectations and follow her own inclinations, which meant getting a job so she could attend college night classes. Over a long period, her cancer appeared to regress; she gained more strength emotionally and physically, began college full-time, and initiated divorce proceedings. Her family continued to hound her, but the satisfactions derived from following the third road carried her through. She became

involved with another man (one whom her parents had always disap-
proved of, because he preached the "wrong religion"), and became a
college librarian. Eventually, she was able to reach an understanding
with her children about why she had left their father and chosen to
travel off the beaten track. Linda summed it up by saying, "They love
me in spite of the fact that they think I'm some kind of nut."

Linda's statement sums up LeShan's "third road" concept. At first,
there seem to be only two roads—both painful. There appears to be no
alternative. But, if one can overcome early fears, and face the possibilities of rejection, the third road becomes a viable option. Ironically, the
more fully one becomes oneself, the greater are the possibilities for
acceptance. It may mean that some friends, family members, or associates whose love was tied to our conformity will be lost, but, according
to LeShan, when we become ourselves, we can accept these losses.
They never really "loved" us to begin with; they only reinforced what
they wanted from us. We will either win new respect and new understanding from those who do love us or we will gain new relationships
with people who see a vital person of passion and intensity.

LeShan believes that this philosophy—and its application in life or
in therapy—can help ameliorate existing cancer and help prevent cancer. We talked recently about how this thinking might be translated
into some practical points for prevention.

LeSHAN: It seems to me that there are different roads for different people. Perhaps you start by saying, Even if I don't believe there's
a new way to live, I'm going to treat myself as if there is. I'm going to
take control of my life intellectually first and act as if there is a way. I'm
going to analyze what I would really enjoy doing. What kind of life
would make me glad to get up in the morning, glad to go to bed at night,
and feel used in my own special way from the tip of my toes to the top
of my head? I'm going to have to develop a fierce and tender concern
for all parts of me so that no part of my being is standing outside the
door, whimpering, "Is there nothing for me?" I will have to ask: Where
do I need feeding on physical levels, emotional levels, spiritual levels?—
and I'm going to have to do my damnedest to feed myself in all those
ways.

DREHER: Is this true, regardless of how much we fall or don't fall
into the Type C category?

LeSHAN: Right. Many of us may feel that we need specialized
help for this, to see more clearly what is blocking us. This is not due to
a weakness on our part. It's due to being in this universe. The best
analogy I can think of is, you may have the most powerful telescope in
the world, and theoretically it can view almost anything in the cosmos
with one exception: itself. For this, it needs a highly specialized mirror.

That's why we decide to work with a therapist.

DREHER: We can agree that psychotherapy is one important possible way to go, but aren't there other ways, too?

LeSHAN: There are a number of paths. There is the path of meditation, if followed with discipline and long, tough work. There's no easy road and no free lunch. It is always difficult to grow and change. Another, for some people, is finding a commitment outside oneself. If you get a new job, or work for a big brother/big sister organization, an ecology or peace organization, it's a way to say that you're concerned with the world outside. *First*, of course, you have to be for yourself; only then can you be for others. But, as part of finding your own special music, it is often necessary to find a noble cause to work for. Hegel wrote that life is only of value if it holds, and works for, an object of value outside itself. There is much truth in this *if* you are *first* concerned about your own personal and unique growth.

There are other paths as well, but underneath it all is full development of the self. It is our task to live our life as a symphony or a tapestry, to make our life more artistic—it's the greatest artistic endeavor we're ever going to have. And each section of the tapestry is different. How do we enrich it, develop the themes? So, as we keep growing, we keep developing new tastes, new enjoyments, and keep responding to and enjoying life more in one five-year period than we did in the last one. Our job is to become more and more ourselves, more and more unique. The question is: do we make this world a waiting room or a living room? In a waiting room, we simply say, "Well, I have achieved my goals and I am going to wait for death." In a living room, we are always increasing our special ways of being, relating, creating: we are working on our individual path.

DREHER: What can you say to people who read the descriptions of emotional states and cancer—those who are depressed and concerned about being so?

LeSHAN: I think if you are depressed it's best to do something about it regardless. Quite apart from whether it leads to despair, you should do something about it. It's a hell of a way to live. It's very unpleasant. It helps to say what can be done about this. For example, sometimes people who are depressed are abrogating responsibility for their own life by saying things like, "I would be happy if only somebody loved me very much," which means they are setting up one hell of a life. Every single morning they put the baby and themselves out for adoption and say, "Does he or she still want me?" Very often people come to me and say, "How can I meet the right person? I'm very lonely. I don't like the singles scene; singles bars are lousy." The personal ads in *New York* magazine are the funniest things I've ever seen. These people come to me and say, "How can I meet the right person?" And I say the answer is very simple: "Stop trying. Make yourself such an interesting person that you thoroughly enjoy your own company and don't give a damn. And, if they come, that's frosting on the cake. Develop those parts of you that you find really fascinating. Find what you enjoy, and then you will be beating them off with a stick!" About 80 percent of the people I tell this to walk away furious. About 20 percent follow it and start having to beat them off with a stick.

DREHER: What about the difference between depression and despair?

LESHAN: They are quite different. With despair, you keep on going. Even though it's hopeless, there is not usually the anger, the strong feelings. Whichever it is—depressed or despairing—is something you should take action on. The best way, in our culture, is to find new interests that will deeply involve you, or see a therapist. Remember, too, that being in despair doesn't mean you are going to get cancer. A person probably has to have a genetic predisposition too, and other factors. The point is that it is simply bad for your body's entire defense system. And it's a lousy way to live.

DREHER: You mention that people in despair—whether they have cancer or not—may need time to get away, to get in touch with their inner forces. On the other hand, they need relationships too.

LESHAN: All persons need both relationships and solitude. The question is how to find the right balance. Each person is different. You must ask, How much solitude do I need? How much relationship do I need? When you can't stand solitude, it means that there's much in your life that is barren. May Sarton, the beautiful novelist and poet, put it very well when she said: "Solitude is richness of the spirit, loneliness is poverty of the spirit."

DREHER: What is the best way for people to recognize if they need psychotherapy?

LESHAN: I would say, one way to know you are in trouble is when, in any five-year period, you are not having more fun and enjoying life more than in the previous five-year period. When you stop growing and changing for a long period. There are two reasons for going into psychotherapy. One is when things have gotten so intolerable that the only thing left to do is therapy. The other reason is that you want as much as possible out of life. The job of the psychotherapist should be to help the person become greedy—and I don't mean greedy as Ivan Boesky means it, greedy for money. That has nothing to do with satisfaction in life. The people I work with, whether cancer patients or not, learn to be greedy for more sensations, colors, ideas, relationships, whatever. I am telling people to be greedy for *life*. This can affect your health in very positive ways.

STEPHANIE SIMONTON-ATCHLEY:
STRESS, IMAGERY, AND THE IMMUNE SYSTEM

During the 1970s, it was the work of radiologist O. Carl Simonton and psychotherapist Stephanie Matthews-Simonton that brought psychological treatments for cancer patients into the limelight. Their Cancer Counseling and Research Center in Ft. Worth, Texas, became a haven for many cancer patients and the focus of great controversy.

With Jeanne Achterberg-Lawlis of the University of Texas Health Science Center, the Simontons developed a special technique of mental imagery to help cancer patients become aware of their bodies, and ally themselves with their immune systems to regain control of their health and fight their malignancy. Jeanne Achterberg's two excellent books detail the use of imagery in the treatment of cancer patients and others (*Imagery of Cancer: A Diagnostic Tool for the Process of Disease*, with Frank Lawlis, and *Imagery in Healing*—see Appendix 4). The Simontons' book, *Getting Well Again*, outlines their approach, which is based on many of the personality findings described here, and describes their therapeutic system, including imagery, psychological counseling, and group support. The Simontons have always recommended their approach as an addition to—not a replacement for—standard medical treatment for cancer. Their aim has been to improve a patient's quality of life and prolong survival to the greatest extent possible.

The Simontons' imagery techniques involve bringing patients into a state of relaxation, then encouraging them to visualize their immune cells, together with the drugs or radiation they are receiving, as attacking their cancer cells aggressively. To tap the full power of imagery, patients are encouraged to find their own symbolic visions: little white dogs attacking, a school of fishes devouring, etc. They are encouraged to see their immune systems and their cancer treatment as strong and powerful and the cancer cells as weak and confused. In the imagery exercise, the victorious scenario culminates with the destruction and flushing out of cancer cells, the revitalization of normal cells, and the return of health and harmony to the body.

The exercise was used to focus the patients' mental energies inward, to align their thoughts with their biological resources, to restore faith in the possibility of recovery, and to strengthen the will to live. The imagery was considered a sensitive probe, both in helping determine the patient's emotional and physical state and in overcoming obstacles to revitalization. In addition to the relaxation and imagery work, the Simontons conducted therapy sessions to help patients deal with old hurts and resentments, develop new goals, and cope with the fear of death.

For years, the Simontons have been in the center of a maelstrom of debate. Their imagery techniques have been either hailed as great innovations or reviled as unproven and uncertain methods.

They have been criticized, too, for not publishing studies that meet the strictest criterion of scientific inquiry. Rather than comparing their group of patients to a control group, they compared their results to statistical averages (cited in the medical literature) for length of survival of a given cancer at a given stage. Using this method, they claimed that in general their patients survived twice as long as patients were expected to survive. In *Getting Well Again,* they state that, after four years of treating 159 patients diagnosed with "incurable" cancer, 63 were alive with an average survival time of 24.4 months after diagnosis. The patients who died averaged 20.3 months after diagnosis, but the average *expected* survival time for these groups was 12 months. Of the 63 still alive, 22.2 percent had "no evidence of the disease," and 19 percent have shown tumor regression.

Several years ago, Carl Simonton formed the Simonton Cancer Center in Pacific Palisades, California, and Stephanie—now Stephanie Simonton-Atchley—founded the Health Training and Research Center in Little Rock, Arkansas. While they were together in Ft. Worth, the Simontons developed a group marathon approach, in part because of the huge demand that had grown for their workshops. Carl Simonton has continued with and expanded this "national treatment"—a five-day group program that attracts cancer patients from all over the world.

Stephanie Simonton-Atchley has gone a somewhat different route. She practices many of the same techniques, including relaxation and imagery, but prefers individual work, in which patients work intensively with a therapist for a year or more. Simonton-Atchley, therefore, does not see patients from other parts of the country or world. Her patients come from the Little Rock area, and all are involved in her clinical research studies. She is following her patients very carefully for emotional and physical progress, and is now monitoring specific immune functions to see if positive changes can be correlated with progress in her treatment methods. Simonton-Atchley emphasizes the benefits of long-term, individual, in-depth psychological work. She continues to train health practitioners from throughout the country, who want to learn her specific therapeutic techniques.

Simonton-Atchley has thought a great deal about how her approach can be applied to prevention of diseases—all diseases—and has made an audio cassette on the subject, "Psychological Strategies for Prevention of Illness." This and other cassettes can be purchased by writing to Simonton-Atchley's Health Training and Research Center (see Appendix 3 for address).

Recently I talked at length with her about prevention and here is part of our conversation:

DREHER: What would you say to people who are healthy, but concerned about their susceptibility to cancer and other illnesses?

SIMONTON-ATCHLEY: What we're talking about are not just those who are susceptible to cancer. In general, the psychological patterns we are talking about are of those people who tend to somaticise [displace emotional conflicts onto the body] when stressed.

If you overstress anybody, you are going to see one of three maladaptive responses: they are either going to show behavioral disruption, a psychiatric disruption, or a physical disruption. Those people in this culture who stay out of prison, who are not alcoholics or drug addicts, who follow the rules and do their best, those people tend to be somaticisers.

Within that group of somaticisers you have a spectrum. You've got people who respond to stress with a cold, you've got people who respond to stress with ulcers, people who develop hypertension and ultimately cardiac disease, and those who end up with cancer. So any person who tends to somaticise should be aware of issues of degree, chronicity, and severity.

This brings up the other issue—denial of feeling and expression of anger. The thing I look for and think is important in prevention is the monitoring of acute stress. LeShan says—and I think it's been borne out by clinical study—that most people who develop cancer have a lifelong depression; but there comes a time frame—from about six months to three years prior to the original diagnosis—when there is an acute clustering of too much stress that overwhelms an already vulnerable system.

One of the stressors is often a real, imagined, or anticipated loss of a primary love object. Even if you have all the other factors in balance, when you lose a primary love object, it can be a very troublesome time for you. Most of our cancer statistics are based on people who never had therapy, have no awareness of stress or how to manage it. If you know you are vulnerable ahead of time—for instance, if you know, as I do, that I am acutely sensitive to loss—then whenever I know there is a loss or an anticipated loss in my life I am more nurturing, more expressive of feelings, I'm more likely to see my therapist and talk it over with her for support, and do the stress-management techniques that we also know will lessen the effects of stress on a person's physiology.

So first—just being aware of the effects of short-term stress is important. Then, it's important to put into play the good healing practices we have for stressful situations. Many people in our culture are apt to deny stress and force a "positive attitude" on themselves, saying they're not really feeling bad, everything is really okay. This process is the exact opposite of what I'm talking about as a healthy procedure.

DREHER: People become frightened or feel guilty when they are stressed out because they think this means they're not up to handling a situation, that therefore they're poorly adjusted. That it's their fault if they get sick.

SIMONTON-ATCHLEY: It's intriguing for me that everyone talks about guilt. I think it's much feared by the medical population but it rarely happens. I have treated thousands of cancer patients, and I can tell you how few of them ever blamed themselves. They say, "Well, I did the best I could, and I never knew about any of this emotional stuff."

I think it's more medicine's punitive attitude of right and wrong, black and white. It's as if they were saying, "If the psyche has something to do with it, then shame on those people." I've seen a lot of physicians get a hold of this work, and use it to beat on patients. They might say something like, "If you did your imaging right, you wouldn't be sick." They use it in a punitive, blaming way.

DREHER: Do you think people who read about your work might misunderstand, and somehow blame themselves for their illness?

SIMONTON-ATCHLEY: *Not* people who have cancer, rather the people who *think* they know how cancer patients respond. In my experience, as I said, it is very rare that patients blame themselves. Very few people in the world would take that much emotional responsibility on themselves. If they've had any experience with trying to get in touch with emotions that have been denied, they know how powerful the unconscious is. They know that consciously they didn't bring about their illness. To assume that cancer patients will blame themselves is ludicrous, but for some reason, it's a great fear to people in established medicine.

DREHER: Susan Sontag, in her *Illness as Metaphor,* said that people positing psychological factors in cancer were "blaming the victim."

SIMONTON-ATCHLEY: I believe just the opposite! I think, if we acknowledged as a culture that people's emotions play a role in their diseases, what would happen would be confrontation with physicians about how they treat patients emotionally. And *they* might feel guilty about how they've made patients feel helpless. I think there's a weird sort of projection going on. If anything, what all of us would do is to be more sensitive, loving, and nurturing to people who have cancer, which is quite the opposite of what these folks say we're proposing. If we psychologists are punitive to anybody, it's to the people who treat patients and are not sensitive to their emotions. It's to the physicians.

DREHER: I would like people to be able to explore these issues without fear, to be challenged to find better ways to handle stress.

SIMONTON-ATCHLEY: I take an interesting approach with cancer patients. We don't spend a whole lot of time discussing whether they will recover from cancer. What we focus on is "How can you and I, together, improve the quality of the next twenty-four hours?" If anyone focuses on how he can keep the quality of his life as high as possible for one day, he would be practicing the best preventive care.

DREHER: When should a person seek psychotherapy because of these issues?

SIMONTON-ATCHLEY: When they know early childhood issues are involved and need to be explored. If they have a problem expressing emotion, if they are self-depriving, or if they don't express anger appropriately.

DREHER: What about specific stress-management techniques for prevention?

SIMONTON-ATCHLEY: There are three I generally recommend. Three that I believe people should incorporate in their lives daily to help prevent almost any kind of disease. I'm not saying everyone should do all three, but these are the major ones which I know from research studies help decrease the effects of stress on the body.

One. The use of regular relaxation technique—including meditation, prayer, or other forms of mental relaxation.

Two. The use of physical exercise, which is an excellent antidepressant (and depression is the issue we're concerned with). People who don't use meditation often use exercise.*

Three. Increasing the intimacy of your social support group.

There is a study from Johns Hopkins Medical Center which looked at social support as a buffer to stress. It concluded that good supports, just like relaxation and physical exercise, decrease the harmful effects of stress. It makes good sense to me that the more intimate and nurturing your support group, the more stress you can withstand.

If you look back at our culture over the past hundred years you notice immediately that we are not only living a more stressful lifestyle, but that we are much more isolated in terms of extended family and community. So people—even if they are single—who have a good support network of close friends and family whom they can turn to when they're troubled—let their hair down and share their troubles with—apparently are able to handle more stress. A close support system functions like the extended family used to.

Another key to handling stress is tied to the issue of therapy—that is, continuing to be aware of what you're feeling in response to stress, and to find appropriate ways of expressing it rather than forcing yourself to be optimistic.

If you're scared, or angry, or sad, you need to express that appropri-

*Michael Murphy of the Esalen Institute has said, "Sport is Western meditation."

ately to get the nurturing and support you need. Those feelings are generally transitory. And, if you are aware of what you are feeling in response to stress, it usually increases your awareness of potential options to solve the problem. If you find difficulty in expressing such "down times" and feelings, then some therapy may be helpful.

DREHER: As for imagery and visualization, can they be of value for prevention as well?

SIMONTON-ATCHLEY: Perhaps. When I talk about relaxation response, some people prefer a sort of TM [Transcendental Meditation, a clearing of the mind]. I am particularly fond of imagery. I have dealt with this question with people I have treated for cancer who are now well—free of disease. Having them work with imagery in the same terms as before means the focus would be imagining their immune system just functioning properly. But that makes about as much sense to me as having to image your breathing, or your heart beating. These are automatic functions.

People who have had cancer and are especially frightened might visualize their white blood cells on a search-and-destroy mission looking for any virus or germs. But, more importantly, what I have these people focus on in their imagery is a constructive set of images that represent three or four different goals that relate to improving their quality of life. For instance, people may see themselves relating to their family in their visualization in a way that is nurturing or supportive. If they have a problem with their spouses or their kids, then they can visually see that problem solved.

So you can use imagery at a psychological level as easily as you can to change your body. It can change your outlook. And that's a way which is *not* blatant denial or forced optimism. But, if you ask your mind to see a problem getting solved, often it jogs memory and many other feelings. People may visualize better relations with their families and, while they're doing the visualization, realize more clearly where they don't feel good about their families.

It's important that people stay in touch with their feelings toward the important objects in their life. They may see family relations being changed in the way they want, or work going in the way they want. If someone's goal is to be a great racer, he might see himself doing that. Using visualization, one focuses on one's life being what one wants it to be. Visualization is also a way to confront and look at the problems one is having.

DREHER: That sounds like a very powerful technique to make someone aware of his own needs—by visualizing what it is he would like to see happen.

SIMONTON-ATCHLEY: Exactly. It can help people become more conscious of underlying needs and feelings.

FEELINGS OUT IN THE OPEN

During my research for this book, I kept coming across—both in the professional literature and in interviews—this issue of repression of feelings, or desires, or "the heart's secret wishes which are seldom explored."*

Without question, there is much in our culture that encourages us to repress feelings of anger, sadness, anxiety, pain—even joy—and much that blocks us from appropriate ways of expressing such feelings, until they explode irrationally or we take them out on ourselves physically.

A large number of therapists are working on this dilemma and are making contributions to the recovery of open expression of feelings in an appropriate way. I include a short discussion of them here because their contributions may be helpful to prevention as well as to recovery.

STEVEN GREER AND SUPPRESSION OF ANGER

Dr. Steven Greer's studies of breast cancer are some of the most precise and conclusive evidence we have that suppression of feelings—in this case, anger—leads to increased risk of cancer. Currently, he is developing a package program of cognitive and psychological change, called "adjuvant psychological therapy," to help breast-cancer patients. The program includes emotional support, counseling for problems in the here-and-now, cognitive and behavioral reinforcement of a positive fighting spirit, and the desire to live and get well. When I went to see Dr. Greer in London, I asked him about the value of psychological changes—such as learning to express anger—to overall health and cancer prevention.

"At the very least it can do no harm," commented Greer. "Even if our predictions turn out to be wrong, and emotional suppression turns out not to be a real risk factor, you haven't lost anything . . . because psychologically it certainly is better for people to be able to express negative emotions rather than bottling them up. You are not doing any harm and it's likely that you're helping them, if only to feel better psychologically."

Greer pointed out that, in his work with breast-cancer patients, he

*Two recent series of studies confirm that repressing emotional turmoil—keeping a stiff upper lip no matter what the circumstances—can increase susceptibility to a whole host of illnesses. In one study at Yale University, Gary E. Schwartz, director of the Yale Psychophysiology Center, found that repressors tended to have lower levels of certain immune cells. Daniel Weinberger of Stanford University uncovered a tendency toward high blood pressure. See the *New York Times* report of March 3, 1988.

is very careful in approaching the subject of suppression of anger. "I talk about suppressing anger, and the importance of letting it out, but am extremely cautious not to make them feel 'Oh dear, I've suppressed anger all my life—therefore, I . . . ,' which might make things worse. Again, if suppression of anger does turn out to be a definite risk factor, then we can gently but definitely advise patients and those at risk to seek ways to express feelings more openly."

DENNIS JAFFE AND THE MESSAGE OF ILLNESS

In his book *Healing from Within,* Dennis T. Jaffe, a leading exponent of psychological approaches to healing, writes cogently about emotional repression and its relation to illness:

> When an emotion is directly experienced in both the body and the mind, it is accompanied by a discharge of psychological tension and arousal. For instance, don't you feel relieved after an emotional cry or an angry exchange? Isn't your body calm and relaxed? Even so, you probably grew up with a degree of distrust or dislike of your emotions. Many families, as well as most school and work environments, encourage the inhibition and control of one's feelings . . . the symptom is actually a veiled expression of the feeling, or perhaps a message from within that the emotion within needs to find a more outward expression.

Jaffe sees most illness as containing a personal message: symptoms are trying to tell us something about our inner selves. We are being signaled by our bodies below the level of consciousness that there is an aspect of our lives that needs exploring and changing, or that emotions are being held in check. One message almost all illnesses contain is that "we need to pay more respect and attention to the demands of our body."

Dennis Jaffe points out that people prone to illness are not taking care of themselves, because they are so often unaware of their physical and emotional needs and hence unable to satisfy them. "So many of my patients have experienced a neglect of their most basic, deepest human needs," writes Jaffe, "for touching and for companionship, for shared inner feelings, for expressing creative energy, for sexual fulfillment, for personal validation, and for the giving and receiving of love. Instead, their lives are characterized by duty and obligation to the very people who gave them little or nothing in return."

Jaffe advocates a form of "self-care" that entails becoming fully reacquainted with the inner voices that bespeak real needs. When these voices have become quiet or even absent, it may take a special effort to amplify them and heed their call. According to Jaffe, one can begin in the simplest ways, just by recognizing the truth of one's current state of affairs and asking the right questions. One can then develop or seek out strategies for cultivating relationships and work that are gratifying and help one express feelings.

REICH AND EMOTIONAL RELEASE

Obviously, anger is not the only feeling that, held in check, compromises our health. Many of LeShan's cancer patients, for instance, lost the capacity for sadness and joy as well; feelings in general may be repressed.

A number of approaches to liberating emotion deal directly with the only receptacle of human feeling—the body itself. Wilhelm Reich, the great but embattled psychoanalyst and natural scientist, was the first Western thinker to give the body its due in terms of its intimate relation to the mind.

In the 1940s, he referred to the profound "resignation" of those who contract cancer and believed that their psychological and physical defenses—which he called *armor*—were especially intense. He found that cancer patients demonstrated an emotional "mildness" and rarely expressed anger. "Chronic emotional calm," Reich said, "must coincide with a bio-energetic stagnation in the cell and plasma system." Reich felt that very early repression of feelings and sexual frustration created the powerful armor that led to a stagnation of the flow of life energy in the body. This stagnation he thought was fertile ground for cancer-cell growth and tumor development. Just as flowing brooks are purified through the continuous movement of water, in stagnant pools the growth of bacteria and other such organisms accelerates.

It's not hard to imagine an allied relationship between the immune system and the energy system that governs internal biological processes. Although this energy system has yet to be defined by Western biological scientists, Reich's concept can be thought of as an early and potentially radical foray into this "other realm" of human functioning. Perhaps the vitality of our immune functions depends in some yet-to-be-established way on the energy functions of the body, which, according to Reich, are the basis of our emotional life. Reich even developed a blood test that sampled the "liveliness" of red blood cells, based on their shape, color, and how long it took them to disintegrate after being drawn from the body. With a reasonable degree of accuracy, he was able to tell, in double-blind tests, which blood had come from cancer patients and which from people without cancer. The "hardier" blood cells always came from the healthy individuals.

If Reich's ideas about emotional repression, the stifling of energy flow in the body, and cancer have validity, then one promising and potent approach to cancer prevention would be a loosening of the body

armor and liberation of the emotions and energy flow this armor ob-
structs. Reichian therapies and several other body therapies are directed toward this goal. I describe Reichian therapies in the last chapter, "New Ways to Mind-Body Health."

CHOOSING A THERAPIST

If you become aware of the psychological factors and life changes
needed to reduce stress, you can often make the necessary changes
without therapeutic help. But, if you feel you need help overcoming
blocks and finding the "third road" described by LeShan, psychotherapy is not a bad idea. But be sure to find a therapist who suits *you*.

Lawrence LeShan advises looking for a therapist who is more concerned with helping you find out what is right about you than what is
wrong with you. The search for your individuality—for what is "your
real name and what has blocked you from knowing it"—is, he says, the
best way to overcome negative feelings and strengthen the body's self-
defense systems.

LeShan advises that you "interview" therapists to determine
whether they will meet your personal needs and special idiosyncrasies.
Does a therapist help you express your real feelings? Do you feel inhibited by the therapist, or does he/she make contact with you in a way
that elicits response? Do you think the therapist will just be a good
"hand-holder," or will he or she challenge you to overcome your blocks?
Do you sense that you will feel safe in expressing negative as well as
positive emotions? An equal, mutually respectful, and open relationship
is most conducive to self-growth.

IDENTIFYING THE PROBLEMS

In *You Can Fight for Your Life,* LeShan sets forth a list of questions that
may help you identify increased susceptibility to cancer:

1. Am I able to express anger when I feel it most strongly?
2. Do I try to make the best of things, no matter what happens, without ever complaining?
3. Do I think of myself as a lovable, worthwhile person?
4. Or have I felt worthless much of the time? Do I often feel lonely,
   rejected, isolated from others?
5. Am I doing what I want to do with my life? Are my relationships
   satisfying? Do I feel reasonably optimistic (or quite hopeless) about
   ever fulfilling myself?

6. If I were told right now that I had only six months to live, would I go on doing what I am doing right now? (Or do I have secret unfulfilled dreams, ambitions, desires of which I am ashamed, and which have plagued me all my life?)
7. If I were told I had a terminal illness, would I experience some sense of relief?

You may answer one or many of these questions on the side of "cancer susceptibility." (If in doubt, see p. 324 in the Epilogue for the "right" answers.) That's no cause for alarm. We all go through times of despair, and certainly none of us can always express our deepest emotions. Rather, it's a lifelong tendency toward depressive or anxious mind states, combined with many other factors, that translates into increased risk.

Use these questions as a simple launching pad toward self-investigation. They will guide you toward areas that need exploring. Whether you feel therapy or stress management or other professional help is needed for change, one thing is certain: you'll need support from real friends or supportive family members. Finding the "third road" need not be a lonely task; finding your "individuality" also means finding people who accept you for who you are.

21

New Ways to Mind-Body Health

*Our essential core is peaceful and whole. The work
of healing is in peeling away the barriers of fear and
past conditioning that keep us unaware of our true
nature of wholeness and love. Discovering our peaceful inner core, in turn brings the body back to wholeness and allows us to live well, in spite of our physical limitations.*

Joan Borysenko
Harvard Medical School
from *New Age Journal,* May/June 1987

During the last twenty years, a large number of relaxation techniques
and mind-body therapies—some new and some as old as China—have
been introduced to the United States and Europe. Many of them are
extraordinarily valuable for reducing the stress of our pressured lifestyles and thereby strengthening our immune systems and revitalizing
bodily functioning. Although the value of these techniques to cancer
prevention has not yet been demonstrated, their capacity to reduce
stress is without question.

In the last chapter, I talked about the psychological changes in
attitude and action that produce a more satisfying and healthier life. In
this chapter, I will discuss stress-reduction techniques that have distinct
physiological effects and psychotherapies that combine body work with
talk therapy. I believe that PNI research will eventually validate the
cancer preventive value of many of the new—and ancient—mind-body
approaches.

What we are learning from the East—from yoga, zen meditation
and the like—is that it is possible for us to learn to control many auto-
nomic-nervous-system processes that we formerly thought were
beyond our command, such as blood pressure, heart rate, blood circulation, digestion, etc. A trained yogi, for instance, can make the temperature of one part of his hand 15 to 20 degrees different from another
point on the same hand. This implies that we have enormous possibilities for controlling our own health. We simply need to tune in more

acutely to our bodies and learn how to modulate them. The next frontier is direct control over our immune functions.

There are a wide variety of stress-management approaches, psychological and physiological therapies, behavioral modification techniques, spiritual practices and social support systems. Each one has its own justification, its own track record, and each targets different aspects of handling stress, emotional suppression, spiritual growth, or behavior change. Choose ones that seem to meet your own needs best.

All of them have one thing in common that relates directly to psychoneuroimmunology research. You will remember the studies mentioned in Chapter 19, "How the Mind Influences Immunity," in which rats were put under stress. Some were given ways to reduce the stressor, others were not. The ones that were powerless to control stressful stimuli were also the ones who were less able to fight an implanted tumor. All of these techniques or therapies encourage more control over your environment—both inner and outer. When you actively engage in an approach that addresses your specific problems, blocks, or fears, you are taking the reins of health into your own hands. You are stepping out of the "helpless cage" and stepping into an environment that has a control lever. You may be exposed to just as much external stress as before, but by finding your own powerful technique— whether it is psychotherapy, TM, yoga, or any combination, you are seizing control.

The approaches that follow are offered *in addition* to the basic concepts of prevention suggested in the preceding chapter. Many of them fall under the umbrella of "behavioral medicine"—the name given to new mind-body methods of treating and preventing disease.

MEDITATION AND RELAXATION

In the 1960s, Dr. Herbert Benson, the renowned cardiologist at Harvard Medical School, was studying animal behavior and its relationship to blood pressure. At the time, a group of people practicing transcendental meditation (TM) challenged Benson with the assertion that they could lower their blood pressure simply by meditating.

Benson wasn't very interested in the challenge until he read a paper in *Science* magazine, establishing the marked physiological effects of meditation, which included lowered blood pressure. Soon Benson was busy measuring biological changes occurring in TM practitioners. He confirmed the physiological benefits to the TM group and then carried his experiments further, finding similar alterations in those who practiced a range of meditative and spiritual exercises, from yoga to zen meditation to Christian prayer.

Benson believed that these various techniques, though practiced differently, had certain common features and one underlying result: they all stimulated similar physiological changes. He realized that this central phenomenon needed a name, so he dubbed it "the relaxation response." Most of the practices evoking this response involve being in a quiet place in a comfortable position, focusing inwardly on breathing, or on God or spiritual thoughts, clearing the mind from the busyness of daily life, and sometimes repeating a simple word or phrase. The key issue is to clear the mind of all outward distractions—worries, plans, desires. As Zen practitioners, who concentrate on breathing, say, "If you have a thought, let it come in the front door and go out the back door, but don't ask it to stop for tea."

Benson describes the relaxation response as "the inborn capacity of the body to enter a special state characterized by lowered heart rate, decreased rate of breathing, lowered blood pressure, slower brain waves, and an overall reduction of the speed of metabolism. It is the counterpart of the 'fight-or-flight;' or stress response."

In researching the biological implications of the relaxation response, Benson has found that it can be applied to almost any physical disorder that has a stress or anxiety component. As a result, some form of the relaxation response is used in most stress-management programs. It has proven its ability to lower hypertension and prevent or ameliorate coronary heart disease.

Benson is Director of Harvard's Division of Behavioral Medicine, a pioneering program in the field, where the relaxation response is used both in a Hypertension Group Program and a Mind/Body Group Program at Beth Israel Hospital in Boston. Both are showing amazing results. The Mind/Body Program, run by the extraordinary psychologist Joan Borysenko, treats people with a wide range of disorders, from headaches and arthritis to gastrointestinal problems and diabetes, using relaxation along with group support and health education. Recently, Benson, Borysenko, and several colleagues have initiated a study to determine the feasibility of treating cancer patients with a similar relaxation-response program.

How could relaxation ameliorate cancer or its symptoms? According to Benson, the relaxation response reduces sympathetic-nervous-system activity. The result is a decrease in the production of stress hormones—catecholamines and corticosteroids—that suppress immune responses. Benson believes that the relaxation response can help bolster immunity through this mechanism, and has set out to study immunological changes that occur during relaxation. Benson and his group are hopeful that relaxation will be a useful adjunct tool in helping cancer patients handle the stresses of their illness, reduce pain, and perhaps lengthen survival.

The rationale behind relaxation for cancer patients applies just as well to cancer prevention. If this simple technique can tap the innate ability of the human organism to reverse the effects of stress, it probably can reduce some of the harm stress does to immunity. Someone who practices relaxation on a regular basis may be strengthening his or her immunological defenses against cancer.

Support for the immune-boosting potential of relaxation comes from studies by researchers Janice Kiecolt-Glaser and Ronald Glaser at Ohio State University. They found that relaxation training given to medical students undergoing exam stress increased the students' T-helper cells, which are critical in fighting infectious diseases. They also found that relaxation taught to patients in a retirement home resulted in the patients' having higher antibody levels and more natural killer cells, which can fight cancer. Since immune functions diminish with aging, leaving the elderly more vulnerable to infections and cancer, they are especially in need of such boosting.

Kiecolt-Glaser and Glaser emphasize the importance of consistent use of the relaxation techniques. Looking back on the evidence, it was clear that those medical students who practiced the exercise on a daily basis received the immune benefits, but those who only used the techniques on an off-and-on basis did not.

Although relaxation as a form of cancer prevention and treatment remains untested, the signs are hopeful. Anyone whose personality or constitution is such that they "break down" emotionally or physically under stress can benefit directly from relaxation techniques. They will feel better and be less prone to a variety of illnesses. Research may someday prove that another unseen benefit is a stronger anticancer defense.

Relaxation, as Benson lays it out in his book *The Relaxation Response* (Avon Books, $3.50), is remarkably easy to learn. You begin by sitting in a quiet environment, adopting a passive mind set and tuning out any distracting thoughts. Then for the next twenty minutes you repeat to yourself a simple word or phrase (Benson suggests the word "one"), and pay close attention to your breathing.

When Benson wrote his book in 1975 he felt that it was unnecessary and perhaps contraindicated to use a religious or meaningful phrase. Later, after studying meditational forms in India and Tibet, he came to believe that the technique was potentially more powerful with the addition of a phrase or mantra that had a personal or spiritual meaning for the meditator. Benson now suggests that everyone—whether Catholic, Jew, Hindu, or agnostic—choose a simple phrase that has special significance to him/her. For example, Christians might choose a line from the Lord's Prayer, Catholics from the Hail Mary. Jews may wish to use the Hebrew word for "peace," "shalom," or for "one," "echod."

Muslims may use "Allah," etc. Benson describes the importance of the "Faith Factor" in healing and meditation in his second book, *Beyond the Relaxation Response* (Times Books, $3.50).

In her recent book, *Minding the Body, Mending the Mind* (Addison-Wesley Publishing Co., 1987), Joan Borysenko provides a series of simple steps to make meditation easy. Her instructions are especially clear and effective:

1. Choose a quiet spot where you will not be disturbed by other people or by the telephone.
2. Sit in a comfortable position, with back straight and arms and legs uncrossed, unless you choose to sit cross-legged on a floor cushion.
3. Close your eyes. This makes it easier to concentrate.
4. Relax your muscles sequentially from head to feet. This step helps to break the connection between stressful thoughts and a tense body. For now, just become aware of each part of your body in succession, letting go as much as you can with the out breath. Take a second now just to take a deep breath in. Let it go. Notice how your body relaxes as you let go. This is the good old sigh of relief. The pull of gravity is always present, encouraging us to let go, but if there is no awareness of being uptight, there can't be any letting go. Notice your shoulders right now. Is there any room to let them down more, cooperating with gravity and your own out breath? Every out breath is an opportunity to let go.

   Starting with your forehead, become aware of tension as you breathe in. Let go of any obvious tension as you breathe out. Go through the rest of your body in this way, proceeding down through your eyes, jaws, neck, shoulders, arms, hands, chest, upper back, middle back and midriff, lower back, belly, pelvis, buttocks, thighs, calves, and feet. This need only take a minute or two.
5. Become aware of your breathing, noticing how the breath goes in and out without trying to control it in any way. You may notice that your breathing gets slower and shallower as the meditation progresses. That's due to the physiological effects of the relaxation response, the fact that your body requires less oxygen because your metabolism has slowed down.
6. Choose a *focus word*—a word or phrase that evokes a sense of meaning that is important to you. This could be anything at all. If you cannot think of your own focus word, you might want to try a very old Sanskrit mantra, *Ham Sah*. (*Ham* means "I am" and *Sah* means "That.")

   Repeat your focus word silently in time to your breathing. In the case of *Ham Sah*, just listen to your breath, imagining that it sounds like *Ham* on the in breath and *Sah* on the out breath.

7. Don't worry about how you are doing. As soon as you start to worry
    about whether you are doing it right, you have shifted from medita-
    tion to anxiety. If you notice that tendency, try labeling it *judging,
    judging,* then let go, coming back to the breath and the focus,
    which are your anchors in the shifting tides of the mind.

    Your mind will not stop for more than seconds at a time, if at
    all, so don't expect it to. What happens is that that part of yourself
    that can watch or witness the shenanigans of the mind is learning
    to flex its muscles. Each time you notice that you've drifted into
    thought, try labeling where you were; for instance, *thinking, think-
    ing* or *anger, anger* or *judging, judging* and then let it go, getting
    back to the anchor. In this way, you begin to train your mind in
    awareness—the antidote to denial and mental unconsciousness.
    The awareness you develop in meditation will begin to carry over
    into life, affording you much more choice in how you respond and
    restoring your ability to enjoy life.

    The most common experience and complaint about meditation
    is "I can't stop my mind from wandering." That's fine. Don't try.
    Just practice bringing it back to concentration on the breath and
    focus whenever you notice it wandering.

8. Practice at least once a day for ten to twenty minutes. Remember
    that practice is indispensable to progress at anything. In meditation
    your goals are twofold. The session itself is the goal. In the true
    sense, the process is the product. Your only goal is to sit and do the
    meditation. Even if it seems that the only thing you're doing is
    chasing after your mind to tie it down again, remarkably, the relaxa-
    tion response is still most likely occurring. Long before patients
    think they know "how to do it," they begin to notice that they are
    generally feeling more peaceful and their symptoms are beginning
    to improve. The second goal is that, of course, it does get easier and
    more deeply peaceful after repeated practice.

    If you can sit twice a day for ten to twenty minutes, so much
    the better. The preferred times are early morning (after a shower
    and exercise if you do it, but before breakfast) or before dinner. The
    only times to avoid are when you're tired—simply because medita-
    tion is a concentration exercise and, if you're tired, you'll fall
    asleep—and just after a heavy meal, since the process of digestion
    makes people sluggish.

OTHER RELAXATION PRACTICES

Progressive Relaxation

This is an excellent and widely used technique developed by University of Chicago researcher Edmund Jacobson. According to Jacobson, an overtired or stressed person "does not know what muscles are tense . . . does not clearly realize that he should relax and does not know how. These capacities must be cultivated or acquired anew."

The progressive relaxation technique involves becoming aware of muscle tension and your ability to relax these tensions throughout the body. As with other relaxation methods, you need to find a quiet place to sit or lie down. You then pay close attention to the sensations in your body, and begin by tensing one muscle group at a time, and then relaxing that group. The exercise usually starts with the hands, arms, and head, and works progressively down the length of the body. You tense each muscle group for several seconds, and then slowly release it so the sensations of relaxation are maximized.

This is just a summary of progressive relaxation. For complete directions, see Jacobson's book, *You Must Relax* (McGraw-Hill, 1962). If it is practiced over a long period, it can be used in real stressful life situations—such as before exams or a difficult business meeting—to relieve anxiety and improve functioning. The technique can also be used to relieve phobias. The particular benefit of progressive relaxation is the body awareness it engenders in the committed practitioner.

Autogenic Training

The German doctor Johannes Schultz developed this form of progressive relaxation of the body, involving a series of verbal suggestions. These suggestions, called "orientations," are a subtle form of self-hypnosis, a way of influencing the body by bypassing the conscious mind. It is a systematic approach. The orientations are six verbal self-directions that gently urge the body to relax: (1) my right arm is very heavy; (2) my right arm is warm; (3) my pulse is calm and strong; (4) my breath is calm and regular; (5) my solar plexus is becoming warm; and (6) my forehead is pleasantly cool. These orientations are used one at a time over a long period, alternating concentration and relaxation, until they are mastered. Slowly, over a few months, all the suggestions are combined into an integrated exercise that calms the mind and the entire body.

Yoga

Yoga is a practice based on Indian philosophical teachings and may be the earliest and most-developed "mind-body technique." It involves meditation, physical exercise and breathing. To describe yoga as an amalgam of techniques, however, does not do justice to this profound and vaunted spiritual system.

There are many different yogic traditions, and I will not try to cover the full range here. Basic elements of most yogic systems include *pranayama*, or breathing purifications; *asanas*, which are stretching postures; along with a variety of meditational practices. Pranayama practices are exercises in directing breath within the body, a key to revitalizing the energy system within. Asana practices help increase body awareness and control of inner processes. Meditations involve inner centering and the development of a spiritual tranquility.

Hatha yoga is one of the yogic systems. "Ha" means sun, and "tha" means moon; Hatha yoga refers to the integration of the sunlike and moonlike aspects of the person. Interpreted in Western terms, this can be viewed as a practice toward integrating the right- and left-hand sides of the brain and body.

As Richard Grossman has written in his book *The Other Medicines,* the principles involved in yoga include "self-regulation, the mental control of physiological processes, and, in a sense, yogic therapy is dedicated to the idea of 'psychosomatic health.'"

Grossman has translated the goals of yogic practice in terms that dovetail with two key aspects of psychological health that may help prevent cancer—mind-body integration and taking control of one's health.

Meditations are so diverse and stem from so many different religious and secular practices that it is impossible for me to do justice to the breadth of choices and possibilities—not to mention their philosophic and theological underpinnings. There are Tibetan, Hindu, Sufi, t'ai chi, zen, Buddhist, and various yogic traditions. There are spiritual teachers and gurus within all of these traditions who claim to be keepers of the flame, with true knowledge and the only path to spiritual growth, inner peace, and healing. One need not accept all of any one system to benefit by the meditational forms they teach. However, it does seem certain, as Benson says, that some form of faith—in a deity, in a living force, in an energy outside oneself—has healing power beyond simple relaxation.

But faith should be found within and not dictated by anyone else. It is unwise to believe that only the teacher possesses true knowledge. In his book *How to Meditate,* Lawrence LeShan makes a point worth heeding: do not proceed with a meditational or spiritual exercise that gives you "a definite and clear feeling that you are doing something to yourself that you should not be doing. This is different from simple anxiety, which is not uncommon in meditation. Rather, it's a feeling that what you're doing does not fit your being."

By taking time to practice a meditational discipline in a tranquil setting, you are reentering the inner world of mind-body. Without relaxed contact with "inner space," free of mental busyness that results from daily stresses, the mind becomes separated from the body, and you can be left with an inexplicable anxiety. This is the state in which health and immunity are easily compromised. Meditation helps undo the split, restores contact with inner reality, and dissolves tensions that make us vulnerable to illness.

Biofeedback

Biofeedback is an ingenious example of the use of modern technology to benefit knowledge of the inner self—a rare occurrence, indeed. It's a form of relaxation with a machine to help.

Many of us walk around unaware of what's going on in our bodies and, what's more, unaware that we *can* be aware and *control* internal body functioning. Put simply, biofeedback is the use of special instruments to monitor interior states.

The concept of biofeedback can be demonstrated without machines. All you need do is take your own pulse, monitor your feelings, and with some practice, you can come to regulate pulse rate.

Biofeedback machines give you a very fine reading of internal processes. Generally, a tone, light or needle reading on a dial indicate tension, and the signal changes when the body relaxes. One learns to relax tense areas or influence bodily processes—like blood pressure—by taking cues from the biofeedback machine. Simply receiving this feedback from instruments gradually trains us to control involuntary processes that were never before believed to be controllable.

Skin temperature is one of the simplest biofeedback readings. It has been shown that stress causes skin to cool, and with relaxation warmth returns. More sophisticated instruments measure galvanic skin response or brain-wave activity that reflects states of tension or relaxation.

Typically, biofeedback trainers will use an electromyograph machine (EMG), which registers muscle tension. Someone with a migraine headache, for example, will have electrodes placed on his or her forehead. The EMG machine will detect muscle tension and will "feed back" this information, and sometimes the trainer will help the person relax his muscles, until the machine tone changes. Reinforcement from the machine helps greatly, and can enable a person to optimize his relaxation response and learn to do so without the machine.

Biofeedback is used to treat many ailments, including hypertension, headaches, back pain, arthritis, gastrointestinal problems, epilepsy, drug withdrawal, asthma, or any form of muscular tension. In essence, biofeedback is a very sophisticated form of relaxation response.

Training is very important, however, and a number of sessions may be needed to learn how to apply the biofeedback information in a way that lessens stress, pain, or other symptoms. If you are interested in using biofeedback, search out an experienced trainer or psychologist who specializes in your particular area of need. Your doctor or hospital should be able to direct you to the appropriate therapists.

How does biofeedback apply to prevention? Almost all of us who are prone to immunological breakdown due to stress receive all sorts of warnings from our bodies that it's "not going to take it any more." These are signs that our immune system is being strained to the limit. By handling these symptoms—whether migraines, asthma, or hives—we are addressing the problem of our stress response. When we solve any mind-body symptom by going to the source of stress, relaxing, and handling underlying tensions, we are giving our bodies a fighting chance to reverse damage to our defenses that creates the fertile ground for further illness.

Biofeedback is an excellent way for some people to handle these stress-related pains and symptoms. An unseen fringe benefit is relaxation and possible restoration of healthy immunity, the sine qua non of cancer prevention.

IMAGERY AND VISUALIZATION

Imagery can be beneficial for treating almost any illness. It is used widely in a fashion similar to the Simontons': the immune defenses are visualized fighting the disease, or the body's healing energies are imagined galvanized at the source of pain or distress. As mentioned earlier, the Simontons have used "guided" imagery successfully with cancer patients.

So how can imagery be applied to prevention? As Stephanie Simonton-Atchley pointed out, a healthy person visualizing his immune system functioning efficiently is a bit like imaging his breathing—it's working just fine, thank you.

However, there are times when we are relatively healthy yet know things are not working just right. We're stressed out, or depressed, or subject to piddling health problems, like nagging colds, and know we're vulnerable to more serious problems. Put simply, we can tell our immune system is in trouble.

Psychologist Howard Hall at Pennsylvania State University conducted a study that addressed the question of the potential value of imagery in healthy people. Hall hypnotized a group of healthy individuals and told them to imagine their white blood cells as strong and powerful (like sharks) attacking any bacteria or other organisms that might be circulating around. He took blood before and after the sessions. What he found was that a number of his subjects—particularly the younger ones and the ones most responsive to hypnosis—had a much stronger immune response after the session.

This does not mean we must hypnotize ourselves, or spend time imaging our own immune systems functioning well, in order to keep them in shape. However, visualizations can be developed in conjunction with relaxation and meditation to expand the possibility of positive mind/body interactions.

Dennis Jaffe, in his book *Healing from Within,* suggests an exercise that is excellent and can be thought of as imagery for prevention:

> Sit quietly, making yourself as comfortable as possible. Next, become aware of the sensations coming from each part of your body, asking yourself at each point if that particular muscle or organ is tense or relaxed. Do you feel any tension in your face or jaw? In your stomach? In your thighs, legs, arms, back, neck, head, or lungs? If you can concentrate intensely on each part of your body, you will probably be able to identify where you habitually carry your tension.
>
> Now, focus your awareness only on that particular part of your body with the most tension. In your mind's eye, try to imagine what that spot looks like when it is tense. Make a mental picture of how the tension feels to you. Is [the spot] all knotted up? Is it being strangled by an outside force? Is it being crushed by heavy weights?
>
> Imagine how you could change that mental picture to relax that part of your body. For example, if you pictured your stomach as a huge, solid knot, tight and wet, you might visualize the knot slowly and gently untying itself, and finally lying limp and loose on a sunny beach to dry.

Jaffe's technique is much like progressive relaxation, although with his system you concentrate on the problem area and add mental pictures to your practice. By using visualization with relaxation, you are bringing your imagination to bear in the quest for health and tranquility.

There is as yet no definitive proof that imagery aids the immune system, though an increasing number of studies suggest that it can. It is not the visual images themselves that might alter immunity, but the intangibles—like a feeling of inner control, or a renewal of hope—generated by the images that induce subtle changes in immune response. From a purely scientific standpoint, it is even more difficult to prove that imagery can aid in prevention. Nevertheless, if the power of imagery in healing is any indication, visualization should also be used to ward off illness. Howard Hall's hypnosis experiment may foretell a future where visualization programs will be devised strictly to maintain health.

An indirect but effective application of imagery for prevention has been suggested by Stephanie Simonton-Atchley: use visualizations to help solve life problems, such as better relations with your family, or the solutions to problems at work. The more you let the mind imagine desired outcomes, the more possibilities will open up. Such imaging also helps identify any current needs and emotions, which is another aspect of staying in touch with your body/mind. Visualization may be seen as a new and important adjunct to relaxation, augmenting the psychological and physical benefits. Some people are using imagery on a daily basis, as part of their meditation routine.

Anyone practicing visualization to meet goals should be as open as possible to the free flow of information from his or her imagination. Be wary of the notion that the only good imagery is positive imagery. Although positive imagery can be very useful to help marshal life-affirmative and healing energies, it can, if used too rigidly, mask negative feelings, which can erupt later.

Listen carefully to what your mind-body tells you. For example, if you ask yourself to imagine having a harmonious and constructive talk with your husband, wife, or child that heals an earlier dispute, let the picture play itself out. If you have trouble imaging a positive outcome, don't worry—just let the "movie" roll on and see where it leads you. If negative feelings or fears appear, don't block them; see what happens and be open to the implications. Then, if you can imagine a positive result, a fuller picture of the problem will have emerged along with a better solution.

You can use imagery to focus in on any area of your life that seems troublesome. If an image of a positive solution seems forced to you, simply go deeper into the problem. If negative images pervade, let them play themselves out over days or weeks, if necessary. Keep exploring until you can imagine a positive scenario, or see an image that completes an unfinished canvas.

ACUPUNCTURE

Acupuncture is a healing practice believed by many to be useful for prevention. This ancient technique of Chinese medicine, involving the insertion of very fine needles into various points on the body, is primarily known as a treatment for a wide range of physical illnesses and as an anesthetic.

But acupuncture is much more than that. It is based on a Chinese view of mind-body interactions, with its unifying principle of qi ("chee"), which is the vital energy that flows through the body. According to Chinese practitioners, this energy circulates in the body along pathways called meridians. The proper, balanced flow of qi along the various meridians is the hallmark of good health.

The major meridians—there are twelve of them—are associated with various organs or organ systems. The vitality of an organ and related structures depends on an unblocked flow of energy through that meridian. Also, organ systems and meridians cross paths and are interdependent; a major weakness along one meridian can create an imbalance that affects other systems as well. Each meridian has points of entry and exit. If you've ever seen an acupuncturist's chart of the body, it looks like a road map with countless criss-crossing paths and points.

The use of needles in acupuncture, which are so fine as to cause little or no pain, are used by trained practitioners in an extremely deliberate and often complex way. They are placed in specified points (there are 360 of them) to stimulate or modify the flow of energy along a particular meridian. These points can be anatomically far away from the problem area. For example, a needle in a person's foot is believed to modulate the flow of energy through the kidneys or lungs.

The acupuncturist, over many sessions, can induce energy flow through depleted areas, reduce flow through overstimulated areas, and thus produce a balance of qi in the body. This balance is often the sine qua non for recovery from a wide variety of illnesses—including all sorts of chronic pain, arthritis, allergies, ulcers, and hypertension. Acupuncture's uses also span a range of behavioral health problems: it can reduce symptoms of withdrawal and anxiety for alcoholics, drug addicts, and those trying to lose weight. There is no greater proof of acupuncture's capacity to regulate bodily sensations than in its use for anesthesia in surgery. People can undergo the most complex brain surgery without pain, with only a number of needles strategically placed in various points on their bodies.

Acupuncture has finally made it to American shores, and typically it is applied here almost exclusively for treatment. But the Chinese philosophy of medicine and the very basis for acupuncture is that balance is required for the *maintenance* of health. Illness is harder to treat than prevent because, once it has set in, a rather pronounced imbalance must be rectified. When minor disruptions in the flow of qi can be rectified through regular acupuncture "tune-ups," there is bound to be less illness and less-severe symptoms when illness does occur. Acupuncture can be thought of as a kind of exercise for our inner organs, blood, and nervous systems. By keeping them "in shape," which involves stimulating and modulating the flow of energy, we can stave off any number of systemic disorders.

Whether regular acupuncture stimulates immunity or prevents cancer is still unanswered. But this ancient practice, dating back thousands of years, certainly promotes inner balance, relaxation, and vigor. With regular treatments, it is believed that energy flow is unblocked and organ systems are vitalized. All these factors contribute to stronger defenses against illness, and Western medicine may one day be able to explain and verify the preventive powers of acupuncture in more "scientific" terms.

There are many other complementary medical practices that have important implications for prevention. Such practices include, for example, therapeutic touch, energy medicine, Feldenkreis, the Alexander Technique, and others. Each one tells us something different about the mind-body connection and the factors—mental, emotional, spiritual, and physical—that all go into maintaining health and well-being. Although these practices seem to be oriented more toward healing existing illness or injury, each has aspects applicable to prevention and to promoting greater health.

From the vantage point of an energy-medicine practitioner, our otherwise healthy bodies need to be replenished with life energy in areas that have been depleted by stress, tension, and emotional conflict. We may not need to go to such a healer unless we are sick, but we should look for activities or therapies that keep our energy flow vibrant. Exercise, body-work programs and movement/dance classes are pleasurable ways to keep our bodies tuned up and our energy moving.

Some of these healing practices can be thought of in terms of prevention in another way. Those of us subject to constant minor but irritating health problems—chronic pains or other symptoms, immunological disorders like allergies, asthma, and arthritis—usually have an underlying problem such as immune malfunction, chronic stress, or both. One way to handle these problems is with medical treatment of symptoms. (We take aspirins for chronic headaches; antihistamines for allergies; bronchodilators for asthma; cortisone for arthritis.) Symptomatic medical treatment is certainly invaluable—the stress caused by symptoms themselves needs to be lessened or we become victims of a vicious circle of symptoms-to-stress-to-worse-symptoms. But many of the complementary or "holistic" therapies address the problems of the "background" itself. When you use relaxation techniques to ease a headache, you are directly cooling down the internal stress-response causing it. From a Chinese standpoint, acupuncture heals by rerouting the flow of energy in the body, which is the background for all health or illness. Imagery can be used to tap the mind's powers to summon a stronger immune response against an incipient bacterial infection. Each in its own way addresses the underlying problem of stress and its effects on our energy and immunity.

EXPRESSIVE BODY PSYCHOTHERAPIES

Certain body-oriented psychotherapies directly address the need to release pent-up emotion. These therapies—which include Reichian orgone therapy, Alexander Lowen's bioenergetics, and Arthur Janov's primal therapy—are possible alternatives for people who believe they need to break through physical blocks in order to express feelings. The best ones incorporate aspects of conventional psychotherapy or psychoanalysis, which allows for talking analysis side by side with physical expression of emotions. Reichian therapies deserve mention here because they are the unacknowledged forerunners of these trends, and because they have forged mind-body connections systematically and powerfully. These therapies remain untested and the only testimony to their effectiveness comes from patients and the therapists themselves. Some of their methods are considered controversial.

According to Wilhelm Reich, the pioneer in body-mind therapy, emotions are held in "rings" or segments of muscular armor that run horizontally around the body, preventing the vertical flow of "life energy." Like his counterparts in Eastern medicine, Reich believed in life energy and, in his role as a scientist, he devoted half of his life's work to demonstrating the objective reality of this energy, which he called "orgone." Emotions were defined by Reich as the expressive movements of life energy within the body. The "muscular armor," in impeding this flow through the body, represses emotional expression as well. Different "character types" have different psychic defenses and particular body attitudes and physical armor which matched their type.

Reich's original therapy is now widely practiced by therapists throughout the U.S. and Europe. It is known by a number of different names: Reichian therapy, orgone therapy, character analysis, or medical orgonomy. The practitioners who adhere to Reich's methods work systematically on the muscular armor, starting from the rings of armor at the top (the eyes, facial muscles, the jaw region) and working down through each segment. The skilled therapist will combine oral work—eliciting the patient's thoughts and feelings—in concert with the physical work, which involves a variety of techniques for loosening and dissolving segments of armor. Some of these techniques are strictly physical: forms of kneading, massaging, rolling, or pressure. Other methods for dissolving armor include the therapist's encouraging expressive movements (or sounds) that help the patient restore energy flow to parts of the body that are blocked, and release repressed anger or sadness.

In *Character Analysis,* Reich's major book describing his technique, he includes a fascinating description of the segments of muscular armor and the specific emotions that are often "held" in these areas. For example, anger is often stuck in the jaw region, longing in the chest segment, and rage and sexual excitation in the pelvis.

Often, when emotion is released from the muscular armor, it carries with it a remembrance of things past. For those, in therapy or not, who have little memory of early events, such loosening of the physical armor can provide a long-sought breakthrough. Usually, such memories involve early hurts inflicted by unaware, unresponsive, or unfeeling parents.

The goals of Reichian therapy are: establishing a free flow of energy throughout the body; reawakening the ability to express the full range of negative and positive feelings; creating a better emotional contact with others; and reinstating the capacity for complete discharge of sexual energy that leads to satisfying sexual relationships.

Bioenergetics is an offshoot of Reichian therapy. It was initially developed by two students and followers of Reich, Drs. Alexander Lowen and John C. Pierrakos. Bioenergetics owes many of its basic tenets and practices to Reich's therapy, with a number of important differences. Unique physical exercises, positions, and stances are used along with touch to soften muscular armor and revitalize the body. Like Reichian therapy, this work is done side by side with talking analysis designed to explore early feelings and emotional conflicts. Lowen has written many books on his treatment methods and philosophy, and Pierrakos has moved to develop his own variant of bioenergetics, called "core energetics," which includes a spiritual aspect. Another important contributor to bioenergetics therapy is Dr. Stanley Keleman, who practices in California.

Because some people are locked into an ongoing stress response in their bodies, Reichian therapy, bioenergetics, or other body therapies are possible options for reintegrating mind and body. They may help to break the stress-response cycle which causes suppression of our immune systems and anticancer defenses.

These therapies, however, are only for people who feel strongly that they require physical as well as emotional breakthroughs to achieve personal growth and physical health. Only therapists who are certified or have trained with a recognized institute or practitioner in their field should be considered. (See Appendix 3 for organizations that will refer you to therapists.)

Other valid alternatives to Reichian techniques and to conventional psychotherapy include: Gestalt therapy, existential analysis, transactional analysis, reality therapy, Rogerian therapy, Jungian analysis, and a host of other mind-body systems. In addition, there are off-shoots of Freudian psychoanalysis; Karen Horney, Harry Stack Sullivan, and Alfred Adler were developers of three major schools. Choose the therapy that seems to suit your psychological needs and personal preferences best. It will be the one most likely to promote your physical health as well.

By handling physical symptoms with mind-body approaches that address and heal background disorders, we are practicing good prevention. Reviving hope, a sense of control, energy flow in the body, and creating a vigorous immune system are critical to cancer prevention. In the final analysis, it may be our capacity for pleasure in life that keeps us healthy.

VI

EPILOGUE: GO FOR THRIVAL

22

Go for Thrival

A sage of human affairs, whose identity escapes me to this day, once said, "We're not talking survival—we're talking *thrival*—going for life all the way."

Diet, lifestyle, and psychological factors are interrelated, just as mind, body, and spirit are interrelated. If we make positive changes in any one of these areas they will affect the others. Any single change represents a renewed commitment to life, and an impetus to make more changes.

When we eat healthfully, we make our present more pleasurable and prolong our future.

When we stop smoking, we are strengthening our minds and spirits as well as our bodies.

When we ask ourselves what we really want to do with our lives, and take steps in that direction, we are battling depression and encouraging better physical health.

When we begin to control our own environment (not other people) and take responsibility for our health and happiness, we strengthen both mind and body.

In "The Psychological Factor," I spoke about the commitment to life that directly strengthens our anticancer defense through mind-body mechanisms. It is the same commitment that provides the motivation for the dietary and lifestyle changes suggested in this book as well. If there is great difficulty in making the necessary behavior changes, consider the issues raised in the psychological section—particularly the search for full meaning and validity in work, relationships, and creativity.

A SELF-ASSESSMENT QUESTIONNAIRE

This questionnaire is to help you identify those areas of cancer risk that need your attention. It is divided into three sections, corresponding with the last three parts of the book: "The Diet Factor," "The Lifestyle Factor," and "The Psychological Factor."

Each section is designed differently and serves a different purpose. The diet section will provide you with a score that will give you a rough idea of how close you are to an ideal cancer-prevention diet. The lifestyle questionnaire is designed to pinpoint specific areas of concern, and refer you to the appropriate chapter for action. The psychological questionnaire is designed to provide food for thought.

Diet and Cancer-Prevention Questionnaire

1.	Do I eat few fresh fruits and vegetables?	Yes	No
2.	Do I consider salads and cruciferous vegetables too boring to consume?	Yes	No
3.	Do I eat fried foods often or dishes with heavy creamy sauces?	Yes	No
4.	Am I perennially overweight, and know I can't control my calories?	Yes	No
5.	Do I drink a lot of whole milk and/or eat a lot of high-fat cheeses?	Yes	No
6.	Are steaks, chops, ribs, roasts, or burgers my daily staples?	Yes	No
7.	Am I someone who rarely eats whole-grain cereals, breads, or bran?	Yes	No
8.	Do I drink more than three cups of coffee a day?	Yes	No
9.	Am I someone who never takes supplemental vitamins and minerals?	Yes	No
10.	Do I delight in cakes, pies, puddings, and ice cream on a regular basis?	Yes	No
11.	When I come home from the supermarket do my bags contain over 80 percent of frozen, boxed, or canned goods?	Yes	No
12.	Do I eat more than once a week in a fast-food joint?	Yes	No

Count your number of "Yes" answers:

0–4: You're eating a diet that does not promote cancer. Shore up somewhat on the few "Yes" answers.

5–6: You're on your way toward cancer-preventive eating; reread the sections of Part III, "The Diet Factor," that refer to your "Yes" answers. And take action.

7–9: You are eating a diet much too high in fat and lacking the essential food allies. Read all chapters of Part III, "The Diet Factor," and follow the recommendations.

10–12: You need to change your diet! It is far too high in fat and low in fiber, and sadly lacking in foods that protect you from cancer. Don't give up; think about how you can introduce dietary changes gradually. And begin as soon as possible. Read Part III, "The Diet Factor," with a close look at "You Can Change Your Eating Habits." Start first with the foods you like best.

Lifestyle and Cancer-Prevention Questionnaire

1.	Do I smoke more than four cigarettes a day?	Yes	No
2.	Have I been smoking for more than five years?	Yes	No
3.	Do I drink more than three or four alcoholic drinks—whether hard liquor, beer or wine—every day?	Yes	No
4.	Do I suntan without using sunblockers or sunscreens?	Yes	No
5.	Have I ever taken immunosuppressive prescription drugs?	Yes	No
6.	Have I been exposed to many diagnostic x-rays in the last five years? (Each procedure includes several pictures.)	Yes	No
7.	Do I smoke marijuana, or take other "hard" drugs on a regular basis?	Yes	No
8.	Do I have or have I ever had genital herpes, papilloma viruses, or HIV?	Yes	No
9.	Do I live in a house with asbestos insulation?	Yes	No
10.	Do I live in a house with building materials that contain formaldehyde?	Yes	No
11.	Do I have old chemical products around the house—such as pesticides, industrial-strength cleaners, spray paints, paint strippers, or thinners?	Yes	No
12.	Do I live in an area where houses are exposed to radon?	Yes	No
13.	Am I an industrial worker exposed to many different chemicals?	Yes	No

14. Do I work in an office and find that I have mild-   Yes   No
     to-severe respiratory discomfort or allergic reac-
     tions that I don't experience elsewhere?

This questionnaire is not as simple as the diet one. Each question corresponds to a specific chapter and, for many of the above questions, a "Yes" answer does not necessarily indicate that you have been exposed to carcinogens. You may not be able to answer several of these questions—such as 10—in which case you should refer to the relevant chapter about ways to find the answer. Others, such as question 13, are launch pads for further investigation.

Here's a guide to "Yes" answers and what to do about them:

Questions 1 and 2. See Chapter 9 on how to stop smoking, a serious risk factor for lung cancer and a proven killer.

Question 3: See Chapter 10 for guidelines on reducing alcohol consumption, a risk factor for cancers of the breast, mouth, esophagus, and liver.

Question 4: See Chapter 12 on how to limit exposure to the ultraviolet rays of sunlight, and how to get a tan safely by use of protective clothing and sunblockers or sunscreens (including which ones work and which don't), so that your risk of skin cancer remains low.

Question 5: See Chapter 11 on which drugs suppress immunity and what to do about this problem. Cancer risk may be elevated through the use of these drugs, and there are precautions you can take. See also Chapter 5 for foods and vitamins and minerals that can help shore up deficient immune systems.

Question 6: See Chapter 11 for the risks associated with x-ray exposure. A "Yes" answer here does not necessarily mean your risk of cancer has gone up appreciably; that depends on a number of variables, including the extent of x-ray exposure you've had. See guidelines for avoiding unnecessary x-rays; questions to ask your radiologist; and methods of protecting yourself from exposure to other parts of the body.

Question 7: See Chapter 10 on recreational drugs and their negative effects on the immune system. These drugs are not direct carcinogens; they may, however, increase risk by suppressing the cancer defenses.

Question 8: See Chapter 14 for the cancer risks associated with specific sexually transmitted diseases.

Question 9: See Chapter 15 to find out what to do if you answer "Yes" or if you're not sure what the answer is. In either case, you need to take action, because asbestos poses a serious health risk and can cause lung cancer.

Question 10: See Chapter 15 to find out what to do if the answer is "Yes," and what to do if you're not sure what the answer is. In either case, you should take action, because formaldehyde can cause irritating health problems and is a possible risk factor for several types of cancer.

Question 11: See Chapter 15 for information on which household chemical products are hazardous—including cleaners, pesticides, spray paints, and other spray products, paint strippers and thinners, etc. Most of the products available pose no risk; some of them definitely do. Find out what's what.

Question 12: See Chapter 15 for a discussion of radon. If you are uncertain about whether or not you live in a house with high levels of radon, find out. This chapter will tell you how, and what to do if the radon count is high.

Question 13: See Chapter 16. Find out what chemicals you are exposed to at work.

Question 14: See Chapter 16. Investigate the possibility of indoor air pollution and investigate which pollutants may be involved.

I am repeating here the questions listed in Chapter 20 because they are the best yardstick I've come across for assessing psychological factors relevant to cancer. They were prepared by the psychologist Lawrence LeShan for his book *You Can Fight for Your Life,* and reflect his concepts of emotional states that may increase susceptibility to cancer. Be ruthlessly honest with yourself.

Psychological Health and Cancer-Prevention Questionnaire

1. Am I able to express anger when I feel it most strongly?   Yes   No

2. Do I try to make the best of things, no matter what happens, without ever complaining?   Yes   No

3. Do I think of myself as a lovable, worthwhile person?   Yes   No

4. Or have I felt worthless much of the time? Do I often feel lonely, rejected, isolated from others?   Yes   No

5. Am I doing what I want to do with my life? Are my relationships satisfying? Do I feel reasonably optimistic about ever fulfilling myself?   Yes   No

6. If I were told right now that I had only six months to live, would I go on doing what I am doing right now? (Or do I have secret unfulfilled dreams, ambitions, desires of which I am ashamed, and which have plagued me all my life?)   Yes   No

7. If I were told I had a terminal illness, would I experience some sense of relief?   Yes   No

Ideally, your answers should be:

1. Yes	5. Yes
2. No	6. Yes
3. Yes	7. No
4. No	

Obviously, these are not simple questions to answer—certainly not as simple as those for diet and lifestyle. Nor is it easy to make the changes necessary to turn a self-destructive answer into a life-affirmative one. Sometimes it requires drastic changes—in jobs, in relationships to "significant others," in personality and behavior. And, not infrequently, some of the people closest to us don't welcome these changes for reasons of their own—often out of fear. But, invariably, life-affirmative changes are well worth the effort—no matter what the inner or outer resistance may be.

Then, if you add any needed changes in lifestyle and diet, you are on your way. Be your own diagnostician. Listen to the quiet signals from your body, mind and spirit, *and go for thrival!*

APPENDIXES

Appendix 1

Fat and Calories from Some Foods*

Food	Serving	Calories	Grams of Fat
Dairy Products			
Cheese:			
American, pasteurized process	1 oz	105	9
Cheddar	1 oz	115	9
Cottage:			
Creamed	½ cup	115	5
Low-fat (2%)	½ cup	100	2
Cream	1 oz	100	10
Mozzarella, part skim	1 oz	80	5
Parmesan	1 tbsp	25	2
Swiss	1 oz	105	8
Cream:			
Half and half	2 tbsp	40	3
Light, coffee, or table	2 tbsp	60	6
Sour	2 tbsp	50	5
Ice Cream	1 cup	270	14
Ice Milk	1 cup	185	6
Milk:			
Whole	1 cup	150	8
Low-fat (2%)	1 cup	125	5
Nonfat, skim	1 cup	85	trace
Yogurt, low-fat, fruit-flavored	8 oz	230	2

*Source: Human Nutrition Information Service, U.S. Department of Agriculture. For fat and calorie values for other foods, see *Nutritive Value of Foods,* HG-72, for sale from Superintendent of Documents, U.S. Government Printing Office, Washington, DC 20402.

(Continued)

Food	Serving	Calories	Grams of Fat
Meats			
Beef, cooked:			
Braised or pot-roasted:			
Less lean cuts, such as chuck blade, lean only	3 oz	255	16
Leaner cuts, such as bottom round, lean only	3 oz	190	8
Ground beef, broiled:			
Lean	3 oz	230	15
Regular	3 oz	245	17
Roast, oven cooked:			
Less lean cuts, such as rib, lean only	3 oz	225	15
Leaner cuts, such as eye of round, lean only	3 oz	155	6
Steak, sirloin, broiled:			
Lean and fat	3 oz	250	17
Lean only	3 oz	185	8
Lamb, cooked:			
Chops, loin, broiled:			
Lean and fat	3 oz	250	17
Lean only	3 oz	185	8
Leg, roasted, lean only	3 oz	160	7
Pork, cured, cooked:			
Bacon, fried	3 slices	110	9
Ham, roasted:			
Lean and fat	3 oz	205	14
Lean only	3 oz	135	5
Pork, fresh, cooked:			
Chop, center loin:			
Broiled:			
Lean and fat	3 oz	270	19
Lean only	3 oz	195	9
Pan-fried:			
Lean and fat	3 oz	320	26
Lean only	3 oz	225	14
Rib, roasted, lean only	3 oz	210	12
Shoulder, braised, lean only	3 oz	210	10
Spareribs, braised, lean and fat	3 oz	340	26
Veal cutlet, braised or broiled	3 oz	185	9
Sausages:			
Bologna	2 oz	180	16

Food	Serving	Calories	Grams of Fat
Frankfurters	2 oz (1 frank)	185	17
Pork, link or patty, cooked	2 oz (4 links)	210	18
Salami, cooked type	2 oz	145	11
Poultry Products			
Chicken:			
Fried, flour-coated:			
Dark meat with skin	3 oz	240	14
Light meat with skin	3 oz	210	10
Chicken, roasted:			
Dark meat without skin	3 oz	175	8
Light meat without skin	3 oz	145	4
Duck, roasted, meat without skin	3 oz	170	10
Turkey, roasted:			
Dark meat without skin	3 oz	160	6
Light meat without skin	3 oz	135	3
Egg, hard cooked	1 large	80	6
Seafood			
Flounder, baked:			
With butter or margarine	3 oz	120	6
Without butter or margarine	3 oz	85	1
Oysters, raw	3 oz	55	2
Shrimp, French fried	3 oz	200	10
Shrimp, boiled or steamed	3 oz	100	1
Tuna, packed in oil, drained	3 oz	165	7
Tuna, packed in water, drained	3 oz	135	1
Grain Products†			
Bread, white	1 slice	65	1
Biscuit, 2½ inches across	one	135	5
Muffin, plain, 2½ inches across	one	120	4
Pancake, 4 inches across	one	60	2
Other Foods			
Avocado	½	160	15
Butter, margarine	1 tbsp	100	12
Cake, white layer, chocolate frosting	1 piece	265	11
Cookies, chocolate chip	4	185	11
Donut, yeast type, glazed	one	235	13
Mayonnaise	1 tbsp	100	11
Oils	1 tbsp	120	14

Food	Serving	Calories	Grams of Fat
Peanut butter	1 tbsp	95	8
Peanuts	½ cup	420	35
Salad dressing:			
Regular	1 tbsp	65	6
Low calorie	1 tbsp	20	1

†Most breads and cereals, dry beans and peas, and other vegetables and fruits (except avocados) contain only a trace of fat. However, spreads, fat, cream sauces, toppings, and dressings often added to these foods do contain fat.

Appendix 2

Checkups for Early Cancer Detection

Here is the American Cancer Society's guidelines for checkups for early detection of cancer. First are the general guidelines, then a breakdown of early warning signals and early detection for the major types of cancer.

Early detection is vital. Finding and treating cancer early is one of the most important ways to control this disease.

CANCER-RELATED CHECKUP GUIDELINES

Guidelines for the early detection of cancer in people without symptoms are recommended by the American Cancer Society as follows:

A cancer-related checkup:

- every 3 years for those 20–40 years of age.
- every year for those 40 and over.

The society advises the public to talk with their doctors and ask how the guidelines relate to them. The checkup should always include health counseling (such as tips on quitting smoking) and examinations for cancer of the thyroid, testes, prostate, mouth, ovaries, skin and lymph nodes.

In particular:

- Ages 20–40—For breast cancer, an examination by a physician every three years, a self-exam every month, and one baseline breast x-ray between the ages of 35 and 39. For cervical cancer, women who are or have been sexually active, or have reached age 18 years, should have an annual Pap test and pelvic exam. After a woman has had three or more consecutive satisfactory normal annual exams, the Pap test may be performed less frequently at the discretion of her physician.
- Ages 40 and over—For breast cancer, a professional exam every year, a self-exam every month and a breast x-ray every 1–2 years for those 40–49; every year for those 50 and over. For cervical cancer, women who are or

have been sexually active, or have reached age 18 years, should have an annual Pap test and pelvic examination. After a woman has had three or more consecutive satisfactory normal annual exams, the Pap test may be performed less frequently at the discretion of her physician. For women at risk, an endometrial tissue sample at menopause should be taken. For colon and rectum cancer, a digital rectal exam every year after 40, and a stool blood test every year after 50 as well as a procto exam every 3–5 years after two initial negative tests one year apart.

Some people are at higher risk for certain cancers and may need to have tests more frequently. See individual cancer sites sections for high risk factors.

Lung Cancer

Warning Signals: A persistent cough; sputum streaked with blood; chest pain; recurring attacks of pneumonia or bronchitis.

Early Detection: Lung cancer is very difficult to detect early; symptoms often don't appear until the disease has advanced considerably. If a smoker quits at the time of early precancerous cellular changes, the damaged bronchial lining often returns to normal. If a smoker continues the habit, cells may form abnormal growth patterns that lead to cancer. Diagnosis may be aided by such procedures as the chest x-ray, sputum cytology test and fiberoptic bronchoscopy.

Colon and Rectum Cancer

Warning Signals: Bleeding from the rectum, blood in the stool, change in bowel habits.

Early Detection: The ACS recommends three tests as valuable aids in detecting colon and rectum cancer early in people without symptoms.

The digital rectal examination is performed by a physician during an office visit. The ACS recommends one every year after age 40.

The stool blood slide test is a simple method of testing the feces for hidden blood. The specimen is obtained by the patient at home, and returned to the physician's office, a hospital or clinic for examination. The ACS recommends the test every year after 50.

Proctosigmoidoscopy, known as the "procto," is an examination in which a physician inspects the rectum and lower colon with a hollow lighted tube. As the site of most colorectal cancers appears to be shifting higher in the colon, longer, flexible instruments are being used as well as the rigid scope. The ACS recommends a procto every 3–5 years after the age of 50, following two annual normal exams.

If any of these tests reveals possible problems, a physician may recommend more extensive studies, such as colonoscopy and a barium enema. Colonoscopes view the entire colon.

Breast Cancer

Warning Signals: Breast changes that persist, such as a lump, thickening, swelling, dimpling, skin irritation, distortion, retraction, or scaliness of the nipple, nipple discharge, pain, or tenderness.

Early Detection: The American Cancer Society recommends the monthly practice of breast self-examination (BSE) by women 20 years and older as a routine good health habit. Most breast lumps are not cancer, but only a physician can make a diagnosis.

The American Cancer Society and the National Cancer Institute, in their joint Breast Cancer Detection Demonstration program, found that mammography—a low-dose x-ray examination—could find cancers too small to be felt by the most experienced examiner.

Besides its effectiveness in screening women without symptoms, mammography is recognized as a valuable diagnostic technique for women who do have findings suggestive of breast cancer. Once a breast lump is found, mammography can help determine if there are other lesions in the same or opposite breast which are too small to be felt. All suspicious lumps should be biopsied for a definitive diagnosis—even when the mammogram is described as normal.

The society recommends a mammogram every year for asymptomatic women age 50 and over, and a baseline mammogram for those 35–39. Asymptomatic women 40–49 should have mammography every 1–2 years. In addition, a professional physical examination of the breast is recommended every three years for women 20–40, and every year for those over 40.

Uterine Cancer

Warning Signals: Intermenstrual or postmenopausal bleeding or unusual discharge.

Early Detection: The Pap test, an examination under a microscope of cells from the cervix and body of the uterus, is a simple procedure, which can be performed at appropriate intervals by physicians as part of every pelvic examination. For the average-risk person, a Pap test is recommended once every three years after two initial negative tests one year apart.

The Pap test is highly effective in detecting early cancer of the uterine cervix; it is only 50 percent effective in detecting endometrial cancer. Women at high risk of developing endometrial cancer should have an endometrial tissue sample at menopause.

The hormone estrogen frequently is given to women during and after menopause to make up for the decline in estrogens formerly produced by the ovaries. Estrogen helps to control menopausal symptoms such as hot flashes or thinning of the vaginal lining, causing painful sexual intercourse. For mature women, there are certain risks associated with such treatment, including an increased risk of endometrial cancer. Women and their physicians should carefully discuss the use of postmenopausal estrogens in terms of the benefit and risk to the individual patient.

Ovarian Cancer

Warning Signals: Ovarian cancer is often "silent," showing no obvious signs or symptoms until late in its development. The most common sign is an enlarged abdomen caused by the collection of fluid. Rarely will there be abnormal vaginal bleeding. In women over 40, vague digestive disturbances (stomach discomfort, gas, distention) that persist and cannot be explained by any other cause may indicate the need for a thorough checkup for ovarian cancer.

Early Detection: Periodic, thorough pelvic examinations are important. *The Pap test, useful in detecting cervical cancer, does not reveal ovarian cancer.* Women over the age of 40 should have a cancer-related checkup every year.

Oral Cancer

Warning Signals: A sore that bleeds easily and doesn't heal; a lump or thickening; a reddish or whitish patch that persists. Difficulty in chewing, swallowing, or moving tongue or jaws are often late changes.

Early Detection: Dentists and primary care physicians have the opportunity, during regular checkups, to see abnormal tissue changes and to detect cancer at an early and curable stage.

Prostate Cancer

Warning Signals: Most signs or symptoms of prostate cancer are nonspecific, and do not distinguish from benign conditions such as infection or prostate enlargement. These include weak or interrupted flow of urine; inability to urinate or difficulty in starting urination; need to urinate frequently, especially at night; blood in the urine; urine flow that is not easily stopped; painful or burning urination; continuing pain in lower back, pelvis or upper thighs.

Early Detection: Every man over 40 should have a rectal exam as part of his regular annual physical checkup. Men over 40 should be alert to changes such as urinary difficulties, continuing pain in lower back, pelvis, or upper thighs, and should see their physician immediately should any occur. The key to saving lives from prostate cancer is early detection and treatment.

Bladder Cancer

Warning Signals: Blood in the urine. Usually associated with increased frequency of urination.

Diagnosis: Diagnosis of bladder cancer is achieved by examination of the bladder wall with a cystoscope, a slender tube fitted with a lens and light that can be inserted into the tract through the urethra.

Skin Cancer

Warning Signals: Any unusual skin condition, especially a change in the size or color of a mole or other darkly pigmented growth or spot. Scaliness, oozing, bleeding, or the appearance of a bump or nodule, the spread of pigment beyond the border, a change in sensation, itchiness, tenderness, or pain are all warning signs of melanoma.

Early Detection: Early detection is critical. Recognition of changes in or the appearance of new skin growths is the best way to find early skin cancer. Basal and squamous cell skin cancers often take the form of a pale, waxlike, pearly nodule, or a red scaly, sharply outlined patch. A sudden or continuous change in a mole's appearance should be checked by a physician. Melanomas often start as small, mole-like growths that increase in size, change color, become ulcerated and bleed easily from a slight injury. There is a simple ABCD rule that will help individuals remember the warning signs of melanoma: **A is for asymmetry.** One half of the mole does not match the other half. **B is for border irregularity.** The edges are ragged, notched, or blurred. **C is for color.** The pigmentation is not uniform. **D is for diameter greater than 6 millimeters.** Any sudden or continuing increase in size should be of special concern.

Adults should practice skin self-examination once a month.

Pancreatic Cancer

Warning Signals: Cancer of the pancreas is a "silent" disease, one that occurs without symptoms until it is advanced.

Early Detection: Research has focused on ways to diagnose pancreatic cancer before it is advanced enough to cause symptoms. Ultrasound and CAT scans are being tried, but to date only a biopsy yields a certain diagnosis.

Leukemia

Warning Signals: Symptoms of acute leukemia in children can appear suddenly. Early signs may include fatigue, paleness, weight loss, repeated infections, easy bruising, nose bleeds or other hemorrhages. Chronic leukemia can progress slowly and with few symptoms.

Early Detection: Leukemia may be difficult to diagnose early because symptoms often appear to be those of other less serious conditions. When a physician does suspect leukemia, a diagnosis can be made through blood tests and an examination of bone marrow.

Testicular Cancer

Warning Signals: The first sign of testicular cancer is usually a slight enlargement and a change in the consistency of the testes. Although these tumors may be painless, there is often a dull ache in the lower abdomen and groin, accompanied by a sensation of dragging and heaviness.

If the tumor is growing rapidly and hemorrhage is present, there may be sharp testicular pain.

Because many testicular cancers metastasize while the primary or original growth is still small, the first indication of the disease is often in the region or organ to which the cancer has spread.

Early Detection: Because of a lack of early symptoms and of pain, patients usually do not go to the doctor for several months after discovering a slightly enlarged testis. This delay in reporting to the physician probably accounts for the fact that in 88 percent of patients testicular cancers have metastasized by the time they are diagnosed.

Self-Examination—A simple self-examination that takes only three minutes once a month is the individual's best hope for early detection of testicular cancer.

Self-examination is best performed after a warm bath or shower when the scrotal skin is most relaxed. Each testicle should be examined gently with the fingers of both hands by rolling the testicle between the thumb and fingers to check for any hard lumps. If a lump, or a nodule, is found, it may not be malignant, but it should be brought promptly to the attention of a physician.

Physical Examination—The physician palpates the testes and surrounding structures as part of a complete physical checkup.

Other Laboratory Procedures—These include a chest x-ray, an x-ray of the urinary tract (excretory urogram), and hormone assay.

X-ray of lymph glands (lymphangiography) aids in detecting metastasis or recurrence.

CANCER INCIDENCE AND DEATHS
BY SITE AND SEX—1988 ESTIMATES

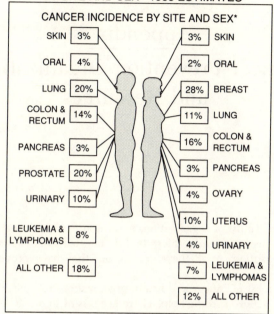

CANCER INCIDENCE BY SITE AND SEX*

SKIN	3%		3%	SKIN
ORAL	4%		2%	ORAL
LUNG	20%		28%	BREAST
COLON & RECTUM	14%		11%	LUNG
PANCREAS	3%		16%	COLON & RECTUM
PROSTATE	20%		3%	PANCREAS
URINARY	10%		4%	OVARY
			10%	UTERUS
LEUKEMIA & LYMPHOMAS	8%		4%	URINARY
ALL OTHER	18%		7%	LEUKEMIA & LYMPHOMAS
			12%	ALL OTHER

*Excluding non-melanoma skin cancer and carcinoma in situ.

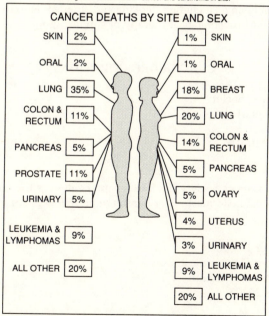

CANCER DEATHS BY SITE AND SEX

SKIN	2%		1%	SKIN
ORAL	2%		1%	ORAL
LUNG	35%		18%	BREAST
COLON & RECTUM	11%		20%	LUNG
PANCREAS	5%		14%	COLON & RECTUM
PROSTATE	11%		5%	PANCREAS
URINARY	5%		5%	OVARY
			4%	UTERUS
LEUKEMIA & LYMPHOMAS	9%		3%	URINARY
ALL OTHER	20%		9%	LEUKEMIA & LYMPHOMAS
			20%	ALL OTHER

Appendix 3

Cancer-Prevention Organizations
and Resources

The following is a list of organizations and resources which may be helpful as guides to a cancer-preventive lifestyle. I do not necessarily endorse the practices or prescriptions of all these groups, but they have proven valuable to many.

There is a list of cancer and health organizations for general information or referrals for more specific help. There are lists of smoking action organizations and groups that help you stop smoking; groups applying alternative methods for behavior change, including smoking and other addictions; holistic health organizations; and psychological therapy or support groups.

CANCER ORGANIZATIONS

American Cancer Society
National Headquarters
90 Park Avenue
New York, NY 10016
212-599-8200

The American Cancer Society has local chapters all over the country. Call or write the national headquarters, or consult your yellow pages for the chapter nearest you.

National Cancer Institute
Office of Cancer Communications
National Institutes of Health
Bethesda, MD 20205

The National Cancer Institute is part of the National Institutes of Health of the U.S. Department of Health and Human Services. You may write to them for specific information at the above address, or you can call their Cancer Information Service. The following toll-free number will connect you automatically to the cancer information office serving your area: 1-800-4-CANCER.

In Alaska call 1-800-638-6070; in Washington, D.C. (and suburbs in Maryland and Virginia) call 202-636-5700; in Hawaii, on Oahu call 808-524-1234 (neighbor islands call collect).

Spanish-speaking staff members are available to callers from the following areas (daytime hours only): California (area codes 213, 714, 619, and 805), Florida, Georgia, Illinois, northern New Jersey, New York City, and Texas.

Cancer Research Institute
133 East 58th Street
New York, NY 10022
212-688-7515

Cancer Care, Inc., of the National Cancer Foundation
1180 Avenue of the Americas
New York, NY 10036
212-302-2400

Cancer Care provides support and referrals for cancer patients and their families.

Leukemia Society of America
733 Third Avenue
New York, NY 10017
212-573-8484

Committee for Freedom of Choice in Cancer Therapy
111 Ellis Street, Suite 300
San Francisco, CA 94102
415-981-8384

Cancer Control Society
2043 North Berendo Street
Los Angeles, CA 90027
213-663-7801

Preventive Medicine

American Health Foundation
320 East 43rd Street
New York, NY 10017
212-953-1900

A nonprofit group that is dedicated to preventive medicine. They support research, education, and practical efforts on causal factors in disease, with an emphasis on nutrition and smoking. They direct a range of health programs, including smoking-cessation groups conducted in hospitals and work-sites.

International Society for Preventive Oncology
217 East 85th Street, Suite 303
New York, NY 10028
212-534-4991

SMOKING ORGANIZATIONS

See the *American Cancer Society,* and the *American Health Association* above. Both have excellent smoking-cessation programs. Refer to Chapter 9, "Smoking: The Most Dangerous Habit," for a description of these and other programs—some of which are run by groups listed below.

Stop Smoking Organizations

American Lung Association
1740 Broadway
New York, NY 10019
212-315-8700

Seventh-Day Adventist Information
12 West 40th Street
New York, NY 10018
212-382-2939

You can contact the Seventh-Day Adventists for information about their 5-Day Plan, and for hospitals that conduct this program.

Smokenders
50 Washington Street
Norwalk, CT 06854
1-800-243-5614

There are many alternative methods to help you stop smoking: acupuncture, hypnosis, behavior therapy, relaxation techniques and others. Refer to the last section here, "Mind-Body Health Organizations," to find groups that either sponsor, or refer you to, the practitioners or groups you are seeking.

Smoking/Environment Action Groups

Action on Smoking and Health (ASH)
2013 H Street NW
Washington, DC 20006
202-659-4310

GASP (Group Against Smoking Pollution) is a nationwide anti-smoking action group devoted to clearing the environment of smoke. They have local chapters throughout the country. Here are a few. If you want to find one closer to you, call or write one of the following and they will help you find your local chapter:

GASP of Massachusetts
25 Deaconess Road
Boston, MA 02215
617-266-2088

New Jersey GASP, Inc.
105 Mountain Avenue
Summit, NJ 07901
201-273-9368

GASP of New York
7 Maxine Avenue
Plainview, NY 11803
516-938-0080

LIFESTYLE FACTORS

AIDS and Safe Sex

AIDS Medical Foundation
230 Park Avenue, Suite 1226
New York, NY 10017
212-949-7410

National Gay Task Force
Hotline for Information:
1-800-221-7044

Gay Men's Health Crisis
Box 274
132 West 24th Street
New York, NY 10011
212-685-4952

Alcoholism

Alcoholics Anonymous
P.O. Box 459
Grand Central Station
New York, NY
212-686-1100

Suntanning and Skin Cancer

The Skin Cancer Foundation
475 Park Avenue South
New York, NY
212-725-5176

CONSUMER AND ENVIRONMENTAL ACTION GROUPS

These groups may help you with a wide range of questions or problems addressed in Parts III and IV, "The Diet Factor" and "The Lifestyle Factor" of this book—including information about foods, drugs, medical procedures, household products, pollutants, occupational and other environmental hazards.

Center for Science in the Public Interest
1501 Sixteenth Street, NW
Washington, DC 20036
202-332-9110

Consumer Federation of America
1314 14th Street NW
Washington, DC 20005
202-387-6121

Consumer Product Safety Commission
Washington, DC 20207
1-800-638-CPSC

Environmental Defense Fund
1616 P Street NW
Washington, DC 20036
202-387-3500

Health Research Group
2000 P Street NW
Washington, DC 20036
202-872-0320

National Public Interest Research Group
1346 Connecticut Avenue NW
Washington, DC 20036
202-546-9707

National Association of 9 to 5 Working Women
614 Superior Avenue
Cleveland, OH 44113

Radon

The first thing you should do with questions or concerns about radon is check your phone book for your local office of the Environmental Protection Agency (EPA). There are also major regional offices of the EPA throughout the country that can refer you to state or local offices. If you can't track down an office serving your area, and need help in doing so, call:

Environmental Protection Agency
Office of Radiation Programs
Radon Division
202-475-9605

or write:

Environmental Protection Agency
Public Information Center
401 M Street SW
Washington, DC 20460

Pesticides

For information about pesticides—at home, at work, in the environment, or in food—call the Environmental Protection Agency's pesticide hotline: 1-800-858-7378.

MIND-BODY HEALTH ORGANIZATIONS

The following groups can help guide you, based on recommendations for behavioral change in Part IV, "The Lifestyle Factor" (especially with regard to smoking cessation); and on discussions in Chapters 20 and 21, "Psychological Health and Cancer Prevention" and "New Ways to Mind-Body Health."

Holistic Health

American Holistic Medical Association
2727 Fairview Ave. E.
Seattle, WA 98102
206-322-6842

Association of Holistic Health
P.O. Box 9352
San Diego, CA 92109
619-425-0618

Health Training and Research Center
P.O. Box 7237
Little Rock, AR 72217
501-224-1933

Training and research on the emotional aspects of disease and health. Write or call for Stephanie Simonton-Atchley's relaxation/imagery cassettes.

For another series of excellent imagery/relaxation tapes write:
Insight Publishing
Box 2070
Mill Valley, CA 14942

Ask for information on Dr. Martin Rossman's imagery tapes. Dr. Rossman is a practicing internist, associated with the University of California Medical Center in San Francisco. He is the author of *Healing Yourself: A Step-by-Step Program for Better Health through Imagery* (Walker, 1987) and one of the nation's foremost instructors on imagery.

Institute for the Advancement of Health
16 East 53rd Street
New York, NY 10022
212-832-8282

This organization is devoted to furthering scientific understanding of mind-body interactions in health and disease (with special emphasis on behavioral medicine and PNI). Its journal, *Advances,* offers articles and reviews on the latest developments in the mind-body sciences.

The following groups sponsor workshops, conferences, and classes on a wide range of "holistic" or "alternative" approaches to health:

Esalen Institute
Big Sur, CA 93920
408-667-2335

Interface
230 Central Street
Newton, MA 02166

The New York Open Center
83 Spring Street
New York, NY 10012
212-219-2527

Omega Institute
Lake Drive, R.D. 2
Box 377
Rhinebeck, NY 12572
914-338-6030

Acupuncture

National Commission for the Certification of Acupuncturists (NCCA)
1424 16th Street NW, Suite 105
Washington, DC 20036
202-232-1404

The NCCA has a national registry of board certified acupuncture practitioners.

Behavior Therapy

Association for Advancement of Behavior Therapy
420 Lexington Avenue
New York, NY 10170
212-682-0065

Society of Behavioral Medicine
P.O. Box 8530, University Station
Knoxville, TN 37996
615-974-5164

Biofeedback

American Association of Biofeedback Clinicians
2424 Dempster
Des Plaines, IL 60016
312-827-0440

Biofeedback Society of America
c/o Francine Butler, Ph.D.
4301 Owens Street
Wheat Ridge, CO 80033
303-420-2889

Hypnosis

International Society for Professional Hypnosis
218 Monroe Street
Boonton, NJ 07005
202-335-4334

American Association of Professional Hypnotherapists
P.O. Box 731
McLean, VA 22101
703-448-9623

Psychotherapy

American Psychoanalytic Association
1 East 57th Street
New York, NY 10022
212-752-0450

American Psychological Association
1200 17th Street NW
Washington, DC 20036

American Psychiatric Association
1400 K Street NW
Washington, DC 20004

American Group Psychotherapy Association
1995 Broadway, 14th Floor
New York, NY 10023
212-787-2618

Body and/or Expressive Psychotherapies

American Society for Group Psychotherapy and Psychodrama
116 East 27th Street
New York, NY 10016

American College of Orgonomy
P.O. Box 490
Princeton, NJ 08542
201-821-1144

The Institute for Bioenergetic Analysis
144 East 36th Street
New York, NY 10016
212-686-2844

The Primal Institute
2215 Colby Avenue
Los Angeles, CA 90064
213-478-0167

Appendix 4
A Short Reading List

PART II. UNDERSTANDING CANCER

CAIRNS, JOHN. *Cancer: Science and Society,* San Francisco, 1978. W. H. Freeman and Co.

DOLL, R., and PETO, R. *The Causes of Cancer,* Oxford, 1981. Oxford University Press.

GOODFIELD, JUNE. *The Siege of Cancer,* New York, 1975. Dell Publishing Co.

ISRAEL, LUCIEN. *Conquering Cancer.* New York, 1978. Random House.

RENNEKER, M., and LEIB, S., editors. *Understanding Cancer,* Palo Alto, CA, 1979. Bull Publishing Co.

WHELAN, E. *Preventing Cancer,* New York, 1980. W. W. Norton & Co.

PART III. THE DIET FACTOR

BALLENTINE, RUDOLPH. *Diet and Nutrition: A Holistic Approach,* Honesdale, PA, 1978. Himalayan International Institute.

BLAND, JEFFREY. *Your Health Under Siege: Using Nutrition to Fight Back,* Brattleboro, VT, 1981. The Stephen Greene Press.

BURKITT, DENIS. *Eat Right—to Stay Healthy and Enjoy Life More,* New York, 1979. Arco Publishers.

CHERASKIN, EMANUEL; RINGSDORF, W. MARSHALL; and SISLEY, EMILY L. *The Vitamin C Connection.* New York, 1983. Harper & Row.

COMMITTEE ON DIET, NUTRITION, AND CANCER. *Diet, Nutrition, and Cancer,* 1982. National Academy Press. (Book-length report of the Committee on Diet, Nutrition, and Cancer of the National Academy of Sciences.)

PAULING, LINUS. *How to Live Longer and Feel Better,* New York, 1986. W. H. Freeman and Co.

——, and CAMERON, EWAN. *Cancer and Vitamin C,* New York, 1979. Warner Books.

SIMONE, CHARLES B. *Cancer and Nutrition,* New York, 1983. McGraw-Hill Book Company.

PART IV. THE LIFESTYLE FACTOR

BERTHERAT, THERESE; and BERNSTEIN, CAROL. *The Body Has Its Reasons: Anti-Exercises and Self-Awareness,* New York, 1977. Avon Books.

CASEWIT, CURTIS W. *Quit Smoking,* Gloucester, MA, 1983. Para Research, Inc.

COOPER, KENNETH H. *The New Aerobics,* New York, 1975. Bantam

CORBETT, THOMAS H. *Cancer and Chemicals,* Chicago, 1977. Nelson-Hall, Inc.

ENVIRONMENTAL DEFENSE FUND, and BOYLE, ROBERT H. *Malignant Neglect,* New York, 1979. Alfred A. Knopf.

EPSTEIN, SAMUEL S. *The Politics of Cancer,* Garden City, New York, 1979. Anchor Books.

GEISINGER, DAVID L. *Kicking It: The New Way to Stop Smoking Permanently,* New York, 1978. New American Library, Signet Books.

NACHTIGALL, LILA, and HEILMAN, JOAN R. *Estrogen,* New York, 1986. Harper & Row.

POCH, DAVID I. *Radiation Alert: A Consumer's Guide to Radiation,* Toronto, Ontario, 1985. An Energy Probe Project, Doubleday Canada Ltd.

SPINO, MIKE. *Beyond Jogging,* Millbrae, CA, 1976. Celestial Arts.

STELLMAN, JEANNE, and HENIFIN, MARY SUE. *Office Work Can Be Dangerous to Your Health,* New York, 1983. Pantheon Books.

PART V. THE PSYCHOLOGICAL FACTOR

ACHTERBERG, JEANNE. *Imagery in Healing,* Boston, 1985. New Science Library. (Write: New Science Library, 314 Dartmouth St., Boston MA 02116.)

——, and LAWLIS, FRANK. *Imagery of Cancer: A Diagnostic Tool for the Process of Disease,* Champaign, IL, 1978. Institute for Personality and Ability Testing.

BENSON, HERBERT. *The Relaxation Response,* New York, 1975. William Morrow and Company.

——. *Beyond the Relaxation Response,* New York, 1984. Times Books.

BORYSENKO, JOAN. *Minding the Body, Mending the Mind,* Reading, MA, 1987. Addison-Wesley.

COUSINS, NORMAN. *Anatomy of an Illness as Perceived by the Patient,* New York, 1979. W. W. Norton & Company.

JACOBSON, EDMUND. *You Must Relax,* New York, 1962. McGraw-Hill.

JAFFE, DENNIS T. *Healing from Within,* New York, 1980. Simon and Schuster.

JANOV, ARTHUR. *Prisoners of Pain,* Garden City, New York, 1980. Doubleday.

LESHAN, LAWRENCE. *How to Meditate,* Boston, 1974. Little, Brown, and Company.

——. *The Mechanic and the Gardener,* New York, 1982. Holt, Rinehart and Winston.

——. *You Can Fight for Your Life,* New York, 1977. M. Evans and Company.

LEVY, SANDRA. *Behavior and Cancer,* San Francisco, 1985. Jossey-Bass Publishers.

LOCKE, STEVEN E., and COLLIGAN, DOUGLAS. *The Healer Within*, New York, 1986. E. P. Dutton.

MANN, EDWARD W., and HOFFMAN, EDWARD. *The Man Who Dreamed of Tomorrow*, Los Angeles, 1980. J.P. Tarcher, Inc.

MONAT, ALAN, and LAZARUS, RICHARD S., editors. *Stress and Coping*, New York, 1985. Columbia University Press.

PELLETIER, KENNETH R. *Holistic Medicine*, New York, 1979. A Merloyd Lawrence Book, Delta/Seymour Lawrence.

REICH, WILHELM. *The Cancer Biopathy*, New York, 1973. Farrar, Straus, and Giroux.

ROSSMAN, M.D., MARTIN L. *Healing Yourself: A Step-by-Step Program for Better Health through Imagery*, New York, 1987. Walker & Co.

SCHULTZ, J.H., and LUTHE, W. *Autogenic Therapy*, 6 vols., New York, 1969. Grune & Stratton.

SIMONTON, O. CARL; MATTHEWS-SIMONTON, STEPHANIE; CREIGHTON, JAMES L. *Getting Well Again*, New York, 1980. Bantam Books.

Appendix 5
Cancer-Prevention Daily Diet

A CUTOUT

This is a simple version of the Diet Guide presented on p. 124. Cut along the dotted lines and post it on your refrigerator or kitchen bulletin board for easy reference. Then do your best to follow it.

MEATS, FISH, AND OTHER PROTEINS
(2 servings per day)

Select Often	Select Occasionally	Select Rarely
Poultry	Lean beef	Pork
Fish	Veal	Ham
Beans	Lamb	Fatty meats
Tofu	Eggs	Hard cheeses

The checklist below tells you which vegetables are high in fiber and vitamins A and C. Many that are high in one category and that are not checked in others may still provide those other nutrients. Brussels sprouts, for example, while high in C and not checked as high in A, do contain a fair amount of vitamin A.

VEGETABLES
(one serving from each group per day)

	High Vitamin C	High Vitamin A	Moderate/High Fiber
Asparagus	✓	✓	✓
Beets			✓
Broccoli*	✓	✓	✓
Brussels sprouts*	✓		✓
Cabbage*	✓		✓
Carrots		✓	
Cauliflower*	✓		
Corn			✓
Eggplant			✓
Leafy greens			
Beets	✓	✓	
Chard		✓	
Collard	✓	✓	
Dandelion		✓	
Kale	✓	✓	✓
Kohlrabi	✓		
Mustard	✓	✓	
Parsley		✓	
Romaine lettuce		✓	
Spinach	✓	✓	✓
Turnip	✓	✓	✓
Watercress	✓	✓	
Peas	✓		✓
Green pepper	✓		
Red pepper	✓	✓	
Soybean products (miso and tofu)†			✓
Sweet potatoes	✓	✓	✓
Tomatoes	✓	✓	
Winter squash		✓	✓

*In addition to their high vitamin content, these cruciferous vegetables contain substances called indoles, which deactivate carcinogens and block them from damaging cells.
†Besides being high in fiber, all soybean products have special properties which block carcinogens.

FRUITS
(one serving from each group per day)

	High Vitamin C	High Fiber
Apples		✓
Avocados	✓	
Blackberries		✓
Cantaloupe	✓	✓
Cranberries		✓
Grapefruit	✓	
Honeydew		✓
Lemons	✓	
Limes	✓	
Oranges	✓	
Papayas	✓	
Pineapple	✓	
Prunes, dried		✓
Raspberries	✓	✓
Strawberries	✓	
Tangerines	✓	
Watermelon		✓

WHOLE GRAINS
(two servings or as many as needed to reach total daily fiber intake of 30–40 grams per day)

Cereals	Grains	Baked Goods
Bran	Barley	Crackers
Whole wheat	Brown rice	Whole wheat
Whole grain	Buckwheat	Rye
Shredded Wheat	Milled oats	Bread
Oatmeal	Rye	Brown
	Whole wheat	Rye
		Whole wheat
		Muffins
		Bran

DAIRY
(1–2 servings per day)

Any low-fat or skim milk product, cheese, or yogurt

DAILY SUPPLEMENT LIST

System 1: Ideal

DAILY SUPPLEMENTS
(Take in A.M.)

Vitamin A	10,000 IU and 15 mg. beta-carotene
Vitamin B	B complex pill (high B50 or B100)
Vitamin C	2–5 grams (2,000–5,000 mg.)
Vitamin E	200–600 IU
Selenium	100–200 mcg.
Calcium	800–1200 mg.
Magnesium	400–600 mg.
Zinc	25 mg.
Copper	3 mg.

Use a multivitamin/multimineral pill, or antioxidant combination, if it helps you to take fewer pills. Try to avoid those that contain iron.

Spread your doses of vitamin C throughout the day.

System 2: Good

In A.M.: Take an antioxidant combination and back this up with a Super B-complex, one or more grams of C, and additional E. (That brings you down to 4 + pills in the morning.)

In P.M.: Take the additional C you need to meet your daily requirement. Divided doses can be taken at noon and after dinner.

System 3: Okay

In A.M.: Take an antioxidant combination with a B-complex and an additional gram of C. This keeps you down to 3 pills in the morning.

In P.M.: Take the additional C you need to meet your daily requirement in one or more additional doses when most convenient.

Let the contents of your antioxidant pill be your guide. Check the values of A, C, E, selenium, and zinc it contains against the ideal recommendations and see how well it fares. Shore up this pill with B, C, or E according to Systems 2 or 3. Try to include calcium and magnesium, zinc and copper. *Your total values should not exceed the recommenda-*

tions in System 1. Of course, if you can swing it, System 1 is ideal. Come as close to it as you can within your pill-taking limitations.

SPECIAL RECOMMENDATIONS FOR:

Smokers and Drinkers

Extra vitamin A and C-rich foods
Add another 15 mg. beta-carotene supplements
Increase your amount of vitamin C to between
  4 and 5 grams

Suntanners

(Whenever you tan, or as a rule if you tan regularly)

Extra beta-carotene rich foods
Add 15 mg. more beta-carotene
Take vitamin E from high end of recommendation (600 IU)

When You Eat Foods with Nitrites

Extra vitamin C and E-rich foods
Increase your amount of vitamin C to between
  4 and 5 grams
Take vitamin E from high end of recommendation (600 IU)

When You Are Exposed to Chemical Carcinogens

Extra vitamin A, C, and E-rich foods
Add 15 mg. more beta-carotene supplements
Increase your amount of vitamin C to between
  4 and 5 grams
Take vitamin E from high end of recommendation (600 IU)

Index